Rheumatoid Arthritis

THE AUTHORS

Dr. Short served as President of the American Rheumatism Association during 1955 and 1956. He holds the posts of Physician at the Massachusetts General Hospital and Instructor in Medicine at the Harvard Medical School. Dr. Bauer holds the Jackson Professorship of Clinical Medicine at Harvard; is Director of the Robert W. Lovett Memorial Foundation for the Study of Crippling Disease, also at Harvard; and is Chief of Medical Services at the Massachusetts General Hospital. Dr. Reynolds was formerly a Senior Research Fellow of the Arthritis and Rheumatism Foundation and an Assistant Professor of Preventive Medicine at Harvard. He is now Professor of Public Health and Preventive Medicine at the University of Washington School of Medicine in Seattle.

Rheumatoid Arthritis

*A Definition of the Disease and a Clinical
Description Based on a Numerical Study of
293 Patients and Controls*

CHARLES L. SHORT, M.D.

WALTER BAUER, M.D.

WILLIAM E. REYNOLDS, M.D.

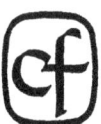

Published for The Commonwealth Fund
BY HARVARD UNIVERSITY PRESS
Cambridge, Massachusetts, 1957

© 1957 BY THE COMMONWEALTH FUND

*Published for
The Commonwealth Fund
By Harvard University Press
Cambridge, Massachusetts*

For approximately a quarter of a century THE COMMONWEALTH FUND, through its Division of Publications, sponsored, edited, produced, and distributed books and pamphlets germane to its purposes and operations as a philanthropic foundation. On July 1, 1951, the Fund entered into an arrangement by which HARVARD UNIVERSITY PRESS became the publisher of Commonwealth Fund books, assuming responsibility for their production and distribution. The Fund continues to sponsor and edit its books, and cooperates with the Press in all phases of manufacture and distribution.

*Distributed in Great Britain
By Oxford University Press
London*

LIBRARY OF CONGRESS CATALOG CARD NO. 57–10706
MANUFACTURED IN THE UNITED STATES OF AMERICA

Preface

This study of rheumatoid arthritis was initiated in 1929 as part of a larger program, the aim of which has been to care for patients with joint disease and to gain knowledge of the anatomy and physiology of articular structures, the diseases which affect them, and the individuals so afflicted. More recently, this program has been extended so as to include a chemical and physiologic characterization of connective tissue, the end-organ or tissue in which the histologic alterations of rheumatoid arthritis and seemingly related diseases are observed.

Initially, this care-of-the-patient and research program was made possible by the income of the Robert W. Lovett Memorial Foundation of the Harvard Medical School, by grants from the Rockefeller Foundation and the John and Mary R. Markle Foundation, and by the hospitalization of patients and the furnishing of much-needed laboratory equipment and supplies by the Massachusetts General Hospital. In September, 1937, the Department of Public Health of the Commonwealth of Massachusetts entered into a contract with the Massachusetts General Hospital for the care and treatment of persons suffering from rheumatic diseases. This contractual arrangement permitted the hospitalization of twenty patients at any one time, most of whom were suffering from rheumatoid arthritis. Since January 1, 1938, a more inclusive care-of-the-patient and research program has been in effect because of a large annual grant from the Commonwealth Fund, and in recent years, this program has been further augmented by substantial research grants from the United States Public Health Service. Without the establishment of the Robert W. Lovett Memorial Foundation by funds raised by Dr. Frank Ober, and without the interest, cooperation, and kindness of Dr. Ober, Dr. James H. Means, and the late Drs. Cecil K. Drinker and S. Burt Wolbach, the pursuit of this work would not have been possible.

This detailed study of patients afflicted with rheumatoid arthritis represents the labors and cooperation of many individuals. We first wish to express our thanks to the patients and control subjects who willingly aided us in our pursuit of clinical facts. We are next indebted to Dr. Marian W. Ropes, Dr. Alfred O. Ludwig, Dr. Nathan R. Abrams, the late Dr. William W. Beckman, Dr. Eric G. L. Bywaters, Dr. John W. Zeller, and other past and present members of the Lovett Fund group for the examination of both the patients and the control subjects. We also wish to acknowledge our gratitude to Drs. E. B. Wilson, Philip E. Sartwell, Ralph E. Wheeler, Herbert L. Lombard, and Morton D. Schweitzer for statistical advice; to Dr. Jacob Lerman for assistance in drawing up the summary statistical sheet used in this study; to the Massachusetts General Hospital house staff and the Metabolism Laboratory for the many tests performed; to Drs. M. S. Strock, E. Ross Mintz, Joe Vincent Meigs, and members of the Otolaryngology Department of the Massachusetts Eye and Ear Infirmary for their painstaking search for foci of infection; to members of the Radiology Department for the many x-ray examinations and their interpretations; to the late Dr. Walter B. Cannon and to Dr. Tracy J. Putnam for their thoughts on the symmetry of lesions observed in the rheumatoid arthritis patients; to Dr. Raymond D. Adams for interpretation of the paresthesias experienced by these patients; to Dr. J. Peter Kulka for advice on pathologic aspects; to Mrs. Dorothy Morgan Bassinor, Mrs. Leonore Bixby Sweeney, and Mrs. Geraldine Sweet Magill as well as to public health nurses of Massachusetts and other New England states and to past and present physician members of the arthritis group for making possible follow-up studies on this large number of rheumatoid arthritis patients; to Miss Rita Nickerson and Miss Katherine Hendrie of the Department

Preface

of Preventive Medicine, Harvard Medical School, for respectively checking calculations and preparing the figures contained in the text; and to Dr. Farahe Maloof for his assistance in the preparation of the chapter on the thyroid. Dr. Nathan R. Abrams tabulated data and assembled them in preliminary form; Dr. Jean M. Beauregard prepared the graphs of the intermittent course exhibited by some of the patients; and Dr. Marian W. Ropes and Dr. Evan Calkins made many helpful comments and suggestions. We are also grateful to Mrs. Magdalene O. Evers, Mrs. Harriet B. Oster, and Mrs. Marjorie E. Martin for their expert secretarial services, to Miss Hope Richardson for assistance in assembling the data, and to Miss Martha Taylor for her painstaking care in the preparation of the bibliography and index. We wish finally to acknowledge again our gratitude to the Commonwealth Fund, whose generous contributions have made possible the continuation of this research project, and to its Division of Publications for most helpful editorial assistance in the preparation of the manuscript for the printer.

It is hoped that this publication concerned with the nature of a chronic disease of unknown etiology will serve as a foundation for future work by ourselves and others. A later report will be devoted to the life-course of rheumatoid arthritis as observed in the patients upon whom the present publication is based, along with additional data on the disease course in patients subsequently seen. The ultimate goal that we and others would like to achieve is a rational therapeutic approach as well as measures designed to control this socially and economically important disease, either in the individual patient or as part of a concerted public health program. Until such objectives are attained, rheumatoid arthritis will continue to be a frequent cause of prolonged morbidity and to rank foremost among the crippling diseases.

C. L. S.
W. B.
W. E. R.

April 1957

Contents

		Page
Preface		v
Chapter 1.	Introduction and Review of Previous Studies	3
Chapter 2.	Diagnostic Criteria for Selection of Patients	14
Chapter 3.	Selection of Patients and Controls and Methods of Analysis	83
Chapter 4.	Scheme of Presentation and Definition of Terms	99
Chapter 5.	Sex Distribution	104
Chapter 6.	Age at Onset	108
Chapter 7.	National Origin	115
Chapter 8.	Family History	118
Chapter 9.	Allergic Diseases	125
Chapter 10.	Illnesses, Operations, and Injuries	128
Chapter 11.	Occupation	137
Chapter 12.	The Menopause	143
Chapter 13.	Prodromal Symptoms	150
Chapter 14.	Precipitating Factors	164
Chapter 15.	Type of Onset	184
Chapter 16.	Joints First Involved	190
Chapter 17.	Unilateral and Bilateral Joint Involvement	206
Chapter 18.	Age of Patients on Hospital Admission and Duration of Disease before Admission	213

Contents

Page

Chapter 19.	Course of Disease before Hospital Admission	222
Chapter 20.	Factors Which Patients Believed to Have Influenced the Course of Their Disease	240
Chapter 21.	Constitutional Symptoms	254
Chapter 22.	Vasomotor Symptoms and Signs	261
Chapter 23.	Neurologic Symptoms and Signs	270
Chapter 24.	Cardio-respiratory Symptoms and Signs	281
Chapter 25.	Gastro-intestinal Symptoms	286
Chapter 26.	Fever	290
Chapter 27.	Pulse Rate	296
Chapter 28.	Blood Pressure	300
Chapter 29.	Eyes	307
Chapter 30.	Lymph Nodes, Spleen, and Liver	311
Chapter 31.	Skin, Nails, and Tongue	318
Chapter 32.	Edema, Varicosities, and Clubbing	323
Chapter 33.	Nodules	326
Chapter 34.	Joint Examination	331
Chapter 35.	Gallbladder	339
Chapter 36.	Colon	341
Chapter 37.	Foci of Infection	344
Chapter 38.	Red-Cell, White-Cell, and Differential Counts	349
Chapter 39.	Urine, Blood Uric Acid, and Blood Non-Protein Nitrogen	357
Chapter 40.	Gastric Acidity	361
Chapter 41.	Basal Metabolism and the Thyroid Gland	367
Chapter 42.	Spondylitis	375
Chapter 43.	Total Disease Severity and Disease Activity on Hospital Admission	382
Chapter 44.	Subsequent Course of Disease	388
Chapter 45.	Summary	401
Appendix		415
Bibliography		421
Index		461

Rheumatoid Arthritis

1

Introduction and Review of Previous Studies

1.1   Over one hundred years, but only a small part of the span of medical history, have elapsed since the introduction by Louis [326] of the numerical method in the study of disease. It is difficult for us to realize now that, before this revolutionary innovation, opinions about the clinical aspects of disease were based largely either upon the authority of the past or upon the personal impression of the physician. Refinements in the handling of observed data, as our knowledge of statistics has grown, have only served to strengthen Louis' conception of the importance of the study of the natural history of disease, as an ally to laboratory experiment. It is fitting, then, that any program directed toward enlarging our knowledge of arthritis should include clinical observations of such a type that general conclusions can be drawn from them, as well as fundamental investigation in the laboratory. In fact, the one method should complement and assist the other. It is our purpose in the following chapters to present detailed observations on 293 patients with rheumatoid arthritis, based on clinical and laboratory data obtained according to a set plan.

1.2   As we shall show below in a brief review of the larger series of cases of rheumatoid arthritis reported in the literature, the problem has been attacked from this aspect before, and conclusions have been drawn from the observations made. At the same time, it must be mentioned that, in a much larger number of instances, mere impressions or generalizations not backed up by numerical data have been presented in an attempt to formulate a composite picture of a disease which assumes an infinite variety of forms. Such impressions have been handed down and have governed, to a certain extent, our concept of the disease. We have therefore made it a part of our study to confirm or disprove these formulations by numerical methods based on careful observations. In addition, we have attempted to avoid, as far as possible, certain factors which have made other numerical studies incomplete or fallacious. We shall mention here only the more important principles which we have tried to follow, referring the reader to Chapter 3 for details.

1.3   In the first place, diagnosis was rigorous and supported by extensive clinical and laboratory study. No doubtful case was included in the series until, through follow-up, the passage of time had made clear the true nature of the patient's illness. In view of the still confused state of classification and nomenclature of joint disease, we propose to define the diagnostic criteria employed, along with our reasons for the selection of patients for a series designed to be representative of rheumatoid arthritis severe enough to warrant hospitalization. A brief description of the disease will also be presented, with attention paid to the rationale for considering rheumatoid arthritis a distinct disease entity. It is our intention by these means to insure that the morbid process dealt with shall be recognizable even to those who use a different terminology.

1.4   The patients chosen represent consecutive admissions to a general hospital and were all questioned and examined as in-patients on the hospital wards. The study was conducted according to a definite plan laid down at the start and the information collected in a systematic manner. This plan avoided a topical survey including only relatively few points in which we might have been interested at the time. Comparison was also made with a control group of 293 individuals without joint disease, selected to correspond with the arthritic patients in sex distribution and age grouping. All the data, both clinical and laboratory, were obtained simultaneously upon the patient's admission to the hospital. By this method a cross-sectional rather than a longitudinal view of the disease emerges, but information was also obtained in regard to factors

Introduction and Review

preceding and associated with the onset, as well as to the type of course pursued before admission. In addition, observations were made on the subsequent course of the patients, who thus furnish the material for the follow-up study which is still in progress.

1.5 In the review which follows, no attempt has been made to cover papers in which only one or a few aspects of rheumatoid arthritis have been treated numerically. Subsequent reference will be made to such work, when applicable to the discussion of our results. We have confined ourselves to those general articles which, to a greater or less extent, derive conclusions from a broad, numerical study of a series of patients.

1.6 The numerical method in the study of rheumatoid arthritis may be said to have begun in Haygarth's [247] *Clinical History of the Nodosity of the Joints,* published in 1805, with a remark upon the preponderance of females in the series—33 out of a total of 34 patients. With the exception of references by Fuller [195] in 1860 to the frequency of ocular inflammation and by Charcot [81] to a family history of joint disease and the proportion of patients with cardiac involvement, no statistical data on rheumatoid arthritis appeared in the literature until A. E. Garrod [199] published his study in 1890. This author gives figures from 500 cases for the frequency of a family history of articular disease, sex distribution, joints most commonly involved, the influence of the menopause and abnormal catamenia, and the etiologic significance of emotional disturbances, as well as a complete tabulation of the age of onset in both sexes. Unfortunately, the basic data from this large series were not obtained from personal observation but from the notebooks of his father, Sir A. B. Garrod, who introduced the term "rheumatoid arthritis." Later on, in a fairly complete description of the constitutional aspects of the disease, the author does give the results of his own examination of 50 patients for muscular atrophy and increased tendon reflexes. From reading the clinical descriptions as given by father and son, we can trust that the cases were in the main properly diagnosed, although the pathologic changes of degenerative joint disease (then called localized rheumatoid arthritis) were still associated with the true polyarticular variety as well. Garrod also introduced the use of control data (which most of his followers omitted) by ascertaining the frequency of a family history of articular disease in 500 nonarthritic hospital patients. In addition he evidenced critical analysis of gross percentages by the statement that family histories of arthritis were not obtained more often from patients in whom the disease began at an earlier age. In 1896 Brabazon [52] analyzed 100 consecutive patients under his personal care over a period of two years. Beside giving the sex distribution and the joints affected in order of frequency, he showed numerically the long duration of the disease as well as the high incidence (29 per cent) of previous attacks described as rheumatic fever, in some occurring as far back as twenty years. Many of the striking constitutional manifestations were listed, but again, with one exception, no figures were given.

1.7   In 1897, at a meeting of the British Medical Association in Montreal, Stewart [502] analyzed, on an etiologic basis, 40 cases of rheumatoid arthritis, "the largest number reported on from any one hospital on this continent." His series is too small to furnish significant conclusions, and the equally divided sex distribution as well as the high incidence (30 per cent) of a history of gonorrhea arouses the suspicion that the author may have included cases of arthritis due to this specific form of infection. In the same year there appeared Still's [504] classical description of rheumatoid arthritis in children, which will be analyzed in detail in a subsequent chapter along with a nosologic consideration of juvenile rheumatoid arthritis, or so-called Still's disease. Bannatyne's [13] treatise on rheumatoid arthritis, published in the following year, supports the theory of a bacterial origin for the disease, of which the author was an early proponent. The frequency of antecedent acute infections was shown by figures, but the time interval between such an infection and the onset of the arthritis was not specified and the data presented do not necessarily establish a causal relation. In this author's 293 cases, the usual tabulations were made of possible etiologic factors (sex distribution, age of onset, influence of exposure, injury, and pregnancy) but the clinical description of the disease, although excellent and detailed, was limited to general statements. Bannatyne clearly distinguished two separate forms then classified under rheumatoid arthritis, the one acute and of microbic etiology, the other chronic and degenerative. For the latter he proposed that the term "osteoarthritis" be reserved. In this paper, then, for the first time, in spite of the still existing confu-

Introduction and Review

sion in pathologic changes, we can feel sure that the observer was not including in his series patients with degenerative joint disease. He also agreed with those who would distinguish rheumatoid arthritis from rheumatic fever, but carefully noted the incidence of antecedent acute or chronic rheumatism (rheumatic fever), as well as the number who developed endocardial or pericardial lesions during their course.

1.8 The first statistical study of patients with rheumatoid arthritis that we have encountered in the twentieth-century literature appeared in 1907. In this year Strangeways and Burt [510] presented tabulated information about 200 patients, equally divided between workhouse cases and those seen with physicians in private practice. The usual etiologic factors were inquired into, and little significant difference was found between the two economic groups. The statistical work was carefully done, but the study can be criticized on two counts: that the patients were not directly under the authors' observation and that their definition of rheumatoid arthritis must be derived from interspersed case histories, which, however, sound typical. In the following year, as part of the same research program, Lambert [307] presented much the same data about 195 patients in metropolitan infirmaries. The material was incidentally obtained in the course of a study of blood pressure in arthritis; hence all points were not covered with respect to each patient, although the number of cases on which the inferences were based was plainly stated under the various headings. In addition, 47 cases of the senile type (degenerative joint disease) were included and, in many instances, figures were drawn from the whole group without differentiation of what are usually regarded today as two distinct disease entities.

1.9 In the year 1909, which marks a real advance in our knowledge of arthritis, Nichols and Richardson [380] published their classical monograph, in which a clear separation was made between the two great types of chronic joint disease on the basis of pathologic anatomy. Although the type that they called proliferative is now known as rheumatoid arthritis, there is much reason to retain their term "degenerative" for the second. In another important treatise, appearing the same year, Llewellyn Jones [286] distinguished the two types partly on the basis of his own clinical observations and partly on the basis of pathologic data derived from earlier, largely neglected German studies. Jones' description of the natural history of rheumatoid arthritis remains unsurpassed, but only the usual etiologic points are backed by figures. Prodromal or pre-articular symptoms are stressed as such, although Bannatyne [13] and others believed that they might constitute the actual onset of the disease.

1.10   In 1915 McCrae [333] contributed the chapter on "Arthritis Deformans" to *Modern Medicine*. This work is full of sound clinical observations but in our opinion represents a regression, since the author expresses the opinion that classification of chronic arthritis of unknown origin into distinct diseases is not justified. We may call this the "unitarian" theory and shall encounter it in our review of more recent studies. McCrae decided upon this viewpoint only after mature reflection and, for purposes of clinical description, did set off periarticular, atrophic, and hypertrophic types. Many of his numerical conclusions, however, were obtained from the entire group of 500 patients, and are thus not suited for comparison with results obtained from series limited to patients with rheumatoid arthritis.

1.11   Only one group study of arthritis derived from the medical work in the first World War has come to our attention, that published by Pemberton [404] in 1920, in which 400 cases were analyzed chiefly for etiologic factors, including foci of infection, and laboratory data, mostly blood chemistry. The author admitted that this was a selected group and that the "factors operating to produce arthritis in young soldiers under stress of warfare differ from those in civil life." Moreover, he presented no diagnostic criteria to determine the type of arthritis studied, and 29 cases were labeled myositis or neuritis without arthritis. It is probably fair to conclude, from the patients' ages (which averaged 28) and the ruling out of arthritis due to specific infections, that the author was dealing largely with rheumatoid arthritis. A control group of 113 nonarthritic soldiers was used in the study to establish the significance of the large percentage of patients in the series who had had previous attacks of "rheumatism."

1.12   In 1922 the growing importance of the rheumatic diseases as a public health problem led the British Ministry of Health to pursue an inquiry into the prevalence of such diseases in the insured population, based on the observations of nearly 50 insurance practitioners [207, 208]. In an insured population at risk of over 90,000, there were 180 cases of rheumatoid arthritis. This group was analyzed as to age of onset, sex

Introduction and Review

distribution, and etiologic factors such as family history of arthritis, previous infections, type of onset, and presence of infectious foci. The value of this study lies largely in pointing out the vast social and economic consequences of rheumatism rather than in actually contributing to our knowledge of rheumatoid arthritis.

1.13 In 1927 Pemberton and Pierce [*403*] supplemented the observations of the first author on the 400 Army cases by presenting data on 700 patients seen in civil practice. None of the points except sex distribution were drawn from a consideration of the entire civilian series, but the number observed ranged from about 150 in regard to certain nervous symptoms to about 620 in regard to distribution of joint involvement. As the authors pointed out, whether certain data were obtained from a given patient or not depended on their approach to the problem at the time or to the exigencies of consultation practice, which made collection of full data difficult. In the latter half of the study only, a printed outline was used for the collection of information. Finally, until the subject of prognosis was reached, no attempt at division into type of arthritis was made, so that the facts listed apply to a heterogeneous group with diagnoses varying from myositis or neuritis to degenerative joint disease.

1.14 About 1930 two valuable monographs on joint disease, by Freund [*192*] and Fischer [*182*], appeared in Germany. In neither of these was an attempt made at a complete numerical study of a group of patients with rheumatoid arthritis and, except for the usual figures for sex distribution and age of onset, the frequency of only a few clinical points was given. These treatises are of great interest, however, in presenting the German point of view in the diagnosis and classification of various forms of rheumatoid arthritis, especially the proper placing of spondylitis, "psoriatic arthritis," and secondary chronic polyarthritis. The last term is seen little in the American literature and warrants explanation. In brief, it is believed that a form of chronic, progressive arthritis, clinically like rheumatoid, follows upon or is secondary to rheumatic fever, with a large percentage—44 per cent of 110 cases (Freund) and 65 per cent of 201 cases (Fischer)—showing organic valvular disease. This concept will be taken up in detail in a consideration of the selection of patients for our series.

1.15 In Stoner's [*508*] study of 300 patients with chronic arthritis treated over seven and one-half years, figures were given for sex distribution, age, associated diseases, type of onset, duration, and results, but no attempt at subdivision into rheumatoid and degenerative types was made. In the same year Vrtiak and Jordan [546] presented an analysis of the clinical records of 102 out-patients with arthritis; 61 of these were placed in the rheumatoid group, but again some of the results were derived from the whole group without differentiation according to type of arthritis.

1.16 *Rheumatoid Arthritis and Its Treatment* by Coates and Delicati [97], which appeared in 1931, although of brief compass and largely devoted to therapy, contained a fairly inclusive tabulation of clinical and laboratory data on 100 consecutive in-patients with carefully diagnosed rheumatoid arthritis at the Royal Mineral Water Hospital in Bath. Douthwaite's [150] treatise is similar in form and content to that of Coates and Delicati [97] but includes a much less complete numerical study of the same number of patients. In contrast to the British studies, Wetherby's [562] analysis of 350 consecutive dispensary cases made no attempt at selection of patients "other than that those chosen had had non-traumatic pain in the joints for at least two months, and no one was included who gave clinical evidence of a specific type of infection such as gonorrhea or tuberculosis." His statistical conclusions were thus drawn from at least two diseases usually considered independent. However, the author did display an advance in method, in his attempt to demonstrate an association between variables, to determine, for example, whether unilateral joint involvement is related to the age of onset.

1.17 In a series of three papers by Millard Smith [477–479] appearing in 1932, data were presented from the first 102 consecutive cases of "atrophic" arthritis of a total series of 612 which had been observed over a period of three years. These papers represent a notable contribution to the conception of rheumatoid arthritis as a constitutional disease manifesting profound generalized physiologic disturbances. In them is seen a return to the careful clinical observation employed by earlier writers such as Bannatyne [13] and Jones [286] which had been largely neglected after the advent of the infectious theory of etiology. From a statistical point of view one might wish that the results from the entire series of 612 had been tabulated and that uniformly complete data had

Introduction and Review 11

been obtained from all patients in the first 102, since the author rightly did not select completely studied cases from the entire series. An interesting descriptive subclassification of types of rheumatoid arthritis was utilized. However, the ability of the author to be sure of the diagnosis of rheumatoid arthritis might be questioned in regard to the "prodromal" type, with constitutional symptoms only, and a type called "muscular rheumatism," with both constitutional and muscular symptoms but no articular involvement. Eight types in all are described, along with the frequency of clinical and laboratory findings in each. The author pointed out that his object in subdividing the data according to descriptive types was not to contrast and set off these types as separate entities, but to show from the wide distribution of common clinical features among them that they merely represent phases of one disease— phases which are not static but change from one to another as the disease progresses. In spite of the absence of suitable control groups for some comparisons and the small number of patients involved in others, this work represents a valuable attempt at an inclusive, numerical view of rheumatoid arthritis based on careful clinical observation.

1.18 In 1932 and 1933 Eaton [*155-160*] published a series of papers on clinical and laboratory observations in chronic arthritis, with one devoted to a study of the habits of 500 patients and another to the symptomatology of 296. In each study rheumatoid and degenerative types were set off and compared. The figures for habits show only differences which might be accounted for by the greater age of the degenerative group. In the paper on symptomatology we have the unexpected finding that certain clinical features we have long associated with rheumatoid arthritis are found with approximately the same frequency in the degenerative type. These include weight loss, vasomotor phenomena, nervousness, exaggerated reflexes, labile pulse, hyperhydrosis, pigmentation, and general weakness. As the data were presented without correction for the patients' ages, it is difficult to express an opinion as to the validity of these findings.

1.19 In a series of papers appearing from 1934 to 1936 [*383-389*] Nissen introduced the life-history point of view into the study of chronic arthritis. His plan was to analyze the life histories of 500 such patients with respect to degrees of functional capacity. The data were obtained partly from follow-up examinations and partly from past medical records. By careful scrutiny of the available records of 95 patients who had died, he classified "life courses" in chronic arthritis into four patterns of functional capacity. These varied from an early restoration to useful activity to a rapid decline over a few years to helplessness and death. Subsequently about 400 living patients were classified into the same four groups, and an attempt was made to determine whether certain extraarticular findings such as weight loss, blood pressure changes, abnormal glucose tolerance, arteriosclerosis, and emotional upsets were of prognostic value. The conclusion reached was that no one of these factors was of assistance in predicting the patient's future course. It should be noted that the group studied represented in no sense a pure strain of rheumatoid arthritis, in that patients with degenerative joint disease, gonorrheal arthritis, and rheumatic fever were included. In this way, although some of the results were subdivided according to the type of arthritis concerned, the figures cannot in general be compared with those from series with types of arthritis other than rheumatoid carefully excluded. In spite of this important criticism, Nissen's approach is unquestionably sound for the study of arthritis and of other chronic diseases as well.

1.20 Dawson's [133] monograph on "Chronic Arthritis" appeared in the *Nelson New Loose-Leaf Medicine* in 1935. In the course of an excellent clinical description of rheumatoid arthritis, only a few figures were interspersed. In most instances these were apparently drawn from separate series, observed for particular purposes, but the figures relating to the frequency of spondylitis, of psoriasis, of tuberculosis, and of the disease in childhood were drawn from a study of the 800 cases seen in the author's clinic over a period of six years. The statistical value of this study is outranked by the author's opinions on classification and nomenclature, to which subsequent reference will be made. In 1939 Monroe [362] contributed a chapter on "Chronic Arthritis" to *Oxford Medicine*. In his description of the atrophic (or rheumatoid) type, he presented figures based on 267 patients observed in his clinic. These were limited to sex distribution, age of onset (unfortunately not divided according to sex), the frequency of a family history of rheumatoid arthritis or rheumatic fever, the joints involved, and the frequency of certain systemic manifestations, including pleurisy, valvular heart disease, and

Introduction and Review

anemia. Prognosis was also discussed in general terms and the proportion specified of those who improved out of the two-thirds remaining under observation.

1.21 In 1943 Sclater [454] reported an analysis of data obtained from 388 patients hospitalized for rheumatoid arthritis. The patients were selected according to explicit diagnostic criteria in order to exclude specific infectious arthritis and degenerative joint disease. This report is the first one in which the age and sex distributions of the patients were compared with data for the population from which the patients had been selected. The relationships of onset of arthritis to preceding infection, pregnancy, and the menopause were also studied.

1.22 Two years later Fletcher and Lewis-Faning [187, 321] published an extensive clinical and statistical description of 1,000 cases of chronic rheumatism, including 254 patients with rheumatoid arthritis. Their report emphasized the clinical and roentgenographic criteria for distinguishing rheumatoid arthritis and degenerative joint disease. Although their study was performed in retrospect on hospital records accumulated during an eight-year period, the authors were careful to point out the limitations of their data and were conservative in their conclusions.

1.23 The last paper to be mentioned in our review is that of Lewis-Faning [320], who presented in 1950 a detailed statistical analysis of data gathered under the auspices of the Empire Rheumatism Council in regard to "Aetiological Factors Associated with Rheumatoid Arthritis." In this study 532 patients, drawn from hospital wards and out-patient departments of nine clinics, were individually matched for age, sex, and civil state with control subjects who did not have any rheumatic disease. Data for both patients and controls were obtained from questionnaires and complete medical examinations. Historical questions put to the patients were asked of the matched controls with respect to corresponding points in time. This device was particularly useful in the evaluation of factors related to the onset of arthritis. All the conclusions drawn from this study were supported by numerical data with appropriate tests for statistical significance. Most of the specific results will be referred to subsequently in comparison with results obtained in the present study.

2

Diagnostic Criteria for Selection of Patients

2.1 The historical development of our knowledge of joint disease has been adequately reviewed elsewhere [13, 150, 286, 436] and need not be repeated in detail here. In order, however, to gain perspective and to aid in the definition of rheumatoid arthritis as applied to our series, it seems worth while to trace briefly in this chapter the steps by which the disease has gradually emerged as an entity. The process has been an interesting one. At one period the method in favor was the analysis or setting off of what seemed distinct diseases from a heterogeneous group; at another, the synthesis or bringing together of conditions regarded merely as clinical or pathologic variants of one disease. Even today there is no common agreement as to what conditions should be included under or excluded from our concept of rheumatoid arthritis. Such being the case, it is insufficient merely to label a given series of patients with the diagnosis of rheumatoid arthritis and expect the reader to visualize the same clinical picture as the authors. We shall therefore attempt in the following pages to set down precisely and clearly the definition of rheumatoid arthritis applied to the series to be analyzed, along with the diagnostic criteria employed for the selection of patients. Although reasons will be presented in detail for the decisions made, it is fully realized that any definition of rheumatoid arthritis must be

Diagnostic Criteria

regarded as provisional until more complete knowledge is attained of the etiology and pathogenesis of the disease.

GOUT

2.2 It is commonly agreed that the first clear setting off of a disease entity from the general group of joint diseases, which, from Hippocrates' time, had existed undivided under various names, occurred in the early seventeenth century, when de Baillou [140] described acute rheumatism, or rheumatic fever. The analytic process was continued by Sydenham [517] in 1683, when both acute and chronic rheumatism were distinguished from gout. From this time on the identity of gout was gradually established, although we find the term "rheumatic gout" applied to chronic arthritis (still not differentiated into rheumatoid and degenerative forms) well into the nineteenth century. While the great authority of Charcot [81] apparently stabilized the separation between gout and acute and chronic rheumatism, in 1881 Hutchinson [269] still looked upon rheumatoid arthritis as a variable blend of the rheumatic and gouty diathesis, in spite of Garrod's [197] having shown conclusively that the excess of uric acid in the blood, so typical of gout, is absent in rheumatoid arthritis. Today, in practically all quarters, gout is sharply separated from rheumatoid arthritis and other forms of joint disease.

2.3 In a typical progressive form, with symmetrical polyarticular involvement, rheumatoid arthritis is usually readily distinguished from gouty arthritis. On the other hand, when the disease occurs in an atypical form, with episodic attacks involving one or a few joints, the differentiation may be more difficult. No patient presenting such a clinical picture was admitted to our series until a decision had been reached by blood uric acid determinations, response to colchicine and, when necessary, prolonged observation. In addition, in order to exclude the infrequently encountered patients with gouty arthritis resembling rheumatoid arthritis in a chronic, progressive stage, roentgenograms of representative joints and blood uric acid determinations were made routinely. The small proportion of patients in the series with a hyperuricemia but no other evidence of gout is referred to in the series analysis (par. 39.4), as is one patient with an elevated serum uric acid in addition to roentgenographic changes somewhat resembling the "punched-out" areas seen in advanced gouty arthritis. This patient's clinical course was that of rheumatoid arthritis, and a synovial biopsy revealed histologic findings consistent with the clinical diagnosis. Some of our other patients, whose roentgenograms showed "punched-out" areas, were carefully studied in regard to the possibility of gout, with negative results. A patient not included in the series but reported elsewhere [329] was proven to have gout resembling rheumatoid arthritis by a synovial biopsy which showed that the pannus responsible for the fibrous ankylosis was caused by urate deposits. A final possibility, the co-existence of gouty and rheumatoid arthritis in the same individual, has been reported by certain authors [73, 97, 519], but without convincing proof including histopathologic studies. We have yet to encounter such a patient either in the selection of patients for the present series or in our subsequent experience.

DEGENERATIVE JOINT DISEASE

2.4 The comparatively late separation of degenerative joint disease from rheumatoid arthritis has been pointed out in the previous chapter. For the first attempt at such division, we are indebted to Adams [2], who in 1857 distinguished constitutional and local forms of what he called chronic rheumatic arthritis. This distinction gradually became generally accepted through the writings of Charcot [81], A. E. Garrod [199], Bannatyne [13], and others, but the pathologic lesions of degenerative joint disease were assigned to both diseases. Not until the first decade of the twentieth century was rheumatoid arthritis definitely distinguished from degenerative joint disease, both clinically and pathologically, by the work of Painter [397], Goldthwait [212], Llewellyn Jones [286], and Nichols and Richardson [380]. Since this time the separation has been generally accepted in the United States, as well as in England and on the Continent.

2.5 In spite of this hard-won victory, the accomplishment of which took years of patient observation and investigation, series analyses have been presented in recent years (as pointed out in the previous chapter) in which all or many of the conclusions have been drawn from

Diagnostic Criteria

observations on heterogeneous groups of patients. The reasons usually given for not attempting to separate the two great types of chronic arthritis are, first, that many patients demonstrate features of both diseases and, second, that rheumatoid arthritis is one of the causes of the secondary type of degenerative joint disease. Since post mortem studies [34] have shown that changes indistinguishable from those of degenerative joint disease appear uniformly from the third decade on, it seems quite reasonable that both types of arthritis should frequently coincide in the same individual. Furthermore, a joint affected by rheumatoid arthritis may acquire many of the alterations characteristic of degenerative joint disease, secondary to varying combinations of mechanical impairment and of cartilage defects from previous inflammation. In any case, regardless of the author's reasons for combining the two types of chronic arthritis, the clinical features should be discussed separately. Accordingly, in the formation of our series, patients who showed unmistakable manifestations of rheumatoid arthritis were included, whether or not changes of degenerative joint disease were present either coincidentally or consequently, while those with pure degenerative joint disease were excluded. In making the distinction, recognition was accorded to the occasional appearance in degenerative joint disease of synovial and periarticular inflammation [294, 494].

RHEUMATIC FEVER

2.6 Over 250 years ago Sydenham [517] set off acute rheumatism from chronic rheumatism. In spite of the antiquity of this distinction, the identity of rheumatic fever and rheumatoid arthritis continues to be maintained by some on clinical as well as pathologic grounds. The evolution of opinion regarding the relationship of the two diseases makes an interesting chapter in the history of rheumatoid arthritis and is well set forth in an article published in 1936 by Dawson and Tyson [138]. As mentioned in the review of previous studies in Chapter 1, German and Scandinavian workers have divided rheumatoid arthritis into primary and secondary forms, the latter group comprising cases in which arthritis supposedly arises as a sequel to rheumatic fever. In Freund's [192] series of 110 patients with "secondary" chronic polyarthritis, 44 per cent showed organic valvular disease, while in Fischer's

[182] series of 201 patients, 65 per cent developed similar cardiac involvement. In a group of 694 patients in Sweden reported by Edström [163] in 1935, only 4 per cent developed chronic arthritis following their first clinical attack of rheumatic fever. With every successive attack, the proportion increased, so that among those afflicted four times, more than half developed chronic arthritis. Altogether 148, or 21 per cent, showed this sequence, of whom 89 acquired valvular lesions. In surveying the whole group, it became apparent that invalidism in younger patients was largely due to cardiac failure, in older patients to chronic arthritis. Ehlertsen [169], however, in a similar study of 215 Danish patients, was unable to confirm these findings. More recently, in 1952, Clemmesen and Arnsø [91] made a distinction between two types of rheumatoid arthritis, the one of insidious onset and the other having an acute onset and developing "after a condition simulating (if not identical with) rheumatic fever." This group was about one-fifth the size of the first one and comprised those cases "arising acutely with a high fever in connection with an upper respiratory infection." The frequency of valvular heart disease is not stated, but the authors assume that rheumatic fever may "precipitate or result in rheumatoid arthritis." Finally, the clinical studies cited above have been supported by observations on the pathologic histology of the two diseases, notably those of Klinge and Grzimek [302], who conclude that they represent different phases of a single disease process.

2.7 In England and the United States the opposite view has predominated [303, 458]. That rheumatoid arthritis may arise in an acute, "atypical" form which simulates rheumatic fever is recognized, but usually, if the patient is observed long enough, he will present the characteristic clinical picture of rheumatoid arthritis. The development of valvular heart disease in such patients has been noted only occasionally, provided care has been taken to exclude from consideration those patients who actually have rheumatic fever but present some of the articular features of rheumatoid arthritis. A distinction can usually be made by means of careful and prolonged observation [172, 486]. Another possibility is the occasional coincidence of the two diseases in the same individual—the most common sequence being the development of rheumatic heart disease secondary to rheumatic fever in childhood, followed

Diagnostic Criteria

at an appreciable interval by the onset of unmistakable rheumatoid arthritis [70, 575]. A follow-up study in this country of a large series of rheumatic fever patients [575] indicates that such a combination occurs infrequently, perhaps not more often than might be expected by chance.

2.8 More difficult to explain are the post mortem findings of what is apparently rheumatic heart disease with gross valvular deformities in a high proportion of patients with typical severe rheumatoid arthritis coming to autopsy [7, 26, 179, 573]. Previous studies in this direction have recently been summarized by Sokoloff [484], who himself found in 105 cases only "a slightly greater than fortuitous coincidence of heart disease in rheumatoid arthritis morphologically indistinguishable from rheumatic heart disease." Space does not permit further discussion of the discrepancies between Sokoloff's results and those of previous workers. While the differences may depend upon the selection of cases or upon the pathologic criteria employed, Mainland [339] has clearly pointed out from a statistical viewpoint the risk of fallacious conclusions, if derived from autopsy data, regarding the relationships of diseases to one another.

2.9 That a pathologic as well as a clinical differentiation can and should be made between rheumatic fever and rheumatoid arthritis, is now generally accepted in this country and England [31, 70]. According to Bennett [31], the differences are so marked that, in the absence of etiologic evidence to the contrary, the two conditions should be looked on as separate entities. Such a distinction applies to the concept of a form of heart disease specific to rheumatoid arthritis, with histologic changes similar to those found in the rheumatoid subcutaneous nodules. Granulomatous lesions of this type have produced valve deformities which can be distinguished grossly and microscopically from rheumatic valvular disease [8, 89, 218, 484]. In addition, aortitis and aortic insufficiency have been recognized as manifestations of rheumatoid spondylitis [89]. What may thus be called rheumatoid heart disease probably accounts for only a small proportion of the cardiac lesions (exclusive of pericarditis) found in rheumatoid arthritis. Although it is conceivable, according to Sokoloff [484], that healed or minor lesions of this nature "may lead to deformities indistinguishable from those of rheumatic heart disease, the proof for this is lacking at present." A last possible source of confusion between rheumatoid arthritis and rheumatic fever lies in what has been termed "postrheumatic fibrous rheumatism," which, according to Bywaters [70], consists in joint deformities simulating those of rheumatoid arthritis but resulting from persistent arthritis due to rheumatic fever. Whether or not, as in one autopsied case [147], patients with these deformities merely have rheumatoid arthritis engrafted upon an antecedent rheumatic fever with rheumatic heart disease, the condition is exceedingly rare and was not encountered in the selection of patients for our series.

2.10   Further knowledge of the etiology or pathogenesis of the two diseases will be necessary before the differing viewpoints in regard to the relationship between rheumatic fever and rheumatoid arthritis can be explained or reconciled, unless we assume that geographic or racial factors are responsible. At any rate, for the purposes of this study, rheumatoid arthritis and rheumatic fever were regarded as separate entities, and every effort was made toward a clinical differentiation between them in the selection of patients for our series. As an aid to weighing the evidence on whether a patient should be included in or excluded from the series, the following working policy was adopted. Patients with a progressive polyarthritis consistent with rheumatoid arthritis were included, even if presenting one or more of the features to be listed: a history of attacks suggesting rheumatic fever or chorea; valvular heart disease, whether present on first examination or developing under observation; electrocardiographic abnormalities, including a delay in auriculo-ventricular conduction; alterations in cardiac size or shape in roentgenograms. Patients entering the hospital with an acute arthritis resembling that found in rheumatic fever were not included until the passage of time had made clear that the attack was merely a precursor of a more typical chronic rheumatoid arthritis. A few patients, who at first showed persistent symmetrical involvement of small joints and were judged to have rheumatoid arthritis, were finally excluded when the arthritis ceased to progress and the diagnosis of rheumatic fever became likely because of the development of valvular disease. In these instances exclusion did not depend upon the development of valvular lesions, but upon their development along with the disappearance of an articular picture resembling that of rheumatoid arthritis. In

Diagnostic Criteria

the final analysis, in patients presenting and holding the clinical features of rheumatoid arthritis, the presence of or development of valvular heart disease was not held sufficient for disqualification.

2.11 The patients making up the present series were admitted to the hospital between 1930 and 1936. By this time a number (300) believed sufficient had been accumulated, and no further patients were added. About two years later the initial status and subsequent course of the 300 patients were appraised by five observers, with a view to finding any in whom the original diagnosis of rheumatoid arthritis could not be substantiated. It was agreed that 7 should be dropped, because of the likelihood that the actual diagnosis was a specific infectious arthritis in 1 patient and rheumatic fever in 6 patients. The series was then arbitrarily "closed," with the understanding that the study should be based on the remaining 293 patients, irrespective of future developments in the course of follow-up which might qualify previous opinions in regard to diagnosis.

2.12 In order to illustrate the considerations which were influential in deciding between a diagnosis of rheumatoid arthritis and rheumatic fever, brief notes are given below on the 6 patients in whom the latter diagnosis seemed likely at the time of re-appraisal in 1938. Following each case summary, reasons are set down which led to exclusion from the series.

1. A woman, aged thirty-two, was admitted in 1933 because of a generalized, migratory arthritis of two months' duration, starting a week after tonsillitis. A bilateral arthritis was found which included involvement of metacarpo-phalangeal joints, but no evidence of heart disease. Over the next five years, the arthritis cleared, except for brief recurrences at rare intervals, and the patient developed definite signs of mitral valve disease with cardiac failure, from which she died in 1939. At autopsy rheumatic heart disease with marked mitral stenosis was present.

This patient was considered to have rheumatic fever and rheumatic heart disease, although the arthritis on admission to the hospital was consistent with rheumatoid arthritis in an acute phase.

2. A man, aged thirty-five, was admitted in 1933 for a generalized arthritis of three weeks' duration, starting five weeks after a sore throat. Findings on admission included a generalized bilateral arthritis and

no signs of heart disease except for prolongation of the P-R interval. Over the next two years, the arthritis and the electrocardiographic abnormalities disappeared. There were no signs of organic valvular disease except for an inconstant grade 2 mitral systolic murmur. When seen in 1938, the patient had articular symptoms and an increased sedimentation rate, but no objective evidence of arthritis. Over the next few years he gradually developed a persistent swelling of the metacarpo-phalangeal joints with interosseous muscle atrophy. When he was last seen in 1950, this was still present to a milder degree, along with the same apical murmur and an increased sedimentation rate.

In spite of a seventeen year follow-up, a differentiation could not be made with certainty between rheumatoid arthritis and rheumatic fever with persistent articular findings. The patient was eliminated from the series in 1938 for this reason.

3. A fourteen-year-old boy was admitted in 1934 for arthritis of eighteen months' duration, following two weeks after scarlet fever. He had had chorea three years before admission. A symmetrical arthritis was found, involving chiefly the interphalangeal joints, but no evidence of heart disease. During the next four years, he continued to have articular symptoms and intermittent fever but signs of arthritis disappeared. Over the next ten years, he had constitutional and vasomotor symptoms suggestive of rheumatoid arthritis, but a normal sedimentation rate and no joint or cardiac abnormalities.

As in Case 2, in spite of a prolonged follow-up, an unequivocal diagnosis could not be made. Exclusion from the series in 1938 was made on account of previous manifestations suggesting rheumatic fever and the patient's failure to develop the clinical picture of rheumatoid arthritis.

4. A man, aged twenty-two, was admitted in 1934 for a persistent polyarthritis starting three months before. At age twelve, he had had scarlet fever, followed by rheumatic fever and rheumatic valvular disease. A symmetrical polyarthritis involving the proximal interphalangeal joints was found, along with signs of aortic and mitral valve disease. For the next four years, he had persistent joint symptoms and recurrent swelling of the proximal interphalangeal and other joints, in attacks lasting up to six months. By 1938 articular symptoms

Diagnostic Criteria

and signs had disappeared. Later he suffered intermittently from bouts of carditis and arthritis and finally died of cardiac failure in 1943. Autopsy showed rheumatic valvular disease with a myocarditis of probable rheumatic origin. Examination of one knee joint showed no abnormalities.

This patient was considered to have rheumatic fever with persistent articular signs simulating those of rheumatoid arthritis and was therefore eliminated from the series.

5. A youth, aged eighteen, was admitted in 1935 for a persistent, febrile polyarthritis of three months' duration. A symmetrical, generalized arthritis was found, along with an aortic murmur at diastole. He improved while in the hospital and was apparently asymptomatic for over two years. When seen in 1937 for a return of symptoms, he had the same aortic murmur and the proximal interphalangeal joints were swollen. Over the next seven years, he had recurrent symptoms, persistence of the murmur, and an elevated sedimentation rate, but no objective changes in the joints.

In this case the diagnostic possibilities included rheumatoid arthritis with a coincidental rheumatic valvular lesion, rheumatic fever with persistent joint swelling, and even involvement of the heart by a rheumatoid process. At the time of appraisal the articular disease was not believed sufficiently characteristic of rheumatoid arthritis to make this diagnosis in the presence of valvular disease.

6. A sixty-year-old woman was admitted in 1935 for arthritis of two weeks' duration. Past history included chorea in childhood, with the development of heart disease, and two attacks of arthritis at long intervals and lasting up to five months. Swelling of the metacarpophalangeal joints and one ankle was found in addition to mitral stenosis and a prolonged P-R interval. The arthritis persisted about three months and then apparently cleared, so that the patient was asymptomatic in 1938. When seen in 1944, her joints were normal to examination and her presenting complaints were due to her heart disease and hypertension. She died in the same year of a myocardial infarction. Autopsy revealed rheumatic valvular disease and myocarditis of probable rheumatic origin. Examination of a metacarpo-phalangeal joint and a knee joint showed a "healed" proliferative arthritis with pannus for-

mation. The pathologist reported that his findings were consistent with rheumatoid arthritis but added, "It remains to be shown that rheumatic fever alone could not have produced the same picture."

In this instance a patient with rheumatic heart disease following chorea did not develop a sufficiently characteristic and persistent arthritis to permit an unqualified diagnosis of rheumatoid arthritis and retention in the series. At autopsy, however, articular changes were present which were consistent with rheumatoid arthritis.

RHEUMATOID SPONDYLITIS*

2.13 According to Jones [286], the earliest detailed study of the morbid anatomy of rheumatoid spondylitis was that of Connor in 1700, entitled "The Bones of a Sceleton United Without Joynting or Cartilage." Although Dr. Connor deduced from the post mortem specimen some of the outstanding clinical features in life, over 150 years passed by before isolated reports of living patients with the disease began to appear. Finally, toward the end of the nineteenth century, the names of Strümpell [511], von Bechterew [545], and Marie [341] became associated with what they believed independent types of spinal arthritis. Strümpell and Marie were probably both describing rheumatoid spondylitis, but von Bechterew's series undoubtedly included patients with a dorsal kyphosis due to a variety of conditions, with rheumatoid spondylitis among them. At present there is general agreement that the term "Bechterew's disease" leads to confusion and should be dropped. On the other hand, opinion is still divided as to whether rheumatoid spondylitis should be considered a form of rheumatoid arthritis which chiefly affects the spine or a disease sui generis. Although this question cannot be settled with the information presently available, both sides of this rather controversial subject will be briefly presented in the following paragraphs along with the authors' decision in regard to the inclusion of patients with spinal involvement in the present series.

2.14 Patients with advanced rheumatoid spondylitis present a distinctive clinical and radiologic picture, which would doubtless be gen-

---

* Synonyms employed in the recent literature include "ankylosing spondylitis," "spondylitis ankylopoietica," and "pelvospondylitis ossificans" [437]. For convenience and for reasons outlined below, the term "rheumatoid spondylitis" will be employed.

Diagnostic Criteria

erally regarded as an independent entity but for one fact: many of them have peripheral joint involvement indistinguishable from that seen in rheumatoid arthritis and including at times the small joints of the hands and feet. In certain series [413, 437] peripheral joint involvement has been found in half or more of the patients and preceding the development of spondylitis in at least half of these. In addition, pathologic examination of such joints has shown changes consistent with a diagnosis of rheumatoid arthritis [4, 108, 540]. As far as the spine and spinal joints are concerned, pathologic studies are incomplete and are based on a relatively small number of specimens obtained post mortem or by biopsy. From the available evidence, Collins [108] has recently concluded that the initial lesion in the intervertebral (apophyseal) and costovertebral joints is an inflammatory arthritis resembling in all respects that found in peripheral joints in rheumatoid arthritis. He does point out the remarkable tendency to ossification of tissues within and around these joints as well as of the disc margins and spinal ligaments. Thus far pathologic data are lacking in regard to the early changes in the sacro-iliac joints. Additional pathologic features which have recently been emphasized [437] are destructive osseous lesions in vertebrae and pelvic bones, which go on to repair and ossification. The chief reasons, then, for regarding rheumatoid spondylitis as a form of rheumatoid arthritis lie in the frequency of peripheral joint involvement and in the evidence found from pathologic examination of both peripheral joints and diarthrodial joints of the spine.

2.15 Certain clinical and laboratory differences between rheumatoid spondylitis and rheumatoid arthritis may next be listed. On the clinical side, rheumatoid spondylitis is distinguished by a preponderantly male sex distribution, an earlier age of onset, an increased frequency of uveitis (par. 29.4) and the failure to find subcutaneous nodules in patients without peripheral arthritis (par. 33.4). The favorable effects of roentgenotherapy [482] and of Butazolidin [533] in spondylitis as well as the lack of response to gold [468] have likewise been cited as differences. Certain laboratory tests have exhibited negative results or a decreased frequency of positive results in rheumatoid spondylitis compared with rheumatoid arthritis. These include: streptococcal agglutinations [47], various serum flocculation tests [240] and, most recently, a hemagglutination test using the euglobulin fraction [576]. Spinal fluid abnormalities are found more frequently in spondylitis [330], with the reverse reported in regard to inflammatory foci in muscle in four reports [142, 193, 296, 470] but not confirmed in a fifth [485]. Of the clinical and laboratory differences presented above, perhaps the most important are the failure to find nodules in spondylitis without peripheral joint involvement other than shoulders and hips and the results thus far obtained with the hemagglutination reaction as modified by Ziff and his colleagues [576].

2.16 Whether rheumatoid spondylitis constitutes a disease sui generis or is a form of rheumatoid arthritis must remain a matter of opinion in the absence of further knowledge. Nevertheless, from experience with the condition in this clinic and from a survey of the literature, the authors have decided to adopt the tentative conclusion that rheumatoid spondylitis constitutes the spinal equivalent of rheumatoid arthritis involving only peripheral joints. For this reason patients with rheumatoid spondylitis have been included in the selection of patients for the present series, whether or not peripheral joints were involved in addition to the spine. Exclusion of such patients, it is believed, would render the series less rather than more representative of rheumatoid arthritis warranting hospitalization. In the series analysis a numerical comparison will be made between patients with and without spondylitis, in order to determine clinical and laboratory similarities and differences between the two groups.

JUVENILE RHEUMATOID ARTHRITIS

2.17 Although rheumatoid arthritis is comparatively rare in children, any definition of this disease must take into account differing opinions as to whether the forms seen in childhood represent a distinct entity or merely a juvenile type. Such a discussion will lead in the next section to a consideration of rheumatoid arthritis in adults with certain features of the juvenile form, chiefly adenopathy and splenomegaly (Still-Chauffard syndrome of Continental authors), and finally to consideration of the so-called Felty's syndrome, the distinguishing points of which are, in addition to the arthritis, splenomegaly and leukopenia.

2.18 Cornil's [119] case history, published in 1864, of a twenty-nine-year-old woman who had had progressive arthritis since the age

Diagnostic Criteria

of twelve, is generally considered the first definite description of rheumatoid arthritis originating in childhood, while the first review of a large series of cases, 35 in number, was recorded by Diamentberger [145] in 1891. Following Still's [504] classical communication in 1896, which will be considered in detail below, single case reports or series of cases appeared in the literature, totaling, according to Byfield [68], several hundred cases by 1925. In recent years several series of children with rheumatoid arthritis have been described in this country and in Europe [112, 121, 325, 409, 513], the largest that of Sury [513], comprising 151 cases. Nevertheless, the disease in children must still be regarded as comparatively rare and as necessarily making up only a small portion of any large series of patients of all ages with rheumatoid arthritis. In Garrod's [199] series of 500 such patients and in McCrae's [333] series of 319 patients, less than 1 per cent and 6.6 per cent respectively were found with onset under the age of ten, while Coss and Boots [121] encountered 56 patients over a period of eighteen years whose disease began at the age of twelve or younger. This last group made up 4.9 per cent of the total number of rheumatoid patients seen during this time. No possible cause for this low frequency has yet been established or even conjectured, although it may be noted in passing that such age distribution is exceptional in diseases known to be of infectious origin.

2.19   On November 10, 1896, Dr. George F. Still [504] read a communication before the Royal Medical and Chirurgical Society of London entitled "On a Form of Chronic Joint Disease in Children." This date marks the origin, not only of the eponym "Still's disease," but also of the conception that a form of arthritis exists in childhood which makes up a distinct clinical and pathologic entity. Up to this time, as Still himself states, the identity of the juvenile and adult forms of the disease was never questioned. As a masterly clinical description of previously unrecognized features of rheumatoid arthritis in children, this presentation should take first rank, but owing to the prevailing confusion of the times about the classification and description of the great nonspecific types of chronic arthritis, the author promulgated a distinction which is now generally regarded as unnecessary and misleading. For a full understanding of the situation, a rather detailed summary and analysis of Still's original paper is requisite.

2.20   In an attempt to demonstrate that the forms of rheumatoid arthritis most commonly seen in children do show a real clinical and pathologic difference from that seen in adults, Still presented 19 personally observed cases of joint disease in children. He defined the newly recognized condition as a chronic, progressive enlargement of the joints, associated with enlargement of the lymph nodes and spleen. These criteria were fulfilled in 12 of the 19 cases. In all but 2 of the 12 cases onset occurred before the age of six; whether gradual or acute, this led to generalized, symmetrical arthritis with limitation of motion. In all cases lymph nodes were enlarged, chiefly those related to the joints affected; they were described as nontender, nonsuppurative, hard, and discrete. In all but 3 cases the spleen was enlarged. The heart was normal, except for hemic bruits and "physical signs suggestive of adherent pericardium" in 2 cases. In 3 others, adherent pericarditis was found at autopsy. Fever, either irregular or continuous, was uniformly found. In some cases growth and development were arrested, but mentality was unimpaired. The joint enlargement seemed to be due to soft tissue swelling, and the *"bony irregularity of the rheumatoid arthritis in adults" was not found.** The course was slow and occasionally remittent but tended to progress relentlessly to complete disability. A few died of complicating diseases, but intercurrent infections (including, of interest to us today, catarrhal jaundice) were sometimes followed by improvement. In all 3 of the cases that came to autopsy adherent pericarditis and pleuritis were present and lymph nodes and spleen were enlarged but grossly normal. The joints showed thickening of the capsules and connective tissue, as well as of the synovia, with fibrous adhesions occasionally present. One case, of three years' duration, showed pitting at the margins of the cartilage with synovial processes in the pits.

2.21   Of the remaining 7 children in Still's series, 6 had rheumatoid arthritis indistinguishable from that seen in adults. There was the same general enlargement of the joints, *"with subsequent bony thickening and lipping and bony grating."** In no case were lymph nodes or spleen enlarged, and there was no evidence of pericarditis. None of these cases came to autopsy. The remaining patient was believed to have chronic fibrous rheumatism (see under rheumatic fever, par. 2.9).

* Italics ours.

Diagnostic Criteria

2.22 In the course of his presentation Still listed what seemed to him to be the important points of difference between the newly recognized children's disease and the rheumatoid arthritis of adults: (1) clinical examination of the joints of the children in his first group showed what felt like extra-articular thickening of soft tissue, "very unlike the irregular bony enlargement of joints found in the advanced rheumatoid arthritis of adults" or in his second group; (2) the pathologic examination of the joints showed "complete absence, even in an advanced case, of the cartilage changes which are seen quite early in the rheumatoid arthritis of adults"; (3) the lymph nodes and spleen were enlarged, which the author believed to be unknown in adults; (4) a large proportion of the children had pericarditis and pleuritis. Finally, the points of distinction mentioned were not regarded as due merely to age differences, because of the existence in children of a condition identical in every respect with the rheumatoid arthritis of adults.

2.23 As mentioned previously, in 1896 the clinical distinction between rheumatoid arthritis and degenerative joint disease was only beginning to be accepted and the pathologic changes of the latter were assigned to both. One is justified in believing, then, that Still's knowledge of joint disease was not in advance of his time and that the criteria which he set up with such pains do not apply to the clinical and pathologic entity which is considered rheumatoid arthritis today. In the absence of roentgenographic evidence, it may be assumed that the bony enlargement which he described in the children with true rheumatoid arthritis was an illusion produced by muscular wasting, as is shown in a photograph illustrating supposed bony thickening of the joints.

2.24 In regard to the second distinction, the absence of cartilage changes, it is probable that the author is again referring to degenerative changes, since in reporting one of his own cases of the new disease he gives a perfect description of early cartilage loss from marginal pannus formation and invasion. In any event, many authors [*141, 192, 262, 406, 416, 554, 563*] have since described pathologic changes with cartilage absorption in cases of so-called Still's disease, although cases of shorter duration [*71, 493*] may present only periarticular and synovial involvement.

2.25 That adults with rheumatoid arthritis often show generalized or satellite adenopathy was probably first mentioned by Chauffard and Ramond [83] in 1896, the year of Still's presentation. Since then the frequency of lymphadenopathy in this disease has been reported in frequencies varying from 19 to 96 per cent [97, 150, 192, 553]. Diverse figures are also given for the frequency of splenomegaly, ranging from 6 [553] to 21 per cent [97]. The occurrence of both is probably more common in children with rheumatoid arthritis than in adults (see Table 30.4). Likewise, pericarditis and pleuritis are apparently less common in adults, although each has been reported, both clinically and at autopsy [13, 81, 119, 333, 388, 418].

2.26   It can thus be seen that the major points of distinction mentioned by Still in his attempt to set off a new syndrome become relatively unimportant in the light of further knowledge. Certainly there is no reason to apply, as is often done, the term "Still's disease" to all cases of rheumatoid arthritis originating in childhood, whether or not the features enumerated by Still are present. Furthermore, as emphasized by Sury [513], it is not reasonable to maintain the concept of "Still's disease" as applicable to a fairly well-defined group of children with rheumatoid arthritis. There are no fundamental clinical or pathologic differences between such a group and the remainder, and borderline cases are often seen. Is there any merit, then, in the use of the eponym "Still's disease," except to honor a keen observer? The present authors are in agreement with Morse [369] that it would be wiser to drop it from the nomenclature and speak only of juvenile or childhood rheumatoid arthritis.

2.27   In the selection of patients for the present series, we adopted the generally accepted principle that rheumatoid arthritis is the same disease in adults and children, with certain minor differences due to peculiarities in response at different ages. These include the increased frequency in childhood of splenomegaly, lymphadenopathy, pericarditis, and pleuritis, as first described by Still, and of both general and localized growth disturbances. It has also been stated that fever and leukocytosis are more common in childhood [133, 513], as well as initial involvement of large rather than small joints [513]. Sury [513] has recently pointed out a difference in the ocular manifestations of the disease, in that "band" keratitis and an indolent form of iridocyclitis

Diagnostic Criteria

have, in his experience, been confined to children. While the differences just listed are of interest and deserve recognition, they hardly merit the separation of rheumatoid arthritis into adult and juvenile disease entities. No patient was therefore excluded from the series because the onset occurred in childhood or adolescence, and a total of 23 were included whose disease began at the age of fifteen or younger.

THE STILL-CHAUFFARD SYNDROME AND FELTY'S SYNDROME

2.28 Reference has been made in the preceding section to the occurrence of splenomegaly and lymphadenopathy in the rheumatoid arthritis of adults. These findings have led to attempts to set off a distinct entity, called Still's disease in adults, or the Still-Chauffard syndrome. The first of such attempts by Chauffard and Ramond [83] in 1896 was based on 5 cases with adenopathy secondary to what sounds like rheumatoid arthritis and 2 cases with enlarged satellite nodes in gonorrheal arthritis. Moltke [359] described 4 rather acute cases of rheumatoid arthritis with adenopathy and, although lymph node biopsies showed nothing specific, wished to classify them with similar cases reported by Bayliss [28] and McCrae [333] as a new clinical entity, "adult Still's disease." In a study of 10 cases of so-called "Still-Chauffard disease," Micheli [354] found a special and constant pathologic picture in the lymph nodes, but on analysis this differs very little from what others [83, 333, 359, 561] have merely described as hyperplasia and mild inflammation of a nonspecific nature. Of interest in this connection is the follicular hyperplasia resembling giant follicle lymphoma recently discovered by Motulsky et al. [370] in lymph nodes biopsied from certain patients with rheumatoid arthritis. Other authors [133, 333] found no reason to separate out patients with rheumatoid arthritis and enlargement of the spleen and lymph nodes. Weil [556] even felt that adenopathy is common to all forms of inflammatory or infectious arthritis and pointed out that the first report of Chauffard and Ramond included two patients with gonorrheal arthritis. Until etiologic evidence is at hand, we shall doubtless continue to encounter in the literature further reports of Still-Chauffard disease or a similar syndrome with some new clinical vagary.

2.29 Such a report was published in 1924 by Felty [178], who described 5 adult cases of chronic arthritis with splenomegaly and leukopenia. All 5 patients showed a brownish pigmentation, 3 had enlarged lymph nodes, and none enlargement of the liver. Since that time reports of at least 30 patients with arthritis, splenomegaly, and leukopenia have appeared [123, 125, 127, 210, 228, 238, 245, 268, 270, 471, 521, 523]. Many of these reports employ the term "Felty's syndrome," although acceptance of the syndrome as an entity has been largely confined to earlier studies. In one of these [471], the observers even essayed a search for a causal agent and arrived at the conclusion that the syndrome represented a special form of sepsis lenta due to *Streptococcus viridans*. More recently, however, the triad of arthritis, splenomegaly, and leukopenia has been considered merely a rather uncommon variant of rheumatoid arthritis. That splenomegaly may constitute a systemic manifestation of rheumatoid arthritis in both children and adults has already been mentioned. When histologic examination of the spleen has been possible in such instances, no specific pathologic picture has been found [123, 228, 238]. Although slight or moderate grades of leukopenia are not unusual in rheumatoid arthritis, severe neutropenia is rare [155]. According to Collins [106], whose criterion for the upper limits of a definitely pathologic leukopenia is a white-cell count of 2,000 or a neutrophil count of 1,000, leukopenia occurs in less than 0.5 per cent of the cases. There seems, then, to be no need to assume that the combination of splenomegaly and leukopenia with rheumatoid arthritis represents a new pathologic entity. In certain recent reports [127, 228, 268, 270], the leukopenia has been considered secondary to the splenomegaly, in accordance with the concept of "hypersplenism." In this way, rheumatoid arthritis may be regarded as an occasional cause of splenic neutropenia. It should also be emphasized that extraneous causes for both splenomegaly and leukopenia have been evident or at least likely in many of the cases reported under the heading of Felty's syndrome [245, 521]. Such causes include liver disease, amyloidosis, diseases of the blood or blood-forming organs, and pyelonephritis and other infections. In addition, lupus erythematosus disseminatus, dermatomyositis, and periarteritis nodosa may present some or all of the features of arthritis, splenomegaly, and leukopenia and must be considered in the differential diagnosis.

Diagnostic Criteria

2.30 It is our conclusion that the term Felty's syndrome, which implies a separate entity, has no reasonable foundation and should be discarded. Rheumatoid arthritis is a generalized disease that may affect with varying frequency the lymph nodes, spleen, bone marrow, and many other tissues besides the articular structures. Perpetuation of syndromes named for Still, Still and Chauffard, or Felty therefore seems undesirable. In the selection of patients for inclusion in our series, the presence of lymphadenopathy, splenomegaly, or leukopenia, either alone or in various combinations, was therefore not considered a valid reason for exclusion. On the other hand, the frequency of these manifestations and their relationship to others will form a part of the numerical study to follow.

PSORIASIS AND ARTHRITIS

2.31 That a relationship exists between psoriasis and rheumatoid arthritis is generally admitted, chiefly because of the frequency with which this skin disease occurs among patients with the clinical features of rheumatoid arthritis. Certain observers even recommend that many cases with this combination should be set apart from rheumatoid arthritis and designated by a term like psoriatic arthritis. The criteria for this diagnosis include: an asymmetrical arthritis, often showing marked articular destruction, with involved joints sometimes isolated and corresponding anatomically to psoriatic lesions; unusually frequent association of terminal interphalangeal joint involvement and psoriatic nails; and synchronous exacerbation and remission of arthritis and dermatitis. Other cases are encountered in which the two conditions seem to be independent in regard to distribution and course. Since there are all gradations between this group and the one labeled psoriatic arthritis, it is suggested in one paper [139] that this term should include all cases presenting features of both diseases. It becomes obvious, then, that in the selection of patients for the present series, the decision had to be made whether or not to exclude any or all patients with psoriasis. The considerations which led to our decision will be discussed in the following paragraphs.

2.32 For an orderly attack upon the problem, it would seem wise to lay down at the start the various possibilities which may determine the relationship of the two diseases. In listing them here, it is realized that, since the causation of neither condition is known, each proposition must stand or fall upon indirect and largely clinical evidence.

1. So-called psoriatic arthritis is an independent entity resembling but not part of either psoriasis or rheumatoid arthritis [390, 461].

2. Psoriasis and rheumatoid arthritis share a common but unknown causation [49, 139, 181, 229, 267, 391].

3. The arthritis accompanying psoriasis is secondary to the skin disease and may properly be labeled an arthropathy rather than an arthritis [196, 250].

4. The skin lesions constitute a manifestation of rheumatoid arthritis and may be called psoriasiform rather than true psoriasis.

5. There is a constitutional, perhaps hereditary, tendency in certain individuals and families for the acquirement of both diseases, resulting in more frequent coincidence than can be laid to chance alone [21]. In certain of such cases the typical picture of the one disease may be modified by the presence of the other.

2.33 The reader will note that we have not included the possibility that the two diseases may exist independently and purely coincidentally in the same individual [57, 175]. The frequency of psoriasis in rheumatoid arthritis is significantly greater than in the control group, as shown by Wassmann's [552] figures of 3.1 per cent in 1,000 rheumatoid patients compared with 0.43 per cent in 10,000 controls. It would therefore be manifestly inaccurate to assign the relationship to chance in every case. In addition, although it has been stated that true psoriatic arthritis can be distinguished from psoriasis coincidental to rheumatoid arthritis [461], such a distinction is often difficult [139] and, even if accepted, does not aid materially in the solution of the problem.

2.34 In order to establish the first proposition that psoriatic arthritis represents an independent disease entity, it should be shown that the skin and joint lesions differ fundamentally from those found in uncomplicated psoriasis and rheumatoid arthritis. The skin lesions in so-called psoriatic arthritis have been variously described, mostly in single case reports or small series, as exudative in nature with the production of waxy, translucent papules and large abundant micaceous scales [139]; as pustular [143, 162, 219, 266, 281]; as exfoliative [162, 391]; and as

Diagnostic Criteria

often involving the nails [12, 49, 139, 162, 219, 250, 251, 391, 462]. All these manifestations occur in uncomplicated psoriasis, although they are admittedly less common and typical. The course of the disease, whether accompanied by arthritis or not, is extremely variable, ranging from sudden remissions and relapses to an inveterate chronicity. It seems fair to state, then, that the skin lesions in so-called psoriatic arthritis are not distinct in morphology or course, although there is a real tendency toward atypical forms. This is evidenced in Dawson and Tyson's [139] series of 26, about three-quarters of whom showed an exudative type of psoriasis, and, in the same proportion, involvement of the nails. In regard to histologic descriptions of the skin lesions in "psoriatic arthritis," the most extensive study encountered is that of Burks and Montgomery [65], who examined biopsies from 24 patients with psoriasis and arthritis, 14 of whom had involvement of the terminal interphalangeal joints. Quantitative differences only were found, in that the process was in general more severe and exudative, with edema and micro-abscesses prominent. Nordin [391] and Plenk [410] also each reported one case in which the findings resembled those in uncomplicated psoriasis.

2.35   The joint lesions in "psoriatic arthritis" have also been variously described. Certain authors [73, 182, 192, 281, 462] believe that the presence of psoriasis foretells an intractable, severe case of arthritis; others believe [49, 250, 507] that the condition is usually mild and may bear a favorable prognosis, especially if the psoriasis is vigorously and successfully treated. Intermittent hydrarthrosis, later going on to a progressive arthritis, has been described in a total of 4 cases of rheumatoid arthritis and psoriasis by Garrod [196] and by Bauer and Vogl [21]. Nearly a fourth of Dawson and Tyson's [139] 26 cases showed asymmetrical involvement of isolated joints. What will be more extensively treated later may be mentioned at this point—that intermittent hydrarthrosis usually represents a phase in the development of rheumatoid arthritis (par. **2.48**) and that an asymmetrical distribution of arthritis is common in early stages of this disease (par. **17.2**).

2.36   On the other hand, the extreme degree of articular and bony destruction [182, 219, 313, 462] and the tendency toward involvement of the terminal interphalangeal joints [139, 251], both of which conditions have been described as characteristic of "psoriatic arthritis," require more prolonged consideration. In regard to the former, it can be said that equally severe loss of bony and cartilaginous substance is found not infrequently in long-standing rheumatoid arthritis without psoriasis. Hench's [251] descriptive terms, "ball and socket, pencil-to-pencil or pencil-to-cup" for the roentgenographic appearance of such joints in "psoriatic arthritis," are matched by Marie and Léri's [342] "la main en lorgnette" (the telescoping hand), which they observed in a patient with severe rheumatoid arthritis without psoriasis. These authors refer to earlier photographs of such cases by Pribram and others, and in 1952 Smyth [481] collected a total of 9 cases from the literature. In addition, he reported 8 patients with rheumatoid arthritis and extensive bone absorption, in the hands, in a single digit, or in the distal end of the ulna. Severe articular destruction, then, may be regarded as an integral, if uncommon, part of the clinical and radiologic picture of rheumatoid arthritis. There seems to be no reason for it to be assigned as a distinguishing mark of "psoriatic arthritis," nor any present way of determining whether its frequency is greater in this condition than in rheumatoid arthritis without psoriasis.

2.37 Several authors [22, 461, 501] agree with Hench [251] that severe involvement of the terminal interphalangeal joints, usually accompanied by psoriasis of the nails, constitutes the most important distinguishing and diagnostic feature of "psoriatic arthritis." Figures from one series of 532 patients with rheumatoid arthritis [320] do indicate that proximal interphalangeal joint involvement is much more common than terminal, but the latter occurred in about one-sixth of the patients. Dawson and Tyson [139] found terminal interphalangeal joint involvement in less than a fourth of their 26 patients with "psoriatic arthritis," but they included in this classification patients in whom the two conditions might be regarded as merely coincidental. Additional data are needed on the frequency of terminal interphalangeal joint involvement in rheumatoid arthritis without psoriasis. At present this feature can be regarded as not more than a minor point of distinction, unless, of course, it is made a requisite for the diagnosis of "psoriatic arthritis."

2.38 Pathologic descriptions of the articular findings in "psoriatic arthritis" are limited to a few studies. In 6 patients with psoriasis and

Diagnostic Criteria

chronic arthritis, 4 of whom had involvement of the terminal interphalangeal joints, Bauer, Bennett, and Zeller [22] observed synovial tissue changes similar to those commonly found in rheumatoid arthritis. The seventh patient, with marked destructive changes limited to the terminal interphalangeal joints, revealed a unique histologic picture at autopsy. The joints showed marginal bony overgrowth with articular and marked bony resorption but without diffuse bony atrophy, while the joint spaces were filled by dense acellular connective tissue showing minimal or no inflammatory changes. Sherman's [461] findings in 33 biopsied joints from patients with "true" psoriatic arthritis varied greatly, apparently according to the age of the lesion. Conspicuous inflammatory changes without specific features characterized the first stage. Later on, granulating tissue produced simultaneous destruction of bone and cartilage, without the pannus formation commonly seen in rheumatoid arthritis. As in the seventh patient reported by Bauer *et al.* [22], cartilage and bone were replaced by fairly dense fibrous tissue showing mild inflammatory changes. Further study is required before a distinctive histologic picture can be established for "psoriatic arthritis." In any event, it is of interest that in two patients of Smyth's [481], who had rheumatoid arthritis with severe articular and bony destruction but without psoriasis, the histologic changes were described as replacement by dense acellular fibrous tissue with minimal or no inflammatory changes.

2.39   The clinical, roentgenographic, and pathologic evidence outlined in the preceding paragraphs appears insufficient to establish a fundamental difference between either the skin or joint lesions in "psoriatic arthritis" and those found in uncomplicated psoriasis and rheumatoid arthritis. One possible exception, to be taken up in greater detail below, is the form of arthritis and psoriasis in which the arthritis is limited to terminal interphalangeal joints in association with psoriatic nails. Otherwise, in the absence of etiologic information, the existence thus far seems unwarranted of "psoriatic arthritis" as an independent disease.

2.40   The proponents of a common etiology for psoriasis and rheumatoid arthritis base their case not only upon the appearance of both in the same individual in a significant number of instances, but also upon clinical, epidemiologic, and pathologic similarities between the two. These have been pointed out chiefly by Hunt [267] and Dawson and Tyson [139]. To begin with, both diseases show variability in severity, extent, site, duration, and periods of remission. But when present in one patient, the anatomical distribution of lesions may correspond most strikingly not only in the fingers but in other places as well. At the same time, as found by Dawson and Tyson [139] in over half of their 26 cases, the courses of the two diseases may be strikingly parallel, especially in the early stages, when remissions are most common. In other cases the two diseases may exist side by side with neither seemingly affected by the other [250, 461]. In both conditions there is a tendency to chronicity or even lifetime involvement, with remissions less complete as the disease progresses. Both are said to be rarely found in tropical regions and are most prevalent in temperate climates. There is also a similar seasonal distribution of exacerbations and remissions. Both show a familial tendency, and both may start after an upper respiratory infection. The symmetrical distribution of both diseases is striking, so much so that in the past a neurotropic etiology has been advanced for each. In each, the course is usually altered favorably by pregnancy [255]. There are also some interesting differences. The average age of onset in one large series of psoriatics [308] was twenty-one years, surely lower than in rheumatoid arthritis, while Ingram [272] found a peak of onset of psoriasis at puberty and another at the climateric. In the same large series about 60 per cent of the psoriatics were of average weight and 30 per cent overweight, a reversal of the situation in rheumatoid arthritis (see par. 21.5). Finally, and perhaps most important, the psoriatic is traditionally a healthy individual with a striking absence of the constitutional symptoms making up so consistently the clinical picture of rheumatoid arthritis. The comparison need not be continued further. It is sufficient to say that the evidence for a clinical and epidemiologic similarity is only suggestive and can readily be opposed by even more striking differences. The pathologic picture in the two diseases is also suggestively similar, in that each shows microscopically both a diffuse and a localized inflammatory infiltration [14, 88, 139], although the resemblance is in no way specific. Finally, no one has ventured to define a common etiology beyond the stage of hypothe-

Diagnostic Criteria

sis, with the older writers leaning toward a neurotropic basis for both, and others [229, 391], more recently, indicting an infection of unknown nature.

2.41 In conclusion, it must appear plain that the etiologic identity of psoriasis and rheumatoid arthritis is hardly established. Furthermore, the apparent influence of one disease upon the course of the other seems well in keeping with the propensities of both to be altered in course by intercurrent disturbances of infectious and noninfectious nature.

2.42 The discussion just preceding may also be applied to the hypothesis that one disease is merely an occasional manifestation of the other. We shall first present the case for those who argue that the arthritis accompanying psoriasis is not rheumatoid arthritis but secondary in some way to the skin disease, in other words, an arthropathy. One leading argument is the fact that the psoriasis precedes the arthritis in the vast majority of recorded individual cases, as well as in the series reported by Bourdillon [49], Guszman [229], and Dawson and Tyson [139]. An increased severity or a change in type of the psoriasis immediately preceding the onset of arthritis is also described. In some closely observed cases [21, 49, 139, 162, 219, 266], however, the articular involvement has come first. The same general rule applies to the onset of exacerbations. Similarly, improvement in the arthritis may be preceded by a fading of the psoriasis, so much so that Hench [251] feels that intensive treatment of the skin is the important factor in clearing up the joint disease. It seems more reasonable to suppose that the terminal interphalangeal joint involvement may be directly connected, in a way not yet demonstrated, to the psoriatic nails. Indeed, in most cases the involved nail and joint are found on the same finger [251].

2.43 If we accept the theory that a condition resembling rheumatoid arthritis may be a manifestation of psoriasis, the frequency of such a sequence is difficult to determine from the literature, since the figures vary from one per cent or less [12, 250, 391] to 32 per cent [308] (the arthritis in a minority of the last group showing a direct association with the psoriasis in onset and course). One author [267] has even stated that 70 per cent of her patients with psoriasis suffer from arthritis or rheumatism. The two authors [267, 308] reporting the highest frequency of arthritis with psoriasis made no attempt to describe the type of arthritis present. It may be assumed, then, that in carefully studied series, a progressive arthritis resembling rheumatoid arthritis occurs in a very small percentage of psoriatics. The best argument against the arthritis being a manifestation of psoriasis lies in the numerous cases wherein the two diseases co-exist without apparent connection, and the even more numerous cases wherein endless gradations occur. It is possible, of course, that arthritis of the terminal interphalangeal joints associated with psoriasis of the nails may be separated off as a secondary arthropathy, but at present the line of division is obscure.

2.44 That psoriatic lesions occurring in rheumatoid arthritis may sometimes be merely a manifestation of the arthritis seems as likely as the reverse but equally incapable of proof. Rheumatoid arthritis is admittedly a generalized disease, affecting many systems of the body beside the joints, including the skin and nails (see Chapter 31). The clinical, epidemiologic, and pathologic comparison between the two diseases as set forth above, applies equally well to either being primary. That the psoriatic skin lesions generally precede the arthritis is not incompatible with the common observation that constitutional and vasomotor symptoms, as well as inflammatory lesions such as uveitis, may precede definite involvement of the joints in rheumatoid arthritis. The decision of course awaits knowledge of the etiology or pathogenesis of both psoriasis and rheumatoid arthritis, but additional studies are indicated on the histopathology of psoriasis accompanied by arthritis.

2.45 In 1931, in a valuable article on psoriasis and joint disease, Bauer and Vogl [21] set forth a theory which supposes an inherited predisposition to both diseases as an explanation of co-existence in the same individual. As evidence, a number of striking examples are cited, from their own observation and from the literature, of the association of psoriasis and rheumatoid arthritis in families, with at least one member suffering from both diseases. Other authors [73, 139, 162, 267] have also commented on the same association. In this way the unexpected frequency of psoriasis in rheumatoid arthritis is explained and no attempt is made to establish "psoriatic arthritis" as an independent entity apart from either psoriasis or rheumatoid arthritis. Furthermore, no suggestion is made for a common etiology for the two diseases except an hereditary and constitutional predisposition. In other words, the

Diagnostic Criteria

relationship between psoriasis and rheumatoid arthritis is a relationship between constitutional factors, with the presence of the one disease perhaps modifying the clinical picture of the other. The objection to this theory is that in neither disease has an hereditary factor been demonstrated beyond criticism [272, 395], although the literature, as well as the experience of many clinicians, includes individual families showing a high incidence of psoriasis or of rheumatoid arthritis (see Chapter 8). Furthermore, as in tuberculosis, the relationship between members of the family afflicted with the disease may be that of contagion rather than inherited predisposition.

2.46 In the foregoing discussion no attempt has been made to advance one theory at the expense of the others, but rather to present the evidence impartially and judicially. At the end it is necessary to admit that few conclusions may be drawn. It is felt that the evidence is against setting off "psoriatic arthritis" as an independent disease; that there is no proof that the two diseases have a common etiology, in spite of interesting resemblances; that there is justification for regarding the arthritis as a secondary arthropathy only when involvement of a terminal interphalangeal joint follows psoriasis of a nail; and finally that the theory of constitutional or familial predisposition is always attractive in obscure conditions but must be backed by carefully planned and controlled investigations along genetic lines.

2.47 In the formation of the present series of 293 patients with rheumatoid arthritis, psoriasis was encountered in 10 cases, or 3.4 per cent. In only 1 of these did the psoriasis and arthritis show a definite relationship in the form of parallel exacerbations and remissions. In all but 1, where complete exfoliation took place, the psoriasis was of the usual variety and, except for 2 patients with spondylitis, the arthritis was not atypical. None developed terminal interphalangeal arthritis following the appearance of psoriatic nails. With the available knowledge, the decision was difficult whether to include these 10 cases in a series limited strictly to patients with unquestioned rheumatoid arthritis. There certainly seemed no reason to exclude them if any one of the following possibilities was accepted: that the two diseases have a common etiology; that their association in the same patient is merely one of chance; that the skin lesions are a manifestation of the arthritis or that there is a constitutional predisposition to both. On the other hand, if "psoriatic arthritis" is regarded as a distinct disease entity, or if the joint lesions can be considered a psoriatic arthropathy, these cases should not be included in a series of patients with pure rheumatoid arthritis. Since, as pointed out above, the evidence is against the first, and since none of these 10 patients had psoriatic nails in association with arthritis of the terminal interphalangeal joints, the decision was made to include them.

INTERMITTENT HYDRARTHROSIS

2.48   The condition termed intermittent hydrarthrosis is generally divided into two types [251, 304, 357, 415]. The first, or idiopathic type, occurs in the absence of demonstrable chronic joint disease, while the second may be called symptomatic and is regarded as merely an interesting phase occurring at the onset or in the course of rheumatoid arthritis. Space does not permit a complete discussion of the first type here, but a brief description seems indicated, in order that a clear distinction may be made between the two forms.

2.49   The first observation of this peculiar disease was made by Perrin [407] in 1845, although Dance [128], who actually described an intermittent form of tetany of unknown origin in 1831, is sometimes given the credit. Perrin's patient also suffered from chronic arthritis, and the intermittent joint swellings were recognized by the author as a part of the chronic disease. The first cases unaccompanied by chronic arthritis were reported by Moore [363, 364] in 1864 and 1867, and the first American case was reported by Fridenburg [194] in 1888. By 1926 about 100 cases had appeared in the literature [251], largely classified as the idiopathic form. It seems clear, then, that we are dealing with a relatively uncommon condition.

2.50   The disease is marked by swelling of the knee joint alone (sometimes accompanied by swelling of other joints), occurring at regular intervals with mathematical precision. Constitutional symptoms are slight during the attack and absent in the intervals of freedom. The usual signs of inflammation and effusion are present in the involved joints during the attacks, with complete restitution to normal in between, except that persistent muscle atrophy has occasionally been described [192, 558]. In a small proportion of cases, trauma, infection, or

Diagnostic Criteria

pregnancy has antedated the onset but in most instances no precipitating causes have been noted. Males and females are affected equally, most commonly in the third, fourth, and fifth decades of life [39]. According to data compiled by Biering [39], the duration of each attack varies in different patients from two to eighteen days and averages four or five, while the free interval, which averages ten to twelve days, may range from four days to thirty. Spontaneous remissions lasting months or years are common, and it has been stated that the chances are good for eventual complete cessation [39, 251]. Such a course makes the evaluation of therapy unusually difficult, although successes have been reported from the use of neoarsphenamine [433], intravenous typhoid vaccine [357], ergotamine tartrate [558], elimination diets [37], roentgenotherapy [424], and synovectomy [304].

2.51 No satisfactory etiologic explanation of this mysterious condition has yet been established, although such knowledge would without doubt assist materially in the study of joint effusions. Possibly some cases which are accompanied by allergic manifestations represent an equivalent of angioneurotic edema. Certain authors [357, 451, 457] have gone so far as to attribute all cases to this cause. The regularity of the attacks and the apparent relief given by quinine led to suggestions for a malarial origin [194, 364], but the proponents offered no confirmation as the true nature of malaria had not become known. In a few cases other infectious diseases have been regarded as responsible, including lymphogranuloma venereum [424] and brucellosis [9].

2.52 Family history of the disease is rare [200, 251], although Schlesinger [451] has reported 5 members of one family thus afflicted, of whom 3 had allergic manifestations in addition. In another interesting family tree [21] diabetes, psoriasis, and intermittent hydrarthrosis were found either alone or in various combinations in 6 members. In this instance the hydrarthrosis in at least 1 individual was of the symptomatic type. Almost uniformly, a complete remission takes place in pregnancy [192, 194, 200, 364, 451], suggesting a relationship to rheumatoid arthritis. Findings have varied in the few synovial biopsies thus far reported. Ghormley and Deacon [204] described only slight thickening of the synovial lining cells, while Krida [304] found that the picture differed in the active and quiescent periods in respect to the degree of edema, proliferative or granulation tissue, and lymphocytic infiltration. In two cases the pathologic findings were consistent with those of rheumatoid arthritis. The first patient [415] went on to develop a progressive polyarthritis and obviously belonged to the symptomatic type. The second [424] was believed to conform to the idiopathic type when examined eighteen months after the biopsy. The pathologic findings reported thus far support the opinion that most patients with intermittent hydrarthrosis, if followed long enough, will eventually develop chronic joint disease consistent with rheumatoid arthritis [439].

2.53   When a patient with intermittent hydrarthrosis is first seen, it may not be possible for the observer to make a distinction between the idiopathic and symptomatic types. If the patient gives a history of previous arthritis clearing without residual, the symptomatic type may be suspected. If persistent arthritic changes are present either in other joints or in the involved joints between bouts of hydrarthrosis, the presence of the symptomatic type may be assumed. Otherwise, the passage of time is necessary to make the differentiation, since a stage of intermittent hydrarthrosis may long precede the onset of what is evidently rheumatoid arthritis. In the selection of patients for the present series, 2 who showed more or less regular intermittent joint effusions in the course of a persistent chronic arthritis were believed to belong to the symptomatic type and were included, while 1 other patient presented the clinical picture of the idiopathic type of intermittent hydrarthrosis of sixteen years' duration at the time that a final selection of patients for the series was made and was therefore excluded. Four years later it became evident that the latter patient actually had rheumatoid arthritis, from the persistence of synovial thickening in one knee, development of arthritis in a shoulder, and continued elevation of the sedimentation rate.

PALINDROMIC RHEUMATISM

2.54   The present status of palindromic rheumatism in relation to rheumatoid arthritis is analogous to that of the subject of the preceding section, intermittent hydrarthrosis. Two forms have been distinguished which again might be termed primary or idiopathic and secondary or symptomatic. In the first, described by Hench in 1940 and 1944

Diagnostic Criteria

[253, 257], the patients have not developed evidence of a chronic rheumatoid arthritis "even after scores or hundreds of attacks and years of disease." A number of cases of the second, or symptomatic form, are now on record in which this syndrome was the first manifestation or the accompaniment of chronic rheumatoid arthritis [45, 69, 439]. Further observations may decide whether or not most or all cases of what seem to be the primary type will, if followed long enough, eventually develop a definite rheumatoid arthritis.

2.55 In any event, a differentiation between rheumatoid arthritis and palindromic rheumatism did not become necessary in the selection of our series of patients (even in retrospect, since it was first described four years after the last patient had been chosen). None of those under consideration presented or developed features of this syndrome.

MENOPAUSAL ARTHRITIS

2.56 About thirty years ago the term menopausal arthritis gradually began to be used in the literature and a succession of papers appeared devoted in whole or in part to a form of joint disease given this name or one of numerous synonyms.* Ten years later, at a time when the patients in the present series were being selected, menopausal, or climacteric arthritis, was even included in one British classification [56] among the chief primary types of chronic arthritis. On the other hand, in two representative American discussions of the nomenclature of the arthritides published in 1935 [133, 251], menopausal arthritis was either put under degenerative joint disease or regarded as an entity not firmly established. There was thus little unanimity when the present series was being formed regarding the place or even the right to independent existence of such a form of joint disease. Since the subject is still confused and somewhat controversial, a detailed discussion seems unwarranted here. Only enough information will be presented to clarify the authors' viewpoint in regard to their selection of patients when confronted with those demonstrating some of the features ascribed to the varying concepts of menopausal arthritis. It should also be mentioned that subsequent data or opinions on this subject have failed to modify

---

* These include climacteric, chronic villous, endocrine, and hypoglandular arthritis and *lipo-arthrite sèche* and *arthrite bilaterale et symétrique des genoux*.

the position taken in 1938, when the series membership was finally established.

2.57 An apparent relation between the climacteric and the onset and development of arthritis in women has been under discussion since the publication of Charcot's [81] observation in 1881. The increased frequency of this form of arthritis in women in the fifth and sixth decades has also been noted. Other factors suggesting that the female reproductive system may influence the disease include the sex distribution, remissions in pregnancy, onset or exacerbation post partum, and increased symptomatology preceding or accompanying the catamenia. Later chapters will present an analysis of our patients in these respects, as well as a survey of the literature. There appears to be no reason, however, for the segregation of such patients from the general group or for applying the term "menopausal arthritis" to those with onset near the climacteric.

2.58 A second possible relationship of joint disease to the climacteric has been described in the literature [20, 120, 206, 340, 371], most completely by Hall [232] in 1938 under the title "Menopause Arthralgia." In his patients symptoms began at the time of physiological menopause or within a few weeks of roentgenotherapeutic or surgical castration. In all, symptoms were out of proportion to signs, but variable amounts of joint swelling were present. All showed the usual mental and physical symptoms common to the menopause and benefited from the use of estrogenic material. The author pointed out that only the passage of time could distinguish these patients from those in the early stages of rheumatoid arthritis before convincing joint signs were present. Relatively little attention has since been paid to this symptom complex but the opinion has been expressed in one paper [226] that painful joints should be more widely accepted "as a complaint of note associated with the climacteric." In the selection of patients for the present series care was taken not to include those with symptoms suggestive of rheumatoid arthritis but without definite signs of arthritis, until the question had been settled by as prolonged observation as necessary. It can thus be stated with assurance that no patients with joint disease which might be classified as "menopause arthralgia" were included.

2.59 A third conception of menopausal arthritis has received the

Diagnostic Criteria

most attention from British authors [56, 66, 94, 216, 260, 529], although a similar picture has been described under various names in France [371], and by Cecil and Archer [77] in this country. The disease is described as essentially limited to females, although some [66] have been willing to make this diagnosis in males with hypothyroidism or at the "male climacteric." It occurs in more or less close relation to a natural or artificial menopause, but an interval of several or more years between climacteric and onset of joint symptoms does not rule out this diagnosis [77, 260]. The knees are universally affected, and occasionally other joints, chiefly the metacarpo-phalangeal joint of the thumb, the shoulder, and the lumbar spine. The first signs in the knees are villous hypertrophy and synovial crepitus, swelling, and tenderness, with eventual relentless progression, unless effectively treated, to a severe degree of degenerative joint disease. Roentgenograms show no bony changes in the early stages, but later on reveal degenerative lesions, including marginal overgrowth and joint narrowing [66, 77]. The patients are usually overweight and frequently exhibit static deformities of the feet. A relationship of the endocrine system to this disease has not been convincingly established. Most authors describe manifestations of hypothyroidism, but there are no detailed studies on the basal metabolism. Others implicate the ovary [206, 420] or even the pituitary [95], again with no quantitative studies of the functions of these organs. The chief arguments in favor of an endocrine etiology in these patients have rested on the relation of onset to the menopause (which, we have stated, need not be close) and the patients' response to therapy with thyroid or ovarian products [95, 260, 420]. Such therapy has been combined with other more general measures which have long proved effective in degenerative joint disease involving weight-bearing joints. These include weight reduction, rest, physiotherapy, and correction of faulty bodily mechanics.

2.60 Why is this condition not merely a form of degenerative joint disease, occurring in women near the menopause, perhaps in response to gain in weight? We read that the disease either quiets down with treatment or leads to definite degenerative joint disease. The chief arguments against this concept are that it occurs chiefly in females at an earlier age, is more amenable to treatment, and is primary in the synovia, not in the cartilage [1, 56, 94, 529]. Only the last point of differentiation seems important, but has not been proven by pathologic studies on typical cases, although inflammatory changes in the synovia are described [260, 530] not differing essentially from those present in degenerative joint disease [4, 380].

2.61 Until further evidence is presented, the authors believe, with others [232, 324], that the proponents of this condition as a disease entity have merely described a common form of degenerative joint disease occurring in women in the fifth and sixth decades and that careful pathologic study would show in most instances early degenerative changes in the cartilage with or without synovitis. The possibility should of course be recognized of confusing such patients and those with rheumatoid arthritis largely confined to the knees, especially if early, coincidental degenerative changes are present. No patient was included in our series unless, as was usually the case, such differentiation could readily be made.

2.62 In summary, patients with evident rheumatoid arthritis were not disbarred from the series because of hypothetical endocrinological relationships. Those with "menopause arthralgia," without characteristic joint changes, were left for the passage of time to decide. Those with degenerative joint disease alone, whether or not related to the menopause, were excluded.

ARTHRITIS DUE TO SPECIFIC INFECTION

2.63 In the evolution of rheumatoid arthritis as an independent disease, the growth of clinical bacteriology made possible the setting off of diseases of the joints due to specific infections. In practice, such separation seems easy and obvious in some patients; in others, the distinction becomes difficult and uncertain. Some of the factors which may be operative in confusing an individual decision can be listed briefly here. In the first place, acute forms of rheumatoid arthritis, involving one or a few large joints, may mimic almost exactly an arthritis due to specific infection. Some evidence has also been presented that a condition resembling rheumatoid arthritis in a chronic, progressive form and involving small joints of the extremities in a symmetrical fashion, may be caused by any one of a number of micro-organisms. This last

Diagnostic Criteria

point will be considered in regard to individual infectious diseases in subsequent paragraphs. Where a bacteriologic or serologic diagnosis is apparently made, the inquiring physician is faced with the question of whether or not the patient is suffering from an infectious disease in addition to rheumatoid arthritis, or, even if micro-organisms are recovered from synovial fluid or articular tissue, whether or not two independent diseases of the joints may be present. For example, a patient with rheumatoid arthritis may have a positive serologic test for syphilis, a bacteriologic diagnosis of genito-urinary gonorrhea, or a superimposed pyogenic infection of one or more joints.

2.64   In the following paragraphs the experience of others as set forth in the literature will be presented, along with the criteria followed in our attempt to exclude from the series individuals actually suffering from forms of arthritis due to specific infections but bearing a clinical resemblance to rheumatoid arthritis. In this attempt it is believed that the index of suspicion was high, so much so that, as will be pointed out in the section on gonorrheal arthritis, it now seems likely that certain patients were excluded who had rheumatoid arthritis precipitated by or coincidental with a gonorrheal infection. In each patient considered for the series, in addition to careful appraisal of the evidence obtained from anamnesis and physical examination, the following tests were performed: pelvic and prostatic smears stained by Gram's method and, in patients seen from 1931 on, gonorrheal complement fixation tests; serologic tests for syphilis; roentgenograms of the chest and of representative joints; and, where suspicion was aroused, joint aspiration with cytologic, chemical, and bacteriologic study of the synovial fluid. In case of doubt a patient was debarred from the series until the passage of time permitted making the correct diagnosis.

2.65   Articular manifestations have been noted in over thirty diseases of known infectious etiology. In most of them, the diagnosis can readily be made and there is little possibility of confusion with rheumatoid arthritis. Such a statement applies to arthritis due to the usual pyogenic bacteria (streptococcus, staphylococcus, etc.), in which the organisms can be isolated from the synovial fluid or articular tissue in a high percentage of instances. When the onset is acute, these conditions are ordinarily easily recognized and the diagnosis can be confirmed by cultural methods, but if the reaction to infection is mild, the diagnosis may not be suspected until joint aspiration has been performed. Certain infections, however, require further discussion and will be taken up in order in succeeding sections. Lastly, the reader must note carefully that we are not concerned at this time with so-called "nonspecific infectious" arthritis, a condition which may bear a relationship to infection of the upper respiratory tract or to a focus of infection but in which bacteriologic proof is wanting of the presence of causative organisms in the joints. Space is reserved later (pars. **2.101–2.104**) for a consideration of the advisability of making a distinction between "true" rheumatoid arthritis and what has been variously called secondary rheumatoid, metastatic, focal, or "nonspecific infectious" arthritis.

PNEUMOCOCCAL ARTHRITIS

2.66 Pneumococcal arthritis forms a rare complication of pneumococcus pneumonia, occurring in approximately 0.1 per cent of the cases reported. Primary forms have also been described [*43*], as well as those accompanying other types of pneumococcal infection. The process is usually acute and involves one or a few larger joints. In two series no mention is made of a chronic, progressive arthritis from this source [*63, 173*]. However, several instances have been reported of long-standing arthritis with superimposed pneumococcal infection in certain joints [*63, 265*]. One patient described by Strangeways [*509*], after ten or twelve years of progressive joint disease conforming clinically to rheumatoid arthritis, died with pneumonia and an exacerbation in his arthritis. Autopsy revealed, in addition to amyloid disease, three joints with a purulent pneumococcal arthritis and the rest showing varying degrees of chronic damage without evidence of bacterial infection. It has been the experience of this clinic that, unless chemotherapy is used, patients with rheumatoid arthritis who develop blood stream infections are likely to acquire one or more septic joints.

2.67 In none of the patients included in our series was the onset associated with pneumonia. However, 1 patient gave a history of arthritis for four years and attacks of septic parotitis for two. A pure culture of pneumococci was grown from the parotid secretion. The joints were not aspirated, but the blood cultures proved to be negative and there appeared to be no chronological relationship between the attacks

Diagnostic Criteria

of parotitis and exacerbations of the arthritis. Since this patient represented a typical case of rheumatoid arthritis in all other respects and since the parotitis, with the evidence at hand, could be regarded only as an intercurrent infection, he was included in the series.

TUBERCULOUS ARTHRITIS

2.68 Tuberculosis of the joints can usually be diagnosed beyond reasonable doubt by recovery of the tubercle bacillus by direct methods or animal inoculation or by the demonstration of a characteristic histologic picture by biopsy. Naturally, such a specific diagnosis is made possible only by clinical suspicion being aroused by the course of the patient's illness, the distribution of joint involvement, the presence of tuberculosis elsewhere, positive tuberculin tests, or, in certain stages only, by characteristic features in the roentgenograms. Certain clinical pictures, however, may cause confusion between tuberculous and rheumatoid arthritis. These include atypical forms of rheumatoid arthritis with persistent involvement of one or a few large joints; polyarticular and even symmetrical forms of tuberculous arthritis; visceral or joint tuberculosis associated with rheumatoid arthritis; and finally, under the concept of a progressive polyarthritis resembling rheumatoid arthritis but due to the tubercle bacillus, the "rhumatisme tuberculeux" of Poncet [414].

2.69 The mistaken diagnoses encountered by always interpreting a persistent monarticular arthritis as tuberculous were emphasized by Smith [474] in 1932 and later by Collins and Cameron [110]. Smith studied 24 cases of this nature, with duration ranging from a few months to ten years. Biopsies were done in all cases, and guinea pig inoculations in 22. In each case pathologic examination excluded tuberculosis and showed gross and histologic changes compatible with rheumatoid arthritis. Later, 5 patients developed polyarthritis. Thus rheumatoid arthritis may begin and persist in one joint, although, of course, the eventual development of polyarthritis, usually symmetrical, is the rule. The articular distribution in our series of patients will be presented subsequently.

2.70 Conversely, tuberculous arthritis may be present in more than one joint. In a series of 168 cases of tuberculous arthritis of the knee, Ghormley and Brav [203] noted tuberculous involvement of two joints in 13.1 per cent and of more than two in 5.4 per cent, while Dawson [*133*] mentioned polyarticular and even symmetrical involvement. Thus, while polyarthritis is occasionally tuberculous in origin, a small proportion of rheumatoid cases are monarticular. Such instances certainly represent exceptions and require rigid standards of diagnosis, including bacteriologic or histologic proof. In addition, an unquestionably tuberculous joint may be associated with rheumatoid arthritis, either preceding, coincident with, or subsequent to the development of polyarthritis. Such a situation is undoubtedly largely responsible for the development of the concept of tuberculous rheumatism and can be applied in criticism to many supposed cases of this condition reported in the literature.

2.71 The finding of visceral tuberculosis with rheumatoid arthritis or a history of exposure to the disease has also been advanced as evidence for the existence of tuberculous rheumatism [*115, 116, 118, 317*]. Such evidence is, of course, entirely indirect and should serve merely to arouse the interest of the physician in the possibility of an overlooked or mistaken diagnosis. In 5 of the patients included in our series active pulmonary tuberculosis was diagnosed at hospital admission, and in 4 others this disease was found active at a later date (par. **24.3**). In each instance, the diagnosis of rheumatoid arthritis was unquestioned and evidence in favor of a tuberculous etiology for the joint disease failed to appear in the course of subsequent study.

2.72 The existence of "tuberculous rheumatism" was first clearly postulated by Poncet [*414*] about fifty years ago. Since then, the idea has continued to hold favor on the Continent, but relatively little attention has been paid to it in England or North America except in the writings of Copeman [*116, 118*], LeSage [*317*], and Cooperman [*115*]. Space forbids a complete discussion or survey of the literature here. For a résumé of the subject up to 1934, the reader is referred to the definitive monograph of Brav and Hench [*54*]. In brief, it is thought that "tuberculous rheumatism" may mimic rheumatoid arthritis, hypertrophic arthritis, or even rheumatic fever. In some cases the diagnosis may be established by the finding of tuberculous changes in tissue or by the recovery of tubercle bacilli from one or more joints. In other cases the histologic picture may be that of "simple inflammation" or "transitional forms" with the demonstration of Koch's bacilli directly or by animal

Diagnostic Criteria

inoculation. With no direct proof, it is assumed that the tubercle bacillus may cause either typical or atypical histologic changes through toxins or an allergic mechanism or while in an attenuated form or in a filterable virus-like phase [115, 146, 317]. In patients for whom bacteriologic or histologic proof is lacking, the diagnosis may be made indirectly from the presence of nonarticular tuberculosis in the patient, from a local or focal reaction to a tuberculin test, from blood cultures according to Lowenstein's method, or even from a history of exposure to the disease [115, 116, 118, 317].

2.73 A critical analysis of the mass of data which has been put forth in support of "tuberculous rheumatism" has been well performed by Brav and Hench [54]. They conclude that there is no incontrovertible proof that such a condition exists. Without denying the possibility that future work may establish the identity of "tuberculous rheumatism," for the present we have decided against the recognition of this condition, especially in regard to the selection of a series of patients with rheumatoid arthritis. The indirect evidence mentioned above merely establishes a past or present tuberculous infection in the patient but not an etiologic relationship to his arthritis. In cases of polyarthritis where the presence of a tuberculous arthritis in one or more joints seems proven, the possibility must be kept in mind of a true tuberculous polyarthritis or of a coincidental rheumatoid arthritis. The latter possibility was probably exemplified by 2 patients admitted to our series. Both showed the accepted picture of rheumatoid arthritis. In one, a tuberculous joint was discovered by biopsy; in the other pulmonary and glandular tuberculosis was proven and roentgenograms of one shoulder showed characteristic tuberculous arthritis. In the first patient the diagnosis of rheumatoid arthritis was further established by typical histologic findings in a subcutaneous nodule. As mentioned above, 9 patients included in the series either entered with or later developed active pulmonary tuberculosis. In these, the relationship between the two diseases was considered that of coincidence rather than cause and effect.

SYPHILIS

2.74 The statement has appeared in the literature [300] that syphilitic arthritis can imitate any form of joint disease. According to McEwen and Thomas [335], this is probably true in rare instances, but the great majority of syphilitic arthritides fall into easily diagnosed categories. These include the symmetrical serous synovitis of congenital syphilis (Clutton's joints), tertiary syphilis involving joints, periostitis causing pain in the region of the joints, and neuropathic (Charcot) joints secondary to luetic involvement of the nervous system. That a polyarthritis simulating the acute and even more chronic forms of rheumatoid arthritis may be caused by syphilis has long been assumed, but bacteriologic evidence was lacking until Chesney and his coworkers [84, 85] demonstrated treponemata in the synovial fluid of 3 such cases by rabbit inoculation. In the following paragraphs will be found a brief discussion of the forms listed, in regard to points applicable to the diagnosis of rheumatoid arthritis.

2.75   Little has been added to our knowledge of the congenital form of syphilitic arthritis since the publication of Clutton's [93] classical description in 1886. This occurs in children from the age of five or six and even in young adults [309]. Almost invariably the knees, and sometimes other large joints, are affected with an indolent, painless effusion. The onset is usually insidious but may follow trauma. The disease is self-limited, so that the response to specific treatment may apparently be rapid [300, 335]. Since the ultimate prognosis is good, whether treated or not, the importance of diagnosis lies in the recognition of syphilis in the patient and his family. The condition has been commonly found among congenital syphilitics and has outranked Hutchinsonian teeth as a stigma [298, 309]. This differential diagnosis, then, may come up in the process of collecting a sizeable series of patients with rheumatoid arthritis. Since the condition can exist with negative serology, it must often be recognized, once clinical suspicion has been aroused, by the demonstration of other features of congenital syphilis in the patient or of syphilis in other members of the family. Furthermore, since rheumatoid arthritis may appear in a congenital luetic, the arthritis must clinically resemble the hydrarthrosis of Clutton's joints, as described above. As far as can be ascertained from the literature, an absolute diagnosis has never been made in such patients by the demonstration of treponemata in the synovial fluid, and biopsy, while sometimes showing miliary gummata, may reveal only nonspecific inflammation of the synovia [298, 300].

Diagnostic Criteria 55

2.76 Tertiary syphilis may involve joints as well as other organs of the body. The process may originate in adjacent bone, in peri-articular tissue or in the joint itself. A presumptive diagnosis may be made by the clinical appearance, roentgenographic evidence of bone destruction with or without periostitis, the demonstration of syphilis in the patient and the response to antiluetic therapy. For a positive diagnosis, biopsy is necessary with the finding of the characteristic histologic picture of tertiary syphilis. If the possibility of this diagnosis is kept in mind by the physician, such cases should rarely cause confusion with rheumatoid arthritis. Gummatous lesions can, of course, coexist with rheumatoid arthritis. This may have been the case in two patients with syphilis reported by Freund [192] to exhibit the clinical picture of primary chronic polyarthritis. Syphilitic periostitis should be recalled as a possible cause of pain in the region of joints, along with other diseases of the osseous system, such as osteomyelitis [547] and pulmonary osteo-arthropathy [290]. McEwen and Thomas [335] surmise that the arthralgia and bone pain so common in secondary syphilis may be due to an unrecognized periostitis, aggravated by tension on the tendon insertions in the periosteum. There seems little reason for difficulty in distinguishing between the neuropathic arthritis due to syphilis and rheumatoid arthritis, except in the rare early case presenting the picture of an acute, painful synovitis [335].

2.77 Mention has been made of the demonstration by Chesney and his coworkers [84, 85] of treponemata in the synovial fluid of 3 patients with polyarthritis accompanying secondary syphilis. Kling's [300] objection that spirochetes may have been carried into the joint from the blood stream seems insufficient to refute the premise that a polyarthritis resembling certain forms of rheumatoid arthritis can thus be caused by syphilis. Other criteria for this diagnosis rest only on a presumptive basis. The demonstration of syphilis in the patient by history, examination, or serologic test does not exclude the coincidence of two diseases. Wassermann tests on the synovial fluid are, unlike the spinal fluid, usually positive along with the blood. Even a positive synovial fluid and a negative blood is not necessarily significant [192, 300]. It is also probable that rheumatoid arthritis, like disseminated lupus erythematosus, may occasionally be responsible for biologic false-positive serologic tests [365]. Periostitis is seen not infrequently in rheumatoid arthritis as well as in syphilis. Neither a prompt response to antiluetic therapy nor a supposed Herxheimer reaction in the joints can be convincing in a disease like rheumatoid arthritis, with variable course and frequent spontaneous remissions and relapses. Osseous or joint syphilis, like bone or joint tuberculosis, may accompany rheumatoid arthritis but not be of etiologic importance. A pathologic picture typical of syphilis has not yet been satisfactorily demonstrated in cases of this type [192, 300, 335]. One must revert, then, to the 3 proven cases reported by Chesney and his coworkers [84, 85], which stand alone at present but point the way for future study. As stated by Slocumb [472], the diagnosis of syphilitic polyarthritis is often loosely made and is used to include almost all cases of progressive arthritis in which the serologic reactions are positive or in which there is a history of lues, with the case proven to the satisfaction of the physician if the patient apparently responds to antisyphilitic treatment.

2.78 In the formation of our series, 4 patients were included with repeatedly positive serology, 1 with clinical tabes but negative serology, and 3 with inconsistent or doubtful reactions. None of these patients showed clinical or roentgenographic evidence suggestive of joint syphilis. In 2 the arthritis developed following treatment for syphilis, and 2 others later received treatment without prompt amelioration in their arthritis. Although no attempt was made to demonstrate treponemata in the synovial fluid of these patients by rabbit inoculation, the evidence at hand was believed to justify their inclusion in the series. One child with an indolent involvement of the knees was finally excluded from consideration for the series when a history of syphilis in the parents was brought to light, although her serology was negative.

SCARLET FEVER

2.79 The frequency of arthritis accompanying or following scarlet fever is variously cited at from 1.8 [51] to 10 per cent [74]. The joint manifestations are commonly divided into three distinct forms: (1) an acute type of polyarthritis representing the activation of rheumatic fever; (2) septic joints due to actual infection with the hemolytic streptococcus; and (3) a nonsuppurative arthritis with sterile joint effusions.

Diagnostic Criteria

2.80 In the first form, which clinically simulates rheumatic fever, the onset may be delayed as long as four weeks from the beginning of the scarlet fever [251]. Paul and his coworkers [401] have brought forward the hypothesis that most of the cases of nonsuppurative postscarlatinal arthritis represent manifestations of rheumatic fever, activated by a *Streptococcus hemolyticus* infection. Their evidence is entirely indirect and rests upon the high incidence of rheumatic fever found in twelve families, one or more of whose members had developed arthritis or endocarditis following scarlet fever. Two other authors [51, 518] believe that such a conclusion is unwarranted and that, while an endocarditis following scarlet fever is presumably rheumatic in origin, only a small percentage of postscarlatinal joint manifestations represent activation of rheumatic fever. It would seem wise, then, to refrain from attributing cases of nonsuppurative postscarlatinal arthritis to rheumatic fever until follow-up studies have demonstrated the presence of endocarditis, which differs clinically in no way from that associated with rheumatic fever, as Faulkner *et al.* [177] have shown.

2.81 The suppurative form of arthritis following scarlet fever may be regarded as a metastatic infection and so takes rank with other forms of sepsis due to hemolytic streptococci occurring in the second or third week [251]. These organisms can be recovered from the synovial fluid, and often a septicemia also develops [51]. Such conditions bear a serious prognosis [74], and, before the advent of specific therapy, the patients usually suffered permanent ankylosis of the joints [518].

2.82 The last and by far the largest group is made up of the cases which do not fall into the two groups described above. The term postscarlatinal arthritis should be limited to this group, which represents a fairly frequent manifestation of the disease. A few cases develop arthritis at the onset of the scarlet fever, over 75 per cent within the first two weeks, and the remainder, according to McClure [332], from the third to the ninth week. On an average three or four joints are affected, often in a migratory fashion, with the small joints of the hands and feet frequently involved symmetrically [51], in contrast to the usual distribution in rheumatic fever. A sterile joint effusion [51] may be present, and the arthritis is usually accompanied by fever. Endocarditis is not present at first [51], but, if it develops, it speaks for a diagnosis of rheumatic fever. The joint involvement is uniformly self-limited [251], with a duration of one or two weeks, but may recur. The mechanism of this form of arthritis, in which no organisms can be demonstrated in the joints, still remains uncertain, but the role of toxins is suggested by the occurrence of arthralgia lasting up to several days in about 3 per cent of healthy individuals actively immunized against scarlet fever [51].

2.83   It will be obvious to the reader that in none of the three types just described should there be confusion with rheumatoid arthritis, if sufficient observation of the patient makes clear either the development of rheumatic fever with or without endocarditis, the suppurative character of the joint lesion, or the self-limited course of the disease. There is, however, a small, rather obscure group of patients in whom chronic arthritis of the rheumatoid type apparently starts following an attack of scarlet fever. McCrae [333] and Strangeways and Burt [510], in their series of patients with rheumatoid arthritis, both cited a few cases whose onset was associated with this disease. Freund [192] stated that, in rare cases, chronic joint disease may follow scarlet fever, but that even these patients run a relatively favorable course, without a tendency to severe progression and ankylosis. In regard to this group of patients, it seems reasonable to assume, with Dawson [133], that scarlet fever may occasionally be numbered among the infections, usually of the upper respiratory tract, which sometimes precede the onset of rheumatoid arthritis.

2.84   In selecting the patients of our series, only one decision on this point had to be made. It was thought best to include a thirty-one-year-old woman with extensive symmetrical joint involvement and marked constitutional symptoms, whose onset dated back to the third week of an attack of scarlet fever five years before. Another patient* was excluded, not because his joint disease had followed scarlet fever, but because a reasonable clinical differentiation could not be made between rheumatoid arthritis and rheumatic fever.

BRUCELLOSIS

2.85   Symptoms referable to the skeletal system form one of the common manifestations of brucellosis. While arthralgia without ob-

* See Case 3, par. 2.12.

Diagnostic Criteria

jective changes is most frequently present, joint swelling, with or without effusion, may occur. Chronic, progressive polyarthritis of the rheumatoid type has been clinically observed in relatively few patients with the diagnosis of brucellosis [209, 355, 459]. In the absence of histopathologic evidence, the most likely possibility remains that such patients had two diseases, rheumatoid arthritis along with a present or past brucellar infection. About ten years ago, brucellergen skin tests were made on a group of patients with classical rheumatoid arthritis as well as on patients with an atypical form of this disease [129]. In the latter group only was the proportion of positive reactions slightly higher than in controls. Similarly, Green and Freyberg [224] found no evidence of brucellosis in 25 patients with typical rheumatoid arthritis, but 12 per cent of an equal number with findings "not typical of any of the common arthritides" were believed to have a brucellar infection. The conclusions from both studies are in agreement as to the absence of data which establish brucellosis as a cause of a form of progressive joint disease resembling rheumatoid arthritis.

2.86 The patients in our series were drawn from a region in which the incidence of brucellosis is relatively low. The usual laboratory tests were not performed, since brucellosis was not suspected in any of the patients included in the series. The only possible exceptions were two patients with intermittent hydrarthrosis as a manifestation of rheumatoid arthritis. On account of Baker's [9] patient with intermittent hydrarthrosis associated with brucellosis, the disease was ruled out as carefully as possible in these individuals.

GONORRHEA

2.87 In recent years gonococcal arthritis has become a relatively rare disease, presumably due to the introduction of specific methods of treatment of genito-urinary gonorrhea. On the other hand, when the patients in our series were being collected, arthritis caused by the gonococcus was still prevalent, forming a complication of gonorrhea in about 3 per cent of the reported cases [314, 526]. For this reason, each patient considered for the series was subjected to careful clinical and laboratory study designed to eliminate the possibility that his joint disease might actually be of gonococcal origin.

2.88 In the large majority of patients believed to have gonorrheal arthritis and thus eliminated from further consideration for the series, the diagnosis was readily suspected from the acute onset, which was often manifested by chills, fever, and a migratory arthritis; from the tendency to final involvement of one or a few large joints; and from a history or signs of a present or past gonorrheal focus in the genitourinary tract. While an absolute diagnosis could be made only from the identification of gonococci in the synovial fluid or joint tissue, a presumptive diagnosis, sufficient for clinical purposes, was assumed if gonococci were found in the genito-urinary tract of a patient with joint disease presenting a history and course consistent with gonorrheal arthritis. Gonorrheal complement fixation tests [274, 550] were also employed, with a positive result adding weight to what was necessarily at times a purely clinical diagnosis of the disease in the absence of bacteriologic proof. Since gonorrheal arthritis starts in a polyarticular form more often than in only one joint [103, 293], the differential diagnosis between it and rheumatoid arthritis with an acute onset was sometimes difficult, as was differentiation between a monarticular form without chills and fever and rheumatoid arthritis involving only one joint. The passage of time usually made the distinction clear, since the principle was accepted that, except for recurrent forms, resulting either from reinfection or exacerbation in the genito-urinary focus, gonorrheal arthritis is a self-limiting disease, tending toward either complete restitution of the joints or to varying degrees of scarring or deformity. Later experience, gained chiefly in World War II [10, 256], has clearly established that chronic, progressive arthritis, resembling rheumatoid arthritis in clinical features and course, may be precipitated or aggravated by a gonorrheal infection but in no sense represents a form of chronic joint disease due to the gonococcus. The authors were aware of the last point, but it now seems likely in retrospect that certain patients were excluded from the series who actually had what has been termed "postgonorrheal rheumatoid arthritis." These decisions may have been influenced by the literature available at the time, in which the opinions were by no means unanimous as to the status of a chronic, progressive form of gonorrheal arthritis.

2.89 As far back as 1890 Charcot [82] and the elder Garrod

Diagnostic Criteria

[198] noted that a chronic form of joint disease "exhibiting all the characters of rheumatoid arthritis" may follow upon an attack of gonorrheal arthritis. Since then certain authors [18, 103, 184, 199, 291, 376, 393] have agreed to this thesis, but without defining their criteria for the identification of chronic gonorrheal arthritis and without presenting case reports or even a general description of the condition. Others [42, 314] have gone so far as to describe two forms, one a chronic hydrops, usually monarticular, and the second a polyarticular deforming type, often involving the fingers with typical spindle swellings. Discussion of these statements will be omitted, since the authors present little or no substantiating evidence.

2.90 The first detailed account of joint disease resembling rheumatoid arthritis, but due to the gonococcus, was presented by Lorain [50] in 1866 before it was possible to make a bacteriologic diagnosis of articular or genito-urinary gonorrhea. Lorain's cases are recorded under the often quoted name of "rhumatisme blennorrhagique à forme noueuse" and indeed apparently justify this designation from the phalangeal joint involvement simulating that seen in rheumatoid arthritis. However, analysis of his two case reports indicates that he was dealing with recurrences of the disease rather than progression and that the finger and toe involvement constituted the sole point of resemblance to rheumatoid arthritis. Since then it has been shown that phalangeal lesions occur in about one-fifth of the patients with undoubted gonorrheal arthritis [293, 526]. Lorain's cases, although of interest from the point of view of differential diagnosis, are thus hardly significant. In 1908 Lindsay [323] analyzed 172 cases of rheumatoid arthritis from the standpoint of sources of infection preceding the disease. Of 138 women in the series, 36 had noted the presence of a vaginal discharge associated with the onset of arthritis. Since there were no data as to the nature and source of this discharge, the author did not attempt to implicate gonorrhea as a cause of the arthritis. In males, on the other hand, it seems likely that the majority of those giving a clinical history of gonorrhea have actually had the disease (although data are lacking in this series to exclude a nonbacterial urethritis as found in Reiter's syndrome). Out of the 34 men in Lindsay's series, 10 reported an attack of gonorrhea preceding the onset of arthritis. Brief case reports were presented for 4 patients. One showed nothing more than recurrent attacks of polyarthritis, presumably due to the gonococcus. In another, an interval of a year elapsed between the urethral infection and the development of a generalized arthritis. In the two others, a definite chronological relationship was present between the gonorrhea and a condition simulating a progressive rheumatoid arthritis, but the gonorrhea may have been merely a precipitating factor. In a study of the value of the gonorrheal complement fixation test in the differential diagnosis of arthritis, Schwartz [453] gave brief outlines of the history of 3 patients with possible gonorrheal arthritis lasting from two to eighteen years. Of these 3 patients, 2 gave histories of gonorrhea in close association with the onset of arthritis, and 1 a history of a two-year interval between the two diseases. All had positive gonorrheal complement fixation reactions, but in none was the organism recovered, either from a joint or from the genito-urinary focus. The patients' histories are not detailed enough for us to tell whether the arthritis was progressive or represented merely residual changes. Thus far the reader should agree that neither Schwartz's [453] cases nor the others described in this paragraph prove the point for the existence of a chronic, progressive arthritis caused by gonorrhea. There should finally be mentioned the theory that a chronic arthritis may be caused by a secondary invasion of the original gonorrheal focus by other organisms [74, 331, 402, 405, 526]. In this way, whether gonococci are still present in the focus or not, a type of joint disease resembling rheumatoid arthritis may be produced. This idea fits in well with the focal infection theory of the origin of rheumatoid arthritis but is equally lacking in direct proof.

2.91 The possibility that the patient may be suffering from two forms of arthritis at the same time applies to gonorrheal arthritis as well as to the other forms of infectious arthritis. Such a circumstance may explain the real nature of certain cases labeled rheumatoid arthritis due to gonorrhea, with the gonorrheal involvement either preceding or following the onset of the rheumatoid arthritis. The opinion has also been given that one may predispose to the other. Lees [314] believed that a still active gonorrheal infection of a joint might favor the onset of rheumatoid arthritis there. Warren [551], opposed by McCahey [331] and Wehrbein [555], has stated that "joints which are already damaged

Diagnostic Criteria

probably offer fruitful soil for the gonococci which are circulating in the patient's blood." Autopsy findings in patients with rheumatoid arthritis who died of septicemia show that one or more already involved joints may become secondarily infected [102]. These considerations must be carefully evaluated before making a diagnosis of joint disease similar to rheumatoid arthritis due to the gonococcus, even though the organisms can be recovered from the joint, which, as far as can be found, has not been done in the cases reported.

2.92 In early stages gonorrheal arthritis can usually be readily distinguished from rheumatoid arthritis on pathologic examination [399]. Such a distinction becomes much more difficult when a stage of fibrous ankylosis is reached [33]. In addition, pannus formation and erosion of cartilage have been noted in advanced cases of gonorrheal arthritis [114]. In 1 patient with bacteriologically proven gonorrheal arthritis, Nichols and Richardson [380] described and illustrated a thin layer of synovial pannus covering the articular surface, with erosion beneath, and granulation tissue of the epiphysis extending upward into the cartilage. Proliferative lesions were noted in 2 other patients, in whom the clinical history did not clearly distinguish between gonorrheal arthritis and "postgonorrheal" rheumatoid arthritis. Allison and Ghormley [4] also confirmed the existence of proliferation of the synovial membrane with pannus formation in arthritis due to specific organisms, including the gonococcus. The conclusion may thus be reached that in gonorrheal arthritis, along with other forms of infectious arthritis of known origin, proliferative changes may be found not unlike those described in rheumatoid arthritis. Such findings are of interest and suggest further study but fail to establish the concept of a chronic, progressive arthritis due to the gonococcus.

2.93 Finally, the opinions may be cited of those who believe that a chronic, progressive gonorrheal arthritis rarely, if ever, occurs. According to Nathan [378] and others [114, 526, 555], gonorrheal arthritis, in the absence of reinfection, is a self-limited disease, tending either toward complete restitution of joint function or varying degrees of disability, due either to scar tissue or secondary degenerative changes in the joints. Strong but not absolute evidence may be derived from the follow-up studies of series of carefully diagnosed cases of acute gonorrheal arthritis. In Cooperman's [*114*] series of 44 infants with gonorrheal arthritis, although some were left with profound structural changes, including dislocation and periarticular fibrosis, no progressive cases were reported. From a study of 610 cases Wehrbein [*555*] concluded that, although complete recovery of an infected joint may require as much as six or even twelve months, the outcome may be a return to normal or any degree of permanent change up to bony ankylosis. Spink and Keefer [*492*] observed 70 patients with gonorrheal arthritis and tabulated the results of therapy. At the time of writing, in about half of these, joint function was completely restored; in the remainder, varying degrees of limitation of motion were present due to fibrosis. Although the disease recurred in association with a urethral infection in two patients, no progressive cases were mentioned. In our clinic [*101*] over 200 patients with gonorrheal arthritis have been followed for periods of up to ten years. In no instance has there developed a chronic, progressive joint disease resembling rheumatoid arthritis. In our opinion the evidence just presented constitutes the most forceful argument against the existence of a chronic, progressive form of gonorrheal arthritis. Furthermore, there is as yet no proof of a second form of joint disease due to the gonococcus, which pursues a chronic, progressive course and never passes through a stage which, by present methods, can be recognized as gonorrheal arthritis. Such cases can much more logically be regarded as instances of rheumatoid arthritis precipitated or aggravated by a gonorrheal infection.

2.94 As mentioned above, an attempt was made to exclude patients with gonorrheal arthritis from the present series by careful laboratory as well as clinical study. In all but one male the prostatic secretion was examined for gonococci and polymorphonuclear leukocytes by stained smears. In about two-thirds of the women smears for gonococci were taken from the cervix and Skene's and Bartholin's glands. (Those in whom this procedure was not performed consisted chiefly in women over fifty years of age or those with a virginal introitus.) Gonorrheal complement fixation tests were performed on 254 of the patients, and in many cases a second test was performed if the first test was positive. Each patient was carefully questioned as to a history of gonorrhea, and pelvic examinations were done on females in addition to obtaining the

Diagnostic Criteria

pelvic smears. Patients with an acute type of rheumatoid arthritis which might at first view be mistaken for gonorrheal arthritis, were tested repeatedly; the synovial fluid was examined if diagnostic joint aspiration was possible. No doubtful case was included until follow-up study had made clear the type of arthritis present.

2.95   Early in our study we adopted the working principle already referred to—that a history or other evidence of gonorrhea in a patient with arthritis does not necessarily establish a gonococcal etiology for the joint disease. Thus no patient with the clinical picture of rheumatoid arthritis was excluded from the series because of a history or other features pointing toward a gonorrheal infection, the one exception being the recovery of gonococci from joint fluid or tissue. Only 2 patients included in the series were believed to have had gonorrheal arthritis in addition to rheumatoid arthritis, in one instance preceding and in the other during the course of the rheumatoid process. This diagnostic opinion was necessarily gained from history alone, since what was believed to be gonorrheal arthritis appeared before the patients came under our observation, at which time no evidence of a gonorrheal infection could be found. Furthermore it is entirely possible that these 2 patients actually had rheumatoid arthritis alone, either precipitated or aggravated by a gonorrheal infection. Both these patients were included in the series, but a third was dropped when the list of patients was finally reviewed in 1938. This patient was a male, aged thirty-six, who developed arthritis in both ankles and one foot three months after an attack of urethritis. The diagnosis of a gonorrheal infection was not established during hospital study, and a gonorrheal complement fixation test was negative. The patient showed gradual but steady improvement under symptomatic treatment. When seen eight months later, he had minor articular complaints but no objective evidence of arthritis. Since he failed to return to the clinic for follow-up observations, and since there was a real possibility that he had gonorrheal rather than rheumatoid arthritis, it was decided to exclude him from the series.

2.96   Following the completion of the series, those patients were sorted out who presented evidence suggesting a past or present gonorrheal infection. Such evidence included: a history of gonorrhea; a history of findings of possible gonorrhea in the past, such as a urethral

Table 2.1

Frequency of possible gonorrheal infection in present series (293 patients) and distribution by type of evidence and sex of patient

Patients with a history or other evidence of gonorrheal infection (total)		No.	Per cent
		51	17.4

		Distribution of evidence	
Type of evidence	Total no.	No. of males	No. of females
History of gonorrhea	24	23	1
Stricture or pelvic inflammation	3	1	2
Prostatitis	21	21	—
Organisms resembling gonococci in smears	3	2	1
Positive complement fixation reactions*	15	6	9

* One positive or, if more than one test was done, the majority of tests positive.

stricture in a male or a history of an operation for pelvic inflammation in a female; prostatic infection demonstrated by the expression of purulent material; the finding of organisms resembling gonococci in stained smears (cultural methods were not available at the time); a positive gonorrheal complement fixation test, or, if more than one test was performed, the majority of them positive. The results are shown in Table 2.1. In 3 patients with a history of gonorrhea the disease appeared after the onset of the arthritis. In the rest the gonorrheal infection was said to have occurred from two to thirty-five years before the arthritis—in all but 1, five or more years before. The males with evidence of prostatitis are included for the sake of completeness, since in only 2 cases were organisms resembling gonococci demonstrated in stained smears. The finding of positive gonorrheal complement fixation reactions in 15 patients out of 254 (5.9 per cent) may indicate that these patients either had nonspecific reactions to the test or coincidental gonorrheal infections [550].

2.97 This analysis is presented in order to make it clear that a definite proportion of the patients considered for the series presented evidence of varying strength of a past or present gonorrheal infection. In the 51 patients in whom some hint was given of a gonorrheal etiology, the joint disease was consistent in clinical features and course with rheumatoid rather than gonorrheal arthritis. To have been entirely on the safe side, some or even many of the 51 patients might have been rejected.

Diagnostic Criteria

Had this been done, it is the authors' belief that they would have failed in their intention to present an analysis of a series of patients with rheumatoid arthritis representing consecutive hospital admissions.

REITER'S SYNDROME

2.98 The clinical triad of nongonococcal urethritis, conjunctivitis, and arthritis has been commonly referred to as Reiter's syndrome. As the etiology of this syndrome has not been established, use of the term to designate patients who show only one or two features of the triad seems unwarranted at present. According to Weinberger and Bauer [557], more than 120 reports on this subject have appeared in the literature, the majority of them since the publication of the first English report in 1942 [24].

2.99 It has recently been pointed out [557] that certain cases fulfilling the usual criteria for the diagnosis of Reiter's syndrome may present features commonly encountered in rheumatoid arthritis. Most important is a symmetrical articular involvement, with clinical and roentgenographic evidence of progression, including sacro-iliac alterations resembling those found in rheumatoid spondylitis. Iritis and vasomotor manifestations have also been observed, while the cutaneous lesions are sometimes indistinguishable clinically and microscopically from pustular psoriasis. Balanced against these are the lack of definite cases of Reiter's syndrome among females, the absence of subcutaneous nodules, and the frequent finding of lesions not encountered in rheumatoid arthritis. These may be listed as purulent conjunctivitis, balanitis, lesions of the buccal mucosa, and severe genito-urinary involvement including urethritis, prostatitis, and cystitis. It therefore does not seem reasonable at present to regard Reiter's syndrome as a possible variant of rheumatoid arthritis, although occasional patients may be encountered in whom it is difficult to make a distinction between this syndrome and rheumatoid arthritis accompanied by a pustular type of psoriasis.

2.100 Patients with Reiter's syndrome were first recognized in our clinic in 1938, the year in which the re-appraisal of the cases selected for the present series was carried out. None was found with a symptom complex corresponding to this syndrome and mistakenly diagnosed rheumatoid arthritis. It was recalled, however, that during the formation of the series several had been encountered who were eliminated from consideration because the diagnosis of gonorrheal arthritis was suspected or because a certain diagnosis could not be made at the time.

"NONSPECIFIC INFECTIOUS ARTHRITIS"

2.101   In the preceding sections an attempt has been made to cover the relationship of rheumatoid arthritis to infectious arthritis due to specific agents or occurring in close association with diseases of known infectious origin. Reference should also be made to the status of so-called infectious arthritis of unproved etiology or related to foci of infection. The concept of this type of arthritis dates back to 1904, when Goldthwait [211] divided chronic nonspecific arthritis into three great types, the atrophic, the hypertrophic, and the infectious. At the time our series was being formed, such a division, with modifications, still held a reasonably secure place in British and Continental nosology but was rapidly losing favor in this country. The identification of the last type of arthritis has depended upon varying criteria according to the authority consulted, but in general distinction has been made by points of resemblance to a type of arthritis known to be infectious. These have included: the history of a preceding infection [78, 472, 514], an abrupt, febrile onset [56, 427], lack of the usual constitutional symptoms characteristic of rheumatoid arthritis [94, 150, 215, 514], asymmetrical involvement of a few large joints [150, 215, 427], and a tendency toward remission, especially after the removal of a focus of infection [56, 97, 124, 150, 427]. The naming of this form of joint disease has shown a similar lack of uniformity, in that the following terms have been used: infectious [211], infective [150], multiple infective [58], multiple nonspecific [94], secondary rheumatoid [56], focal [58], and metastatic [427].

2.102   At present it is generally believed that the terms "infectious" or "infective" should be restricted to cases in which the connection between the joint disease and infection is indisputable. "Metastatic" implies that organisms can actually be demonstrated in the joints, a finding which should automatically throw such a case into the group of arthritides due to specific infections. The demonstration of a focus of infection in a given patient fails to establish a relationship between the

Diagnostic Criteria

focus and the involved joints. Even if the arthritis clears following the removal of a focus, there is no proof that a similar result might not have ensued had the focus not been treated. As Dawson [*133*] has suggested, such instances may represent abortive cases of rheumatoid arthritis. In addition, it has been recognized that a chronic, progressive stage of rheumatoid arthritis may be preceded by one or more attacks of the "infectious" variety followed by complete remissions [*74, 131*]. Such attacks may be preceded by infections, exhibit slight or no constitutional symptoms, and involve a few large joints in an asymmetrical fashion [*550*]. In the early days of roentgenology it was believed that bony atrophy was absent in the "infectious" type [*211*]. Statements have also appeared that rarefaction was present only in the parts of the bones adjacent to the joints, rather than generalized, as in true atrophic arthritis [*56, 58, 472*]. Further study [*524*] has failed to furnish evidence which would warrant a subdivision of rheumatoid arthritis according to roentgenographic changes. Finally, a conclusive description of pathologic differences which would set apart an "infectious" type of rheumatoid arthritis has not appeared.

2.103 One may speculate as to the explanation for the long persistence of this division of rheumatoid arthritis into types. As put by one author [*419*], stages rather than types should be referred to. What has been called the "infectious" type of rheumatoid arthritis more likely represents an early stage in the course of the arthritis, one in which the prognosis is much more favorable for at least a temporary remission, so that the connection may easily be lost between the acute attack and the chronic disease [*131*]. Similarly, many patients with a well-established, progressive type of rheumatoid arthritis will recall an acute attack of arthritis, often far in the past and perhaps labeled rheumatic fever. Llewellyn Jones [*286*] noted the resemblance between "acute" cases of rheumatoid arthritis and arthritis arising from a specific type of infection, but he included the acute as well as the classical variety under the general heading of rheumatoid arthritis—chiefly because of the endless number of transitional forms. It may thus be concluded that rheumatoid arthritis, at certain stages, may resemble arthritis arising from a specific infection, but the evidence is against setting up this clinical variant as an independent disease or even as a subtype. The term "infectious stage" may be legitimately used [4, 550] for descriptive purposes, or as an aid to prognosis. It should be understood, however, that further observation, if carried on long enough, will sooner or later reveal, except for the small proportion that go into a lasting remission, the development of a progressive rheumatoid arthritis. If such follow-up is not performed, as exemplified in one paper [548], a false picture may be gained of the course of rheumatoid arthritis.

2.104 No patient believed to have rheumatoid arthritis was finally excluded from the present series unless there was reasonable proof of a causal relation between the joint disease and a specific infection. When the clinical features could not be interpreted in terms of the "infectious" stage of rheumatoid arthritis, decision was left to the passage of time. In the analysis to follow the features usually assigned to the "infectious" stage of rheumatoid arthritis will be discussed in respect to their frequency in our series of patients. Their inter-relationships will also be outlined in an attempt to determine whether or not an atypical "infectious" form of rheumatoid arthritis emerges (pars. 16.13, 16.14, 16.15).

CHRONIC ULCERATIVE COLITIS

2.105 Arthritis is stated to be the most common systemic complication of chronic ulcerative colitis of undetermined origin [17]. Ranging from 4 to 8.3 per cent of the cases in various series [17, 251, 275, 336], the frequency must be regarded as higher than can be explained by coincidence alone, but the exact nature of the relationship between the two diseases is as yet undemonstrated. The writings of Hench [251] have been largely responsible for the thesis that in some instances the arthritis represents a specific complication of ulcerative colitis and indeed an independent type of arthritis secondary to the disease of the colon. The evidence for this point of view rests entirely upon the relationship of the arthritis to the colitis in time of appearance, activity, and recovery. Clinically it is distinguished from rheumatoid arthritis by a greater tendency to periodicity and to more complete remissions, at least after the earlier bouts [251]. On the other hand, both Bargen [15, 16] and Hench [251] admit that there are many cases where the arthritis long precedes the colitis and others where each condition follows

Diagnostic Criteria

an entirely independent course. Furthermore, since the disease admittedly bears a general resemblance to rheumatoid arthritis, a periodicity with complete remissions in the early stages can hardly be counted a significant difference. As will be pointed out in the series analysis, this type of course is not unusual in the early stages of rheumatoid arthritis. It has been possible thus far to quote only from general statements, since no detailed clinical analysis has been made of the large amount of material studied by Hench [251] and Bargen [15, 16]. More important, no mention has been made in the literature at hand of the demonstration by pathologic examination of a type of arthritis distinct from the usual picture seen in rheumatoid arthritis. In our clinic a synovitis consistent with rheumatoid arthritis has been uniformly found in biopsy and autopsy material from patients with arthritis accompanying ulcerative colitis. Without more information, the authors hesitate to accept the existence of a specific type of arthritis secondary to ulcerative colitis and prefer to assume the presence of a coincident, although perhaps related, rheumatoid arthritis.

2.106 Among the successive ward admissions from whom the patients in our series were selected, 3 patients were encountered with chronic ulcerative colitis and the clinical features of rheumatoid arthritis. The first gave a history of having colitis four years before admission. The attack subsided after four months, but about two years later he developed arthritis of the knees and then gradually acquired typical spondylitis in severe form. On admission proctoscopy showed healed lesions of ulcerative colitis. During follow-up observation over the next twelve years, the arthritis steadily worsened so that he became bedridden, but no further evidence of colitis appeared. In this patient the arthritis progressed in the face of a remission of the colitis. In a second patient the reverse was true. Chronic ulcerative colitis appeared nearly four years after the onset of rheumatoid spondylitis without involvement of the peripheral joints. From that time on, with the exception of one exacerbation, his arthritis steadily improved to the point of quiescence. This exacerbation was followed by increased symptoms in his colitis, which had progressed steadily despite an ileostomy. A colectomy was performed just before his death. In the third patient a typical rheumatoid arthritis appeared six months after her first attack of ulcerative colitis two years before admission. Both diseases then pursued an essentially unrelated course, with exacerbations and remissions only occasionally coinciding. Pathologic findings obtained from a synovectomy of the knee were those of a chronic synovitis consistent with rheumatoid arthritis. Following discharge from the hospital, a more definite association was noted between flare-ups in her colitis and in her arthritis, but the latter continued active and progressive in spite of an ileostomy, a subtotal colectomy, and removal of the rectum. It is evident that the first two cases fall outside the usual criteria for a specific type of arthritis associated with chronic ulcerative colitis. In the third patient the two conditions pursued an independent course at least as often as a parallel one. From these considerations, in addition to the as yet unproven existence of a separate type of arthritis accompanying ulcerative colitis, it was believed justifiable to label all three cases rheumatoid arthritis and include them in the series.

FIBROSITIS AND PSYCHOGENIC RHEUMATISM

2.107   The term "fibrositis" was introduced into the nomenclature of disease in 1904 by Gowers [217] and Stockman [506] to apply to "chronic inflammation of white fibrous tissue" in any part of the body. The structures most commonly affected, according to Stockman [507], include "fasciae, aponeuroses, sheaths of muscles and nerves, ligaments, tendons, periosteum, articular capsules and subcutaneous tissue." A division of fibrositis into primary and secondary forms has been commonly employed [473], the latter being found in association with diseases of the joints, including rheumatoid arthritis. Clinical evidence of involvement of extra-articular supporting structures is present, if looked for, in nearly all cases of rheumatoid arthritis and may form a dominant feature, especially in early stages. In such cases recognition and diagnosis of the underlying arthritis may necessarily be long postponed.

2.108   That it is possible occasionally to make a provisional diagnosis of rheumatoid arthritis in patients with characteristic symptomatology, including constitutional manifestations, but without objective joint changes, will be pointed out in the series analysis (par. 34.1). In 4 patients included in the series neither joint limitation nor swelling was evident on admission, but both developed during follow-up ob-

Diagnostic Criteria

servation. It seems likely that in these patients the disease process was largely located in extra-articular connective tissue at the time of hospitalization.

2.109 While the term "primary fibrositis" is still commonly used in England, it has gained relatively little acceptance in this country. It may be said without qualification that the etiology of this condition is unknown [534]; pathologic studies are meager and rest entirely upon the work of Stockman [507]. Recent writers have pointed out that, except for the more localized forms associated with strain, trauma, occupation or posture, most patients whose conditions have been labeled primary fibrositis are in reality suffering from a psychosomatic disorder [220, 234, 559]. Diagnostic terms believed to be more accurate have accordingly been suggested and include "psychosomatic" [235] or "psychogenic" [44] rheumatism. Further discussion of this still controversial subject seems irrelevant; the details are available in the references cited. It should be mentioned, however, that Army experience in World War II led Hench and Boland [256] to the conclusion that a certain number of patients had a true primary fibrositis and that they could differentiate such patients from those with a purely psychologic basis for their symptoms.

2.110 Whatever the classification or terminology employed, the patient in an early stage of rheumatoid arthritis may be given a diagnosis of neurosis (or of fibrositis). Conversely, one whose symptoms turn out to be entirely of psychologic origin may be regarded for a time as a candidate for the development of a manifest rheumatoid arthritis. In forming our series, these points were recognized and no patients were finally included until observation had clearly disclosed objective findings of articular involvement.

THE CONNECTIVE TISSUE DISEASES

2.111 The concept of connective tissue disease was introduced by Klinge [301] about twenty-five years ago in relation to rheumatic fever. In the last ten or fifteen years, largely through the work of Klemperer [299], the term "collagen" (or better, "connective tissue") disease has come to be applied chiefly to rheumatic fever, periarteritis nodosa, rheumatoid arthritis, lupus erythematosus disseminatus, dermatomyositis, and scleroderma. On a pathologic basis these diseases may be grouped together on account of a common attribute, the widespread involvement of connective tissue throughout the body. In the majority of cases, sufficiently characteristic features are present at autopsy to enable the pathologist to distinguish among them on histologic grounds and supply a specific anatomic diagnosis to the clinician. Nevertheless, exceptions are not infrequently encountered in which overlapping features are present or even typical pathologic lesions of two or more of these diseases. Similarly, although the individual connective tissue disorders usually sooner or later conform to distinct disease patterns, clinical manifestations of more than one may appear in the same patient, either simultaneously or in sequence. For the above reasons, a relationship among these diseases in regard to etiology or pathogenesis has been postulated, but it remains as yet unproven. While the possibility of a common etiology should continue to be entertained from an investigative standpoint, it seems best to regard each disease as distinct, with the full understanding that in certain patients it may be impossible to apply a single diagnostic label either at the onset, throughout the course, or even at autopsy.

2.112 The patients of the present series were selected between 1930 and 1938, before the establishment of the concept of connective tissue disease. Nevertheless, early in the study clinical overlappings between rheumatoid arthritis and other diseases in the connective tissue group began to appear, with occasional difficulties in the formation of exact diagnoses. Such situations were probably encountered most frequently in the case of patients with features of both rheumatic fever and rheumatoid arthritis, a subject already discussed in a previous section. Since synovitis may appear during the course of diseases in this group other than rheumatoid arthritis and rheumatic fever, a few patients were tentatively included in the series on account of articular changes which seemed consistent with those of rheumatoid arthritis but were later rejected when the actual diagnosis became clear. One such patient, whose case history has been given in detail elsewhere [25], was a young man of nineteen who reported persistent symmetric articular swellings of two years' duration. The joints involved included those of the ankles, wrists, and fingers. Constitutional symptoms, fever, splenomegaly, and subcutaneous nodules were also present at the time of

Diagnostic Criteria

hospital admission. A year later, the finding of a well-marked eosinophilia led to the biopsy of a nodule, which showed typical findings of periarteritis nodosa. In spite of the development of renal involvement, the patient was still in fair health sixteen years after his first hospital admission. This case was regarded as one of periarteritis nodosa which for a time simulated rheumatoid arthritis, although the possibility remains that the arteritis was an unusual manifestation of the rheumatoid arthritis [11].

2.113   The series was finally reviewed in 1938 and a few patients were discarded about whom there was a reasonable doubt as to the diagnosis of rheumatoid arthritis. Follow-up observations have continued as far as possible, and in only one patient have signs of another connective tissue disease appeared. This was a woman who entered the hospital at the age of twenty-six with a polyarthritis, involving multiple joints in a symmetrical fashion, of about two years' duration. She also had severe constitutional manifestations, including vasomotor symptoms resembling Raynaud's syndrome. Her arthritis continued to progress over the next five years, with the development of extensive deformities of the fingers. She then improved symptomatically, but in 1948, twelve years after her first hospital admission, a persistent erythematous eruption appeared over the face, neck, and arms. When the case was studied in the hospital in 1950, the diagnosis of scleroderma was established by skin biopsy, although the rash on the face was suggestive of lupus erythematosus disseminatus. The cutaneous picture was that of well-marked scleroderma and the arthritis was relatively quiescent when the patient was last seen in 1955.

2.114   This patient must be regarded as one who developed classical manifestations of scleroderma following fourteen years of what was apparently typical rheumatoid arthritis. The diagnosis of two diseases now seems possible in this patient, but the clinical evidence pointing toward scleroderma did not appear until long after the series was "closed."

RHEUMATOID ARTHRITIS AS A DISEASE ENTITY

2.115   The preceding sections of this chapter have been devoted to an account of the development of the concept of rheumatoid arthritis as a disease entity in order to furnish a foundation for the principles employed in the selection of patients for the series. As mentioned before, the process has been twofold and the disease has assumed its present generally well-recognized status both by the separation of other, unrelated forms of joint disease and by the reinstatement of conditions which probably represent clinical variants of rheumatoid arthritis rather than separate entities. To illustrate this point, a brief résumé is in order. To begin with, there is no present opposition to the setting off of gout as an independent disease of metabolic origin, with the realization that a rare case may mimic the clinical appearance of rheumatoid arthritis [329]. Degenerative joint disease deserves equal autonomy but has not received it from all quarters, largely owing to the fact that it may be associated with rheumatoid arthritis coincidentally or in a secondary role. With the evidence at hand, at least one form of so-called "climacteric arthritis" should be classified under degenerative joint disease. There continues to be some opposition to the separation of rheumatic fever and rheumatoid arthritis. For practical purposes, we believe with the majority that separation on clinical and pathologic grounds is justified for the present, in spite of borderline cases and the finding of valvular disease in a certain number of patients with rheumatoid arthritis. Types of infectious arthritis which can either be traced to organisms demonstrable in the joints or which occur in unmistakable association with infectious diseases, form a group which is admittedly distinct from rheumatoid arthritis. Some of the difficulties which crop up in making this distinction have been outlined, and the evidence has been presented against the existence of "tuberculous rheumatism" and of a chronic, progressive arthritis due to the gonococcus or to brucellosis. The secondary type of fibrositis may be a manifestation of various forms of joint disease, including rheumatoid arthritis, while so-called "primary fibrositis," whether or not of psychogenic origin, may present difficulties in diagnosis in respect to rheumatoid arthritis in a mild or early stage. Finally, although both clinical and pathologic relationships exist between rheumatoid arthritis and other connective tissue diseases, it seems best to regard this group as made up of distinct diseases unless a common etiology or pathogenesis should come to light.

2.116 There should next be considered the somewhat artificially created syndromes which merit restoration to their proper position as

Diagnostic Criteria

variants of rheumatoid arthritis. These include Still's disease (both juvenile and adult) and Felty's syndrome. There seems no reason for separate classification of the type of rheumatoid arthritis starting in women at the menopause or for the failure to recognize that most cases of intermittent hydrarthrosis represent merely one stage in the clinical course of rheumatoid arthritis. The status of the arthritis associated with ulcerative colitis awaits further clinical and laboratory study, but at present there are insufficient data for the creation of an independent type of joint disease. The same may be said of the articular manifestations accompanying psoriasis, with the possible exception of destructive lesions of the terminal interphalangeal joints associated with psoriatic nails. Evidence has also been outlined against partition of rheumatoid arthritis into primary and "infectious" types. Opinion is still divided in regard to the status of rheumatoid or ankylosing spondylitis. For reasons already set forth the authors adopted the working decision to include such patients in the series analysis, whether or not peripheral joints were involved in addition to the spine. An attempt has thus been made to define and limit the diagnosis of rheumatoid arthritis without ignoring the fact that in not a few points the boundaries of this disease cannot be accurately delimited with our present knowledge. In such instances we have tried to weigh the evidence judicially and adopt temporary criteria, which we realize may be later over-ruled. "An opinion yields later to the impact of facts unforeseen." [261]

2.117 There has been no intention of leaving the reader of the preceding sections of this chapter with the impression that the diagnosis of rheumatoid arthritis is made chiefly by exclusion. On the contrary, when this disease has reached a well-developed stage, it presents an unmistakable appearance, so that, with rare exceptions, the diagnosis can be made with reasonable certainty at a glance. As will be outlined below, a patient with well-marked rheumatoid arthritis can be identified by characteristic symptoms, physical signs, articular roentgenograms, and histopathologic findings, at least in the subcutaneous nodule and synovial membrane. Proof of the identity of rheumatoid arthritis on etiologic grounds is of course still lacking. However, recent studies [64, 576] suggest that a laboratory test of diagnostic significance may in time be available. As detailed description of the disease would be premature at this point, the following paragraphs will be devoted chiefly to summarizing the evidence for the concept of rheumatoid arthritis as a distinct disease entity.

2.118 In the first place, rheumatoid arthritis is a generalized chronic inflammatory disease of familial nature, with well-marked constitutional manifestations which are not merely secondary to the articular lesions. Females are more commonly affected, except in cases where the spine is involved. The onset is not limited to any age group and may occur from infancy to the ninth decade. Constitutional symptoms often develop before objective changes in the joints, so that a prodromal stage may be arbitrarily set off if desired. Various potentially disturbing events may precede the onset of arthritis, most commonly mental or physical strain or infections, and apparently act as precipitating factors in some instances. The type of onset ranges from the insidious to the explosive, with endless variations in between. Either large or small joints may be initially affected, at first perhaps in a migratory fashion, but later usually with unrelenting persistence. Loss of weight and appetite, fatigability, and symptoms referable to the nervous system and the vasomotor apparatus are the most common of the extra-articular complaints. Examination of the joints reveals no early changes specifically differing from other forms of arthritis; periarticular inflammation, often with effusion, usually precedes the development of limitation of motion and deformity. The latter includes subluxation and ulnar deviation and may present a characteristic appearance, especially in the hands. Although involvement of one or a few joints is not uncommon in early stages, the arthritis usually eventually assumes a symmetrical polyarticular distribution. Muscular atrophy is prominent, and involvement of tendons, bursae, and fasciae is frequently present. Subcutaneous nodules form a characteristic part of the picture in about 20 per cent of the cases observed. Fever and tachycardia are common findings, and involvement of other organs of the body is evidenced in certain cases by pigmentation and atrophy of the skin, lymphadenopathy and splenomegaly, pericarditis and pleuritis, and ocular changes, including uveitis, keratitis, and scleritis. Vasomotor instability and signs suggesting involvement of the nervous system are commonly present to some degree and may dominate the picture.

Diagnostic Criteria

2.119 On the laboratory side, an anemia is often found. Variations in the white blood cell picture are not diagnostic and may vary from a polymorphonuclear leukocytosis to a normal or low white-cell count, with a relative lymphocytosis. The sedimentation rate of the red cells is useful in following the progress of the disease and occasionally in differential diagnosis, but it is entirely nonspecific. With our present knowledge, alterations in blood chemistry are not as helpful in distinguishing rheumatoid arthritis from other forms of joint disease as is the elevated serum uric acid in gout. While quantitative changes in the plasma proteins are revealed chemically and in electrophoretic patterns, such alterations may be duplicated in other joint diseases [*442*]. Amyloidosis is a not infrequent necropsy finding in long-standing cases but the significance is not yet apparent of intermediate values found in Congo red tests on rheumatoid subjects [*148*]. Systematic examination of the synovial fluid, although of help, does not yield specific diagnostic criteria for rheumatoid arthritis. Cases of traumatic arthritis or of degenerative joint disease with articular effusions can be distinguished in this way, as well as arthritis with a purulent type of effusion due to a specific infection, but, in the latter, cultural methods will often reveal the causative organism. Otherwise, chemical and cytologic features of the synovial fluid in rheumatoid arthritis may often be duplicated in various forms of joint disease, including gouty arthritis, rheumatic fever, and arthritis due to specific infections [*440*].

2.120 The search for a serologic test for rheumatoid arthritis goes back at least twenty-five years, to the finding in 1929 by Cecil, Nicholls, and Stainsby [*79*] that hemolytic streptococci recovered from the blood and synovial fluid of patients with rheumatoid arthritis were uniformly agglutinated to a high titer in the serums obtained from patients with this disease. It was later found that similar reactions were given by streptococci obtained from other sources [*137, 334*] and by R forms of the pneumococcus [*137*]. Furthermore, in the case of the hemolytic streptococcus, positive agglutinations could be obtained in a large proportion of patients with rheumatic fever [*292*]. The fact that the test is usually negative in children with rheumatoid arthritis and during the first six months of the disease in adults, has also made it of limited practical value. Furthermore, the relatively small percentage of positive results obtained in subsequent series of patients with rheumatoid arthritis [379, 469] has tended to diminish the importance of this reaction as characteristic of the disease. On the other hand, discovery that rheumatoid sera have the capacity to agglutinate sheep erythrocytes sensitized by rabbit antiserum has led to the development of two serologic tests with a higher degree of specificity for the identification of rheumatoid arthritis [64, 248, 576]. These are outlined in detail in a recent review and consist essentially in "the measurement of either the agglutinating or inhibiting activity of the euglobulin fraction" of the serum [576]. Such tests have given positive readings in children with rheumatoid arthritis and in adults with disease of less than six months' duration but have thus far been consistently negative in cases with spondylitis or psoriasis. Further experience is required with these modifications of a hemagglutination reaction before their diagnostic significance can be finally evaluated. It can at least be said that such advances have enhanced the concept of rheumatoid arthritis as a disease entity.

2.121 The oft-repeated maxim that in any disease roentgenograms must be interpreted in the light of the clinical picture is equally applicable to rheumatoid arthritis. Given a few facts, however, about duration, severity, and articular distribution, accurate roentgenologic diagnosis of the disease is usually possible except in early cases. The more typical features seen in articular roentgenograms in this condition include: juxta-articular and generalized bony decalcification; circumscribed areas of rarefaction (some of which are due to granulomatous invasion of bone); narrowing, irregularity, and even obliteration of the joint space; marginal erosions and, finally, gross bony destruction and subluxation. No single feature constitutes a diagnostic criterion, but unless the patient is seen too early for the development of roentgenographic changes in bone and cartilage, observations on representative joints, especially if repeated at intervals, make up an important part of the clinical picture in rheumatoid arthritis.

2.122 It has been mentioned above that rheumatoid arthritis is a disease of characteristic morbid anatomy. This statement can thus far be applied only to the synovial tissue and to nodules, whether subcutaneous or in other parts of the body. That "very large lymphoid foci and follicles" in synovial tissue occur only in rheumatoid arthritis has been

Diagnostic Criteria

stated by Collins [109]. Others have questioned the specificity of these lesions [32] and have mentioned their appearance in association with chronic articular irritation caused by juxta-articular tumors or old fractures with severe degenerative joint disease [460] and with osteo-arthritis of the hip [202]. In such cases a coinciding rheumatoid arthritis remains a possibility [305], although lymphocytic collections may be produced in animals by the intra-articular injection of irritating substances [297]. Lymphoid follicles are also frequently absent in cases of short duration [305], where the tissue reaction often shows a closer resemblance to that of various stages in nodule formation [64, 305]. Although admittedly not entirely specific and perhaps representing "at best a quantitative diagnostic criterion" [305], such lesions can reasonably be considered an outstanding and characteristic pathologic feature of the disease. There is general agreement, on the other hand, that the fully developed rheumatoid nodule constitutes a unique morphologic lesion which is not found in other forms of joint disease or, in fact, in diseases predominantly involving other bodily systems. The one exception is the dermal lesion of granuloma annulare, which also shows a focus of destroyed connective tissue surrounded by palisaded cells [108]. The nodule of rheumatoid arthritis differs fundamentally in microscopic appearance from that of rheumatic fever [35, 108]. In diseases of connective tissue other than these two, the nodules which may be encountered can usually be distinguished histologically from a typical nodule of rheumatoid origin. Thus the histologic findings in the nodule, as well as in the lymphoid follicles of synovial tissue, lend substantial support to the disease identity of rheumatoid arthritis.

2.123 In certain diseases a favorable response to a particular form of therapy constitutes a diagnostic point of great importance. Examples are furnished by the response of pernicious anemia to vitamin B_{12}, scurvy to ascorbic acid, and acute gouty arthritis to colchicine. No curative treatment is yet available for rheumatoid arthritis, while the suppressive action of cortisone and other steroids applies equally to many other inflammatory and noninflammatory diseases. In addition, the ameliorating effect of jaundice and pregnancy is not limited to rheumatoid arthritis [255].

2.124 In view of the evidence presented in the preceding paragraphs, is it reasonable to consider rheumatoid arthritis a distinct disease entity? A definitive answer can hardly be given to this question until its etiology or pathogenesis has been solved. As brought out in the section on connective tissue diseases, it is entirely possible that the disease represents only one type of response to a single agent or disease mechanism which is shared by other pathologic disorders. One may equally speculate that multiple causes or mechanisms are responsible for the varied and at times seemingly unrelated clinical pictures included under a single diagnostic heading. That the present clinical description was undertaken does not necessarily assume the authors' belief in the identity of rheumatoid arthritis, since such a description might be justified of a syndrome with multiple causes or of a fairly well-defined type of response to a single disease mechanism also causative of other illnesses with different clinical patterns. Thus far, the weight of medical opinion favors an independent status of this disease, although certain of its boundaries are still in dispute. From the considerations already set forth, the authors are willing to commit themselves, with reservations, to the majority opinion and to the belief that the present evidence favors the concept of rheumatoid arthritis as an independent disease of unitary though unknown etiology.

3

Selection of Patients and Controls and Methods of Analysis

SELECTION OF PATIENTS

3.1   The present study is based upon patients with the clinical findings of rheumatoid arthritis among admissions to the medical wards of the Massachusetts General Hospital between 1930 and 1936. The series was terminated after 300 consecutive patients had been selected according to the diagnostic criteria which have been discussed in detail in Chapter 2. In 1938, two years after the series was closed, the initial findings and subsequent course of each patient were carefully reviewed by five observers in order to verify the diagnosis of rheumatoid arthritis. As a result of this re-appraisal, 7 patients were removed from the study—6 with findings suggesting rheumatic fever (par. 2.12), and one whose course resembled that of arthritis due to specific infections (par. 2.95). It was then agreed to make no further changes in the composition of the series. It is of interest that several subsequent reviews of these cases have necessitated modification of the primary diagnosis in only 1 of the 293 patients (see par. 2.113). On the other hand, some patients who were admitted to the hospital with joint disease during the years 1930 to 1936, but excluded from the study group for diagnostic reasons, are known to have subsequently developed findings characteristic of rheumatoid arthritis.

3.2   It is our opinion that the patients studied are representative of individuals over twelve years of age with rheumatoid arthritis who were referred for diagnosis or treatment to a general hospital affiliated with a medical school. Although the majority of them were residents of Massachusetts, a number of the patients were referred from communities scattered throughout the New England States. Most of them had been under the care of family physicians and many had been hospitalized previously for their rheumatic complaints.

3.3   There are, of course, many selective factors which operate to distort the clinical concept of a disease when information is obtained from samples of hospitalized patients [37a, 339a]. So little is known about the occurrence and distribution of rheumatoid arthritis in the population at large that we cannot even make intelligent guesses about the extent to which our patients might depart from the characteristics of a random sample of rheumatoid arthritics drawn from New England communities. Two specific factors are known to have influenced the formation of the series owing to the admitting policy of the hospital: (1) patients under twelve years of age were not admitted to the medical services, and (2) admission to the medical wards was reserved for patients with relatively low levels of income.

SELECTION OF CONTROLS

3.4   In order to attempt an evaluation of the occurrence of certain signs and symptoms of rheumatoid arthritis, it was necessary to study a group of nonarthritic persons with whom the patients in the series could be compared. The controls were chosen so as to correspond to the sex and age distribution of the arthritics when the latter were arranged in five-year groups according to age on admission to the study. The 300 controls were examined during 1936 and 1937, after the series was closed. After the diagnostic re-appraisal of the patients in 1938 and the exclusion of the previously mentioned 7 patients, 7 other persons were dropped from the control group by random selections from the appropriate sex and age groups.

3.5   It was originally intended to enlist other patients from the hospital in order to balance some of the unknown factors which determine admission to the hospital. The first 92 control subjects were drawn from patients admitted to the out-patient departments or wards of the Massachusetts General Hospital and Massachusetts Eye and Ear

Selection and Analysis

Infirmary for minor medical and surgical procedures, such as refraction, extraction of cataracts, repair of hernia, and ligation of varicose veins. Because of slowness in finding suitable control subjects, attention was shifted to the only other large and readily available segment of the hospital population, the employees and staff. Thus, the remaining 201 controls were drawn from secretaries, social workers, nurses, maids, porters, kitchen workers, and other hospital employees. Persons who showed evidence of joint disease by history or physical examination were excluded from the control group, except when this consisted merely of a slight degree of degenerative joint disease.

COLLECTION OF DATA

3.6 The study to be reported may be considered in two parts: (1) a cross-sectional description of rheumatoid arthritis, which includes information in regard to factors preceding and associated with the onset as well as to the type of course pursued before admission, and (2) a long-term follow-up study of the course of rheumatoid arthritis in patients treated with simple medical and orthopedic measures. The plan of observations for the cross-sectional description was established before the study began, and a printed check list of possible findings became a part of each patient's study record (see page 94). The check list was a modification of the forms described and illustrated by Lerman and Means [315] for use in clinical descriptive studies. Each patient admitted to the study was carefully observed during a period of hospitalization by one of six physicians of the Arthritis Unit.* Two of the observers (C. L. S. and W. B.) participated in the study throughout the six-year period in which patients were selected. Data were recorded for more than 300 items arranged in the following major categories:

Sex	Marital history
Age	Habits
Race	Past history
Civil state	Menstruation
Occupation	Menopause
Family history	Present illness

* Drs. Nathan R. Abrams, Walter Bauer, Howard C. Coggeshall, Alfred O. Ludwig, Marian W. Ropes, and Charles L. Short.

86   Rheumatoid Arthritis

Dietary history	X-ray examination
Past treatment	Treatment used
Physical examination	Diagnoses
Laboratory findings	

Two of the observers (C. L. S. and N. R. A.) assumed responsibility for checking the records in order to assure their completeness and uniformity and to decide upon equivocal findings.

3.7   Information about the control subjects was obtained from single interviews and physical examinations by members of the clinic staff, including those who had selected the arthritic patients. The data were recorded on mimeographed check lists of 130 items under the following major headings:

Sex	Past history
Age	Present history
Occupation	Physical examination
Family history	Diagnoses

3.8   A follow-up clinic was organized for continued observation and management of the patients in the study. Special effort was made to obtain data on each patient at least once a year. Oral temperature, pulse rate, and body weight were recorded at each clinic visit. The following laboratory tests were obtained at frequent intervals: hematocrit and hemoglobin determinations, erythrocyte sedimentation rate, white blood cell count, and urinalysis. Interval histories and physical findings were recorded in detailed progress notes but were not obtained according to a pre-arranged schedule. Typewritten copies of all progress notes, laboratory findings, x-ray reports, correspondence, summaries of hospital admissions, and autopsy reports were included in the permanent study records.

ANALYSIS AND INTERPRETATION OF DATA

3.9   Most of the numerical comparisons made in this study, whether between the arthritic patients and the control subjects or among subgroups of the arthritic patients, require the interpretation of a difference between two percentages. In most instances, a standard error of the difference has been computed, and a difference that is large enough to exceed two standard errors is called *significant*. Occasionally, more than

Selection and Analysis

two percentages are compared simultaneously, in which case a chi-square test has been computed and evaluated at the 5 per cent level of significance.

COMPARISONS OF ARTHRITIC AND CONTROL GROUPS

3.10 The arthritic and control groups are compared with respect to seventy-three historical and physical findings. While each finding is presented in the appropriate chapter to follow, the results are tabulated for ready reference in Table 46 in the Appendix. The validity of these comparisons rests largely on the extent to which the controls reflect the effects of the many variables, unrelated to the occurrence of rheumatoid arthritis, which might have influenced the findings in the patients. Some possible sources of bias related to the selection of the patients and controls have been mentioned previously. These and other limiting factors will be discussed further in the presentation of results. In general, one must be cautious in the interpretation of probability statements about differences between the patients and the controls. If a difference in percentages is not greater than would commonly occur under conditions of random sampling from a homogeneous population, then there is not sufficient evidence to conclude that the difference is characteristic of rheumatoid arthritis. A statistically significant difference, on the other hand, may be the result of a hidden bias in the composition of the two groups or in the method of making the observations.

3.11 Thus, the conclusions to be drawn from these comparisons are *statistical impressions,* which closely resemble ordinary *clinical impressions*. The distinguishing feature of a statistical impression is its greater objectivity, which renders it more readily subject to confirmation or refutation by other investigators but does not confer upon it any special authority as an explanation for observable facts. In brief, simple numerical description does not constitute a controlled experiment.

CLASSIFICATION OF PATIENTS BY VARIABLES

3.12 The arthritic patients were classified according to the presence or absence of thirty-nine attributes chosen because of their clinical interest or importance. All possible pairs of these attributes were then examined systematically for the presence of association by methods illustrated in the example to follow. The results are summarized in Appendix Table 47. In a few instances of particular clinical importance the relationships among three variables were studied.

3.13 Difficulties in the interpretation of comparisons among the arthritic patients arise from several related sources:
1. The large number of variables investigated.
2. The qualitative nature of many of the variables.
3. The limited amount of information afforded by the small number of individuals in many of the subcategories.
4. The retrospective nature of the observations, i.e., the inability of the observer to control or manipulate the variables.

3.14 In a descriptive study comparisons among variables are made by manipulating the data rather than the variables. The data may establish the fact that variables A and B are related, but this fact does not reveal what effect, if any, upon variable B would result from changes in variable A. Nevertheless, much of the knowledge upon which the practice of medicine is based has accrued from the discovery and further investigation of such associations.

3.15 As an illustration of the methods used and the difficulties encountered, consider the comparison of *duration of arthritis before admission* and *infection as a precipitating factor*.* The latter is a qualitative variable, the effect of which is most simply measured by classifying patients into two mutually exclusive groups—those with and those without a history of infection as a precipitating factor in their illness. For comparative purposes it was convenient in this instance to reduce the quantitative variable, "duration of disease before admission," to a dichotomy of short and long durations by arbitrarily calling a duration of one year or less "short" and any of more than one year "long." The classifications of the 293 arthritic patients in regard to these two variables may be expressed in a fourfold table. As shown in Table 3.1, a history of infection as a precipitating factor was found twice as often among patients having a short duration of illness before admission as among those with a long duration. If the two variables were independent, in a statistical sense [574], in the hypothetical population from which the sample of 293 patients was drawn, the percentage of the

* See definitions, pars. 4.7 and 4.12.

Selection and Analysis

Table 3.1
Infection as a precipitating factor in relation to duration of rheumatoid arthritis before hospital admission among patients of present series

		Infection			
		Absent		Present	
Duration	No. of patients	No.	Per cent	No.	Per cent
Total	293	244	83	49	17
Short (1 year or less)	86	64	74	22	26
Long (more than 1 year)	207	180	87	27	13
		Difference in percentages: 13 ± 4.9			

population with infection as a precipitating factor among those with a short duration of illness before admission would equal the corresponding percentage among patients with a long duration before admission. Any difference between the percentages observed in a random sample would be the result of chance fluctuations. In order to conclude from a single sample that two variables are not independent, i.e., are "associated," the statistician requires that the observed difference be one which would occur only rarely by chance if repeated samples were drawn at random from a population in which the variables were independent. To appraise this chance occurrence, the standard error of the difference of percentages is estimated from the sample data under the assumption that the two variables are, in fact, independent. If the observed difference is greater than twice the standard error, the assumption of independence is rejected on the grounds that a difference as great as the observed one would be a rare chance occurrence, to be expected less than 5 per cent of the time. The observed difference is then said to be statistically significant at the 5 per cent level.

3.16   When this method is applied to the data in Table 3.1, the standard error of the difference is found to be 4.9 per cent. Hence the observed difference of 13 per cent exceeds two standard errors and is significant at the 5 per cent level. In the absence of any other information one may conclude that the duration of illness before admission is associated with history of infection as a precipitating factor. When, as in the present study, it is not possible to select the sample strictly at random from a well-defined population, the generalization of such a conclusion is simply a documented clinical impression rather than a scientifically validated hypothesis. In either case the bare fact of association is seldom interesting unless it provides an answer to a preconceived question or unless it suggests a question worthy of further study.

3.17 It is important to notice that the statistical test of significance alone does not offer an explanation for the association. One plausible explanation for the findings in Table 3.1 could be a tendency for those patients who were examined shortly after the onset of arthritis to recall an infectious episode more often than those who were examined after one or more years of illness. However, the present study does not provide any direct evidence on this point. Many hidden variables, other than memory, might also account for the association, but since none of them could be controlled in the study, there are no experimental criteria for excluding some and considering others.

3.18 Of course it is possible that one or more of the several variables actually studied might explain the association. For example, it was also found that both a short duration of illness before admission and a history of infection as a precipitating factor were associated with a third attribute, an acute onset of arthritis,* as shown in Tables 3.2 and 3.3.

3.19 To examine the influence of the type of onset on the association in Table 3.1, it is necessary to make separate comparisons of duration before admission with infection as a precipitating factor for patients who had an acute onset and for those with a gradual onset, as in Tables 3.4 and 3.5, respectively. In both cases the observed differences are in the same direction as the original association, but in magnitude they are small, relative to their standard errors, and thus might readily result from sampling fluctuations alone. Hence, the available data suggest that the apparent association of "duration" and "infection" in Table 3.1 can be largely explained by the hidden variable "type of onset."

3.20 A closer look at Tables 3.4 and 3.5 will help to clarify this result. Notice that, apart from chance fluctuations, only 11 per cent of the patients with a gradual onset gave a history of infection as a precipitating factor, regardless of the duration of their illness before admission, but 38 per cent of patients with an acute onset gave such a history. When Table 3.1 is broken down into Tables 3.4 and 3.5 most of the patients with

* See definition, par. 4.8.

Selection and Analysis

Table 3.2
Duration of rheumatoid arthritis before hospital admission in relation to type of onset among patients of present series

Onset	No. of patients	Duration			
		Long		Short	
		No.	Per cent	No.	Per cent
Total	293	207	71	86	29
Acute	64	31	48	33	52
Gradual	229	176	77	53	23
			Difference in percentages: 29 ± 6.4		

Table 3.3
Infection as a precipitating factor in relation to type of onset of rheumatoid arthritis among patients of present series

Onset	No. of patients	Infection			
		Absent		Present	
		No.	Per cent	No.	Per cent
Total	293	244	83	49	17
Acute	64	40	62	24	38
Gradual	229	204	89	25	11
			Difference in percentages: 27 ± 5.3		

a long duration, 176, are those with a gradual onset contributed by Table 3.5. The patients with short durations are more evenly divided between those with acute and gradual onsets, 33 and 53 respectively. Thus, in effect, Table 3.1 is a comparison of "infection as a precipitating factor" with "type of onset" rather than with "duration before admission." It is in this way that a spurious association may arise through the influence of a hidden variable.

3.21 In order that this conclusion be consistent, it is necessary to demonstrate that (1) the association of acute onset with short duration (Table 3.2) is not influenced by the history of infection, and (2) the association of acute onset with a history of infection (Table 3.3) does not vary with the duration of illness. The first statement is verified by the data in Tables 3.6 and 3.7, and the second assertion is supported by the comparisons in Table 3.8 and 3.9.

3.22 Hidden variables can also give rise to spurious independence

Table 3.4
Infection as a precipitating factor in relation to duration of rheumatoid arthritis before hospital admission *among group with acute onset*

Duration	No. of patients	Infection			
		Absent		Present	
		No.	Per cent	No.	Per cent
Total	64	40	62	24	38
Short	33	18	55	15	45
Long	31	22	71	9	29

Difference in percentages: 16 ± 12.1

Table 3.5
Infection as a precipitating factor in relation to duration of rheumatoid arthritis before hospital admission *among group with gradual onset*

Duration	No. of patients	Infection			
		Absent		Present	
		No.	Per cent	No.	Per cent
Total	229	204	89	25	11
Short	53	46	87	7	13
Long	176	158	90	18	10

Difference in percentages: 3 ± 4.9

Table 3.6
Duration of rheumatoid arthritis before hospital admission in relation to type of onset *among group with infection as a precipitating factor*

Onset	No. of patients	Duration			
		Long		Short	
		No.	Per cent	No.	Per cent
Total	49	27	55	22	45
Acute	24	9	37	15	63
Gradual	25	18	72	7	28

Difference in percentages: 35 ± 14.4

of variables. It is partly for this reason that there is no satisfactory statistical criterion by which an investigator can decide what variables he should be interested in comparing, or to what extent he should subdivide his data in a search for possible explanations of observed associations. Finally, if one is particularly interested in all of the inter-relationships

Table 3.7
Duration of rheumatoid arthritis before hospital admission in relation to type of onset *among group without infection as a precipitating factor*

Onset	No. of patients	Duration			
		Long		Short	
		No.	Per cent	No.	Per cent
Total	244	180	74	64	26
Acute	40	22	55	18	45
Gradual	204	158	77	46	23

Difference in percentages: 22 ± 7.6

Table 3.8
Infection as a precipitating factor in relation to type of onset *among group with short duration before hospital admission* (1 year or less)

Onset	No. of patients	Infection			
		Absent		Present	
		No.	Per cent	No.	Per cent
Total	86	64	74	22	26
Acute	33	18	55	15	45
Gradual	53	46	87	7	13

Difference in percentages: 32 ± 9.7

Table 3.9
Infection as a precipitating factor in relation to type of onset *among group with long duration before hospital admission* (more than 1 year)

Onset	No. of patients	Infection			
		Absent		Present	
		No.	Per cent	No.	Per cent
Total	207	180	87	27	13
Acute	31	22	71	9	29
Gradual	176	158	90	18	10

Difference in percentages: 19 ± 6.6

among several qualitative variables, there is the additional difficulty introduced by the small numbers of observations usually available in the subcategories. For example, inferences about associations in the subpopulations are hampered by the small amount of information contained in comparisons such as those of Table 3.4.

MASSACHUSETTS GENERAL HOSPITAL
ARTHRITIS SHEET

Hosp. No. _____
O. P. D. No. _____
X-ray No. _____
Clinic No. _____

Name_____ Date_____

Check as follows:
    v=Present   o=Absent   ?=Doubtful   x=Unobtained

___Sex   Color   Civil State   Race_____
  (1)_____Male   (3)_____White   (5)_____S   Age_____
  (2)_____Female   (4)_____Colored   (6)_____M
                                            (7)_____W

___Occupation:
  Past_____ Present_____

FAMILY HISTORY

___(1, 2)_____Tuberculosis, exposure to   (5, 6)_____Cancer   (11, 12)_____Allergic Condition
   (3, 4)_____Cardio-Renal   (7, 8)_____Diabetes   Urticaria
            Apoplexy   (9, 10)_____Arthritis—Indicate Type   Asthma
            Nephritis   Parents   Hay fever
            High blood pressure   Grandparents   Eczema
            Heart trouble   Cousins   Migraine
                                                                         Brothers, sisters
                                                                          Aunts, uncles
                                                                          Children

MARITAL HISTORY   HABITS

___Years of marriage_____   ___(1, 2)_____Sleep, adequate
   Number of pregnancies_____   (3, 4)_____Alcohol
   Interval between onset and last pregnancy_____   (5, 6)_____Tobacco
                                                                          (7, 8)_____Lead

PAST HISTORY

___(1, 2)_____Serious Illness_____   (7, 8)_____Rheumatic fever, chorea_____
   (3, 4)_____Venereal disease_____   (9, 10)_____Allergic conditions_____
   (5, 6)_____Operations_____   (11, 12)_____Injuries_____

Cardio-Respiratory Symptoms   **Gastro-Intestinal Symptoms**
___(1, 2)_____Palpitation   ___(1, 2)_____Nausea
   (3, 4)_____Dyspnea   (3, 4)_____Vomiting
   (5, 6)_____Pain   (5, 6)_____Abdominal Pain
   (7, 8)_____Cough   (7, 8)_____Flatulence
   (9, 10)_____Sputum   (9, 10)_____Jaundice

MENSTRUATION
___(1)_____Early Onset of Cta.
   (2)_____Late Onset of Cta.   } Age_____
   (3)_____Normal Onset of Cta.
   (4)_____Irregular: Duration_____   (7)_____Profuse
   (5)_____Regular: Duration_____   (8)_____Normal flow
   (6)_____Scanty   (9)_____Amenorrhea { Duration_____
                                                            (10, 11)_____Dysmennorrhea { Days between_____

MENOPAUSE   Severity of Menopause Symptoms:
___(1)_____Artificial   (8)_____Mild
   (2)_____Natural   (9)_____Moderate
   (3)_____Early Onset   (10)_____Severe
   (4)_____Late Onset   } Age_____   Duration_____
   (5)_____Normal Onset
   (6, 7)_____Association with P. I.   Character_____

PRESENT ILLNESS
       Prodromal Symptoms   (7, 8)_____Muscle and Joint Aching
___(1, 2)_____Fatiguability   (9, 10)_____Crepitus
   (3, 4)_____Sensory Changes   (11, 12)_____Association of Above
   (5, 6)_____Appetite Loss   with Weather Changes
Other Symptoms:_____

       Onset
___(1)_____Acute   (2)_____Gradual

Figure 3.1 Check list of possible findings utilized in the study of the patients of the present series

Associated with

(3, 4, 5) _____ Strain _____   (1, 2, 3) _____ Operation _____
(6, 7, 8) _____ Exposure _____   (4, 5, 6) _____ Acute Trauma _____
(9, 10, 11) _____ Acute Infection _____ (7, 8, 9) _____ Chronic Trauma _____

Course

(10) _____ Progressive   (11) _____ Exacerbations and Remissions   (12) _____ Improvement
Duration: _____   Age of onset: _____

Joint Symptoms   Joints First Involved
(1, 2, 3) _____ Migratory   (6, 7) _____ Small Joints of Extremities _____
(4) _____ Mon-articular   (8, 9) _____ Large Joints of Extremities _____
(5) _____ Poly-articular   (10, 11) _____ Joints of Trunk _____

Joints Finally Involved
(1, 2) _____ Phalangeal   (7, 8) _____ Shoulders   (1, 2) _____ Knees   (7, 8) _____ Toes
(3, 4) _____ Wrists   (9, 10) _____ Spine   (3, 4) _____ Ankles   (9, 10) _____ Jaws
(5, 6) _____ Elbows   (11, 12) _____ Hips   (5, 6) _____ Metatarsal (11, 12) _____ Other joints:

Symptoms Prominent
(1, 2) _____ Pain   (5, 6) _____ Redness   (9, 10) _____ Stiffness   (1, 2) _____ Locking
(3, 4) _____ Swelling (7, 8) _____ Heat   (11, 12) _____ Ankylosis (3, 4) _____ Crepitus

Associated Symptoms
(5, 6) _____ Fever   (11, 12) _____ Muscular pains   (7, 8) _____ Retro-bulbar aching
(7, 8) _____ Appetite Loss (1, 2) _____ Pallor   (9, 10) _____ Thyroid swelling
(9, 10) _____ Headache   (3, 4) _____ Weakness   (11, 12) _____ Muscular wasting
                          (5, 6) _____ Exophthalmos

Other symptoms: _____

Weight
(1) _____ Loss   (2) _____ Gain   (3) _____ Maintenance
Degree: _____   Duration: _____

Skin Conditions
(4, 5) _____ Psoriasis   (6, 7) _____ Herpes   (8, 9) _____ Urticaria   (10, 11) _____ Scleroderma
                                                       Other conditions: _____

Neurological Symptoms
(1, 2) _____ Nervousness   (5, 6) _____ Vertigo   (9, 10) _____ Tinnitus
(3, 4) _____ Twitchings   (7, 8) _____ Tremor   (11, 12) _____ Emotional Upsets
Other symptoms: _____

Vasomotor Symptoms
(1, 2) _____ Paraesthesiae   (5, 6) _____ Vascular spasm   (9, 10) _____ Changes in skin or nails
(3, 4) _____ Coldness of Extremities (7, 8) _____ Sweating   (11, 12) _____ Cyanosis
Other symptoms: _____

Course Affected by
(1, 2, 3)* _____ Pregnancy   (1, 2, 3) _____ Allergy   (1, 2, 3) _____ Altitude
(4, 5, 6) _____ Menstruation   (4, 5, 6) _____ Cold   (4, 5, 6) _____ Latitude
(7, 8, 9) _____ Strain   (7, 8, 9) _____ Heat   (7, 8, 9) _____ Proximity to water
(10, 11, 12) _____ Acute Infections (10, 11, 12) _____ Moisture (10, 11, 12) _____ Season
*v=Favorably   o=Not affected   x=Unfavorably

Foci
(1, 2) _____ Sinus Symptoms   (5, 6) _____ Sore Throats   (9, 10) _____ Urinary Symptoms
(3, 4) _____ Dental Symptoms (7, 8) _____ Gall Bladder Symptoms (11, 12) _____ Genital Symptoms

Bowels
(1) _____ Diarrhea   Cathartics used _____
(2) _____ Constipation   No. movements daily _____
(3) _____ Normal Bowel Action Consistency _____

DIETARY HISTORY

Protein: Carbohydrate: Fat:
(4) _____ Low   (7) _____ Low   (10) _____ Low
(5) _____ Adequate   (8) _____ Adequate   (11) _____ Adequate
(6) _____ High   (9) _____ High   (12) _____ High

Vitamins: Minerals:
(1, 2) _____ A   (9, 10) _____ Iron
(3, 4) _____ B   (11, 12) _____ Calcium
(5, 6) _____ C
(7, 8) _____ D

TREATMENT TRIED*

- (1) _____ Removal of foci _____
- (2) _____ Salicylates _____
- (3) _____ Iodides _____
- (4) _____ Physiotherapy _____
- (5) _____ Bed Rest _____
- (6) _____ Vaccines _____
- (7) _____ Colonic Irrigation _____
- (8) _____ Low Protein Diet _____
- (9) _____ Low Carbohydrate Diet _____
- (10) _____ High Vitamin Diet _____
- (11) _____ Orthopedic Manipulation _____
- (12) _____ Operation _____

*More than one can be checked.

PHYSICAL EXAMINATION

General Appearance

- (1) _____ Over-developed
- (2) _____ Under-developed
- (3) _____ Normal
- (4) _____ Older than actual age
- (5) _____ Younger than actual age
- (6) _____ Appearance of actual age
- (7) _____ Obese
- (8) _____ Under-nourished
- (9) _____ Normal
- (10) _____ Febrile
- (11) _____ Afebrile

Type: _____

Hair:
Abnormalities: _____

Eyes:
- (1, 2) _____ Exophthalmos
- (3, 4) _____ Arcus Senilis
- (5, 6) _____ Abnormalities of Pupils _____
- (7, 8) _____ Arteriosclerosis of Fundi _____
- Other abnormalities: _____

Nose:
- (1, 2) _____ Obstruction
- (3, 4) _____ Deviated Septum
- (5, 6) _____ Pus
- (7, 8) _____ Sinus Tenderness
- (9, 10) _____ Faulty Transillumination

Mouth:
- (1, 2) _____ Poor Hygiene
- (3, 4) _____ Cavities
- (5, 6) _____ Pyorrhea
- (7, 8) _____ Apical Absorption
- (9) _____ Cyanosis of Lips
- (10) _____ Pallor of Lips
- (11) _____ Normal color of Lips

Tonsils:
- (1, 2) _____ Absent
- (3, 4) _____ Tabs
- (5, 6) _____ Inflamed
- (7, 8) _____ Cryptic
- (9, 10) _____ Pus Expressed
- (11, 12) _____ Glands

Tongue:
- (1, 2) _____ Coated
- (3, 4) _____ Atrophic

Thyroid:
- (5) _____ Normal
- (6) _____ Nodular
- (7) _____ Colloid
- (8) _____ Exophthalmic

Heart:
- (1, 2) _____ Enlargement
- (3, 4) _____ Arrhythmias
- (5, 6) _____ Sounds poor quality
- (7, 8) _____ Valvular Disease
- (9, 10) _____ Accentuated A_2

Vessels:
- (1, 2) _____ Arteriosclerosis. Evidence _____
- (3, 4) _____ Dorsales pedis pulsate
- (5, 6) _____ Posterior tibials pulsate
- (7, 8) _____ Popliteals pulsate

Blood Pressure:
- _____ Systolic _____
- _____ Diastolic _____

Chest:
- (1) _____ Barrel
- (2) _____ Flat
- (3) _____ Normal

Lungs:
- (4, 5) _____ Signs of Consolidation
- (6, 7) _____ Emphysema
- (8, 9) _____ Rales without Consolidation
- (10, 11) _____ Pleurisy

Abdomen:
- (1, 2) _____ Relaxed wall
- (3, 4) _____ Ptosis

Organs palpable:
- (5, 6) _____ Spleen
- (7, 8) _____ Liver
- (9, 10) _____ Kidneys
- (11, 12) _____ Colon

Extremities:
- (1, 2) _____ Edema
- (3, 4) _____ Clubbing
- (5, 6) _____ Tremor
- (7, 8) _____ Heberden's Nodes
- (9, 10) _____ Lymphadenopathy
- (11, 12) _____ Varicosities

Skin:
- (1) _____ Dry
- (2) _____ Moist
- (3) _____ Hot
- (4) _____ Cold
- (5) _____ Warm
- (6) _____ Coarse
- (7) _____ Normal texture
- (8) _____ Atrophic
- (9) _____ Cyanotic
- (10) _____ Pale
- (11) _____ Red
- (12) _____ Normal

Figure 3.1 (cont.)

- (1, 2) ___ Subcutaneous Nodules
- (3, 4) ___ Skin Disease ___
- (5, 6) ___ Nails Atrophic

Prostate:
- (1) ___ Normal Size
- (2) ___ Large
- (3, 4) ___ Tender
- (5) ___ Soft
- (6) ___ Hard
- (7) ___ Normal Consistency

Pelvic:
- (1, 2) ___ Lacerated cervix
- (3, 4) ___ Infected cervix
- (5, 6) ___ Leukorrhea
- (7, 8) ___ Vaults Abnormal
- (9, 10) ___ Peri-vaginal Infection
- (11, 12) ___ Other Abnormalities ___

Neurological:
- (1) ___ Over-active
- (2) ___ Under-active
- (3) ___ Normal Activity
- (4) ___ Depressed
- (5) ___ Good Reaction to Illness
- (6) ___ Deep Reflexes exaggerated
- (7) ___ Deep Reflexes absent
- (8) ___ Deep Reflexes normal
- (9, 10) ___ Organic Signs ___

Joints Involved:
- (1, 2) ___ Phalangeal ___
- (3, 4) ___ Wrist ___
- (5, 6) ___ Elbow ___
- (7, 8) ___ Shoulder ___
- (9, 10) ___ Jaw ___
- (11, 12) ___ Spine ___

Indicate Side.
- (1, 2) ___ Hip ___
- (3, 4) ___ Knee ___
- (5, 6) ___ Ankle ___
- (7, 8) ___ Metatarsal ___
- (9, 10) ___ Toes ___
- (10, 11) ___ Others ___

Joint Signs:
- (1, 2) ___ Tenderness ___
- (3, 4) ___ Peri-articular Swelling ___
- (5, 6) ___ Fluid ___
- (7, 8) ___ Pain on Motion ___
- (9, 10) ___ Limitation of Motion ___
- (11, 12) ___ Heat ___
- (1, 2) ___ Redness ___
- (3, 4) ___ Muscular Wasting ___
- (5, 6) ___ Deformity ___
- (7, 8) ___ Crepitus ___
- (9, 10) ___ Palpable Fringes ___
- (11, 12) ___ Osseous Overgrowth ___

LABORATORY

___ Pulse ___ Weight, o/o of normal ___ Basal Metabolism ___ Height, inches ___

Urine:
- (1, 2) ___ Albumin
- (3, 4) ___ Pus
- (5, 6) ___ Red Cells
- (7, 8) ___ Casts

- ___ Hemoglobin ___
- ___ Red count ___
- ___ Blood Uric Acid ___
- ___ NPN ___
- ___ White count ___

- ___ Gastric Analysis ___
- ___ Urine Creatin (24 hour) ___
- ___ Hinton ___
- ___ Prostatic Smear ___
- ___ Sugar tolerance ___

X-RAY EXAMINATION

Joints:
- (1, 2) ___ Narrowing of Spaces
- (3, 4) ___ Irregularity of Spaces
- (5, 6) ___ Atrophy of Bone
- (7, 8) ___ Soft Tissue Swelling
- (1, 2) ___ Cysts
- (3, 4) ___ Loose Bodies
- (5, 6) ___ Peri-articular Lipping
- (7, 8) ___ Osteophytes

Teeth:
- (1, 2) ___ Apical Absorption
- (3, 4) ___ Abscesses
- (5, 6) ___ Marginal Pockets

Sinuses:
- (7, 8) ___ Thickening
- (9, 10) ___ Retained Secretion
- (11, 12) ___ Cysts

Chest:
- (1) ___ Normal
- (2) ___ Questionable
- (3) ___ Abnormal

Gall Bladder:
- (4) ___ Normal
- (5) ___ Questionable
- (6) ___ Abnormal

Barium Enema:
- (1, 2) ___ Atonic Colon
- (3, 4) ___ Low Position
- (5, 6) ___ Kinks
- (7, 8) ___ Loss of Haustration
- (9, 10) ___ Diverticuli
- (11, 12) ___ Other Abnormalities ___

TREATMENT USED

- (1, 2) ___ Removal of Foci ___
- (3, 4) ___ Heat
- (5, 6) ___ Massage
- (7, 8) ___ Active Motion
- (9, 10) ___ Passive Motion
- (11, 12) ___ Splinting
- (1, 2) ___ Specific Vaccines
- (3, 4) ___ Postural Exercises
- (5, 6) ___ Colonic Irrigations
- (7, 8) ___ Orthopedic Correction of Deformity
- (9, 10) ___ Operations on Joints
- (11, 12) ___ Operations on Sympathetic System
- (1, 2) ___ High Vitamin Diet
- (3, 4) ___ Low Carbohydrate Diet
- (5, 6) ___ Salicylates
- (7, 8) ___ Luminal
- (9, 10) ___ Amidoxyl
- (11, 12) ___ Non-specific Vaccines

DIAGNOSIS:

Primary: Secondary:

SUMMARY

3.23 The 293 patients chosen for this study represent consecutive admissions to the medical wards of a general hospital of persons who satisfied our diagnostic criteria for rheumatoid arthritis. A control group of 293 persons without joint disease was selected from patients and hospital employees to correspond with the arthritic series in sex and age.

3.24 Historical, physical, and laboratory data were obtained from both patients and controls at the time of their admission to the study. These data were systematically recorded according to a prearranged plan to provide a cross-sectional view of the disease. Information was also obtained in regard to factors preceding and associated with the onset of arthritis as well as to the course of the illness before admission. In addition, the subsequent course pursued by the patients has been observed in a follow-up study which is still in progress.

3.25 Numerical comparisons were made between the arthritic patients and the control subjects and between subgroups of the patients for many variables of particular clinical interest. Interpretation of the results has been guided by appropriate tests for statistical significance of the observed differences.

3.26 Several sources of difficulty in the interpretation of the data are discussed. These include comparability of the arthritic patients and the control subjects, the retrospective nature of the observations, the influence of hidden factors on an association between two variables, and finally the fact that the information was obtained from a sample of hospitalized patients.

4

Scheme of Presentation and Definition of Terms

PRESENTATION

4.1 The analysis of the present series of patients has been divided into forty chapters, with the order of subjects in general corresponding to that customarily employed in a description of a disease. Factors of possible etiologic significance are first considered, including sex, age, national origin, family history, past or associated illnesses, and occupation (Chapters 5–11). Next are taken up aspects of the disease associated with the onset, such as prodromal symptoms, possible precipitating factors, and time of menopause, as well as the type of onset and the initial distribution of the arthritis (Chapters 12–17). The course of the disease before hospital admission follows, including its duration, type (whether intermittent or progressive), and a description of factors believed by the patients to have influenced it (Chapters 18–20). The next five chapters (21–25) are concerned with extra-articular symptoms, especially those of a constitutional nature and those pertaining to the nervous system and vasomotor apparatus. For convenience and unity, the physical findings are included in the appropriate chapter rather than in the next group of chapters (26–33), which deal with observations disclosed by examination of the patients. The following four chapters (34–37) have to do with the joint examination and the status of the gall bladder and colon and of foci of infection. The results of laboratory tests are next considered and include determinations of the basal metabolism and gastric acidity as well as data obtained from examination of the urine and blood (Chapters 38–41). Chapter 42 is concerned with a comparison between patients with spondylitis and the remainder of the series, while the two next chapters deal with disease activity and severity as estimated on hospital admission and with the subsequent course of the patients derived from long-term follow-up observations (Chapters 43–44).

4.2   Each paragraph in the series analysis as well as in the introductory chapters has been numbered to permit cross reference according to a system which allows ready recognition of its chapter location, e.g., paragraph 5.3 is the third paragraph in Chapter 5. Tables and figures have been included in the text and numbered according to a similar plan, e.g., Table 8.4 is the fourth table in Chapter 8.

DEFINITIONS

4.3   Certain terms used in the series description, although usually explained when first mentioned in the text, are given below, along with brief definitions of their meaning as employed in this study. Where indicated, reference to these definitions is made in the text, but it is hoped that the reader will acquaint himself with them at this point. For this reason, the definitions are listed in an order which corresponds with that employed for the chapters in the text.

4.4   ONSET: The first appearance of persistent pain, swelling, or limitation of motion of one or more joints. In patients with a remittent course the beginning of the initial attack, not of the one preceding hospital admission, was regarded as the onset of the disease.

4.5   MENOPAUSE, DATE OF: When artificial, the time of irradiation or surgical castration was utilized; when natural, the date of the last period.

4.6   PRODROMAL SYMPTOMS, OR PRODROMATA, refer to symptoms, not necessarily related to the joints, which precede the actual "onset" (see definition of onset). Those utilized in the present study were fatigue, musculo-skeletal pain, sensory disturbances, appetite loss, and crepitus.

Presentation and Definitions

The controls were questioned in regard to the presence or absence of these symptoms at the time of, or preceding, examination.

4.7 PRECIPITATING FACTORS: Events or conditions preceding the "onset" (q.v.) of a potentially disturbing nature, e.g., infection, surgical operation, or physical or emotional strain.

4.8 ACUTE ONSET: One in which the arthritis not only began suddenly but also was so incapacitating that the patient was forced to bed, with fever and marked joint inflammation often present.

4.9 SMALL JOINTS: The joints of hands, feet, and wrists and the temporo-mandibular joint.

4.10 LARGE JOINTS: The joints of the shoulders, elbows, hips, knees, and ankles.

4.11 ONSET—MONARTICULAR: Initial involvement of a single joint for at least a week.

4.12 DURATION OF ARTHRITIS BEFORE ADMISSION: The time elapsing between the "onset" (q.v.) and admission to the hospital.

4.13 COURSE BEFORE ADMISSION was called INTERMITTENT, if the patient enjoyed one or more periods lasting at least one month of complete or nearly complete freedom from arthritic symptoms, along with cessation of disease activity (q.v.), as far as could be judged by history alone. The course was considered PROGRESSIVE, if the general trend was unfavorable, although showing minor fluctuations or variations.

4.14 CONSTITUTIONAL SYMPTOMS: Each patient and each control was questioned in regard to weakness or fatigability, anorexia, weight loss, and headache. For the patients such symptoms were tabulated only if they occurred between the onset of the arthritis and the time of questioning; for the controls the time of occurrence was not specified.

4.15 VASOMOTOR SYMPTOMS: Each patient and each control was questioned in regard to four such symptoms: cold extremities (from a subjective standpoint), cyanosis of extremities, paresthesias of hands or feet (numbness and tingling, stinging, burning, or sensation of pins and needles), and vascular spasm resembling Raynaud's syndrome. For the temporal criteria, see par. 4.14.

4.16 VASOMOTOR SIGNS were considered present when the examiner found hands or feet both cold and moist.

4.17 NEUROLOGIC SYMPTOMS: Each patient and control was questioned in regard to muscular twitching, vertigo (or, more properly, giddiness), tremor, tinnitus, and nervousness or emotional upsets. For the temporal criteria, see par. 4.14.

4.18 FEVER: Patients were classified as febrile or with "frequent" fever whose oral temperature while in the hospital was 99° F. or over more than once a week.

4.19 TACHYCARDIA: A pulse rate over 90 was considered a tachycardia, the reading in most instances being made under basal conditions.

4.20 LYMPHADENOPATHY: Lymph nodes were considered enlarged if, according to the judgment of the observer, they were of a size not ordinarily felt in an individual of similar age and habitus.

4.21 SPLENOMEGALY: If palpable, the spleen was considered enlarged.

4.22 JOINT INVOLVEMENT: The extent of articular involvement was estimated on admission by more than one observer. Three divisions, mild, moderate, and marked were used. Patients with spondylitis were deemed to have mild involvement if only the spine was affected, moderate if shoulders or hips or both were also affected, and marked if arthritis was found in other peripheral joints.

4.23 ANEMIA was considered present if the red-cell count was below 4.5 million per mm^3 in males and 4.0 million per mm^3 in females.

4.24 GASTRIC ANACIDITY was deemed present when no free acid was found after a test meal of 7 per cent alcohol and the injection of 0.5 mg. of histamine phosphate.

4.25 SPONDYLITIS: A diagnosis of spondylitis was made if at least one of two conditions was fulfilled: (1) persistent objective findings of spinal arthritis, chiefly in the form of limitation of motion not due to other forms of spinal disease or (2) characteristic roentgenographic changes, usually in the sacro-iliac joints. Symptoms referred to the spine, without persistent signs of arthritis or characteristic roentgenographic changes, were not regarded as sufficient to make this diagnosis.

4.26 TOTAL SEVERITY was estimated for each patient by two or more observers on the basis of his condition on admission. The factors taken into consideration included the degree of constitutional symptoms and signs, the speed of progression of the disease, the amount of disability,

Presentation and Definitions

the extent of involvement, and the activity of the process. Three classes of severity were used, mild, moderate, and marked.

4.27 ACTIVITY: The degree of disease activity on admission, whether mild, moderate, or marked, was also estimated for each patient. Both articular and extra-articular manifestations were taken into account.

4.28 IMPROVEMENT: Whenever possible, contact was maintained with each patient discharged from the hospital. Those considered improved manifested definite objective changes of a favorable nature in addition to subjective improvement, the base line in all cases being the patient's condition on admission to the hospital.

5

Sex Distribution

5.1 The present series of 293 patients was composed of 107 males (36 per cent) and 186 females (64 per cent). Although figures for the sex distribution of rheumatoid arthritis in the general population are not yet available, it seems unlikely that this striking sex difference was influenced by the fact that the series was made up entirely of patients hospitalized for arthritis. The group was selected from consecutive admissions to the Medical Service, which contains an equal number of male and female beds. As far as can be ascertained, males and females have enjoyed an equal opportunity for hospital admission. No data are available which suggest that males evidence less willingness than females to enter a hospital for the treatment of rheumatoid arthritis [320]. Table 5.1 demonstrates that a significantly higher prevalence of rheumatoid arthritis in females is generally agreed to in the literature. The underlying cause or causes of this finding are unknown. One possible explanation, that the disease attacks females at a much earlier age than males, is not borne out by the figures presented in Table 5.1 for median age at onset.*

---

* In the analysis of clinical and laboratory data to follow, the frequency of each factor under consideration will be presented with the patients divided according to sex and the presence or absence of significant differences noted. To avoid repetition, such results will not be discussed in this chapter but will be listed under the appropriate heading in Appendix Table 47.

Sex Distribution

Table 5.1
Sex distribution of rheumatoid arthritis and median age at onset—present series compared with representative series from the literature

Source	No. of patients in series	Percentage of females in series	Median age at onset		
			All patients	Males	Females
Garrod [199]	500	82		51	45
Strangeways and Burt [510]	200	73		37	39
Jones [286]	150	85		33	29
Freund [192]	280	71		46	42
Thompson, Wyatt, and Hicks [531]	343	55		37	37*
Smith [477]	102	60		30	33
Hartfall, Garland, and Goldie [241]	750	78	43		
Monroe [362]	267	75	35		
Sclater [454]	388	69		41	39
Lewis-Faning [320]	532	64			
Present series	293	64		32†	37

* Mean.
† 34 if spondylitics are excluded.

5.2   With spinal involvement, a reversal of the sex ratio in rheumatoid arthritis has been consistently observed. The present series furnishes no exception, in that 33 of the 41 patients with definite clinical or roentgenographic evidence of spondylitis were males (80.5 per cent). This reversal of the sex ratio has been cited as an argument for regarding rheumatoid spondylitis as a separate disease entity. Reasons influencing our decision to include such patients in the series under consideration have been presented above (pars. 2.13–2.16), but, by way of analogy, it is of some interest to point out that a similar situation exists in other diseases of both known and unknown etiology. For example, syphilis involving the cardio-vascular and nervous systems shows a predilection for males out of all proportion to the sex distribution of the disease as a whole [539]. On the other hand, chorea and mitral stenosis occur much more frequently in females, although the incidence of all manifestations of rheumatic fever does not favor either sex [567]. In any case, if the 41 patients with spondylitis are deducted from the present series, the percentage of females rises from 64 to 70. Varying criteria in regard to the placement of patients with rheumatoid spondylitis may account for some of the differences in the sex ratios listed in Table 5.1.

5.3   As already mentioned, a reasonable explanation for the sex ratio in rheumatoid arthritis has yet to be substantiated. The suggestion that females inherit a susceptibility to the disease, possibly through sex linkage, has not been verified by genetic studies [496]. The frequency of onset of rheumatoid arthritis in women near the usual time of the menopause has suggested an influence of the female endocrine system. Similarly, the increased tendency to vasomotor instability shown by women has been thought to determine the sex ratio in rheumatoid arthritis [570]. Wherever the explanation may lie, the sex distribution in this disease remains of more than passing interest and must be taken into account in any discussion of its etiology and pathogenesis.

5.4   The sex distribution in many other diseases is equally interesting and unexplained. Males are generally more liable to serious infectious, degenerative, and neoplastic diseases [3, 87]. These include lobar pneumonia, tuberculosis, leprosy, and syphilis of the cardio-vascular and nervous systems; most malignant tumors, with the notable exception of cancers of the gall bladder and thyroid; leukemia and malignant lymphoma; coronary artery disease, cerebral vascular disease, and obliterating arteriosclerosis of the legs. Diseases due to allergy (hay fever and asthma) show no predilection for either sex. Among metabolic diseases, gout and hemochromatosis are preponderant in males and certain lipidoses in females, with diabetes nearly equally represented in both sexes. In this country at least, pulmonary tuberculosis in childhood and young adulthood constitutes the only exception to the greater morbidity of this condition among males. Important diseases which, like rheumatoid arthritis, occur predominately in females include: all disorders of the gall bladder and thyroid, hypochromic anemia, certain lipidoses, Raynaud's disease, migraine, hysteria, manic-depressive psychosis, scleroderma, and disseminated lupus erythematosus. This is certainly at first glance an ill-assorted and heterogeneous group. In only a minority of this list can we in any way indict the female reproductive system as a causative or predisposing factor. In fact, there seems to be no common attribute which binds them together except for their sex distribution, although migraine and Raynaud's disease may be termed vasomotor neuroses and disseminated lupus and scleroderma are usually grouped with rheumatoid arthritis as diseases of vascular and connective tissue. Since we lack more extensive knowledge either of the several causes of

Sex Distribution

this group of diseases or of the role of heredity in their production, we may summarize our ignorance by the concept of constitutional susceptibility in females for certain diseases. In the case of diseases of the thyroid and gall bladder, this susceptibility may be called organ-specific, since morbid conditions of differing pathogenesis but affecting either organ are much more common in the female. If we regard the joints as an organ-system, constitutional susceptibility as related to sex now becomes disease-specific, since the sex distribution of the arthritides varies in respect to the individual disease.

SUMMARY

5.5 The sex distribution in the present series, which is composed of nearly twice as many females as males, is in agreement with that obtained in other similarly selected series of patients with rheumatoid arthritis. Many other diseases of both known and unknown etiology and diversified in type also show an equally obscure predilection for one sex or the other. In rheumatoid spondylitis a reversal of the sex ratio accompanies a special localization of the morbid process, analogous to what takes place in certain forms of syphilis and rheumatic fever.

5.6 Objectives for further study:

1. The sex distribution of rheumatoid arthritis in the population.
2. Reasons for the preponderance of females in hospital and clinic patients with this disease and, if confirmed, in the population.

6

Age at Onset

6.1 Opinions and figures vary widely in regard to the frequency distribution of the age at onset in rheumatoid arthritis. In three series [*133, 286, 333*] the highest frequency was found to be between the ages of 20 and 40 in both males and females, but in two others [*192, 199*] the disease began more often at a later period of life, between the ages of 40 and 55. Such data mean little unless the age distribution of the population at risk is taken into consideration. To facilitate analysis our patients were divided into five-year groups according to the age at onset, or stage at which definite joint involvement appeared.* The actual frequencies and the percentage age distribution in these groups were then compared with expected frequencies based on the U.S. Census figures for the age distribution of the population of Massachusetts in 1930. In the interpretation of these comparisons, shown in Tables 6.1 and 6.2 and Figures 6.1 and 6.2, it is necessary to assume that our patients were representative in respect to age at onset of all persons with rheumatoid arthritis in the Massachusetts population.

6.2 In males, although a higher than expected frequency of onset was found between the ages of 20 and 35 and a decline from the popula-

---

* See definition of onset, par. **4.4**. Patients with onset before age 15 were not tabulated because so few of them were available for inclusion in the study.

Table 6.1

Age at onset of rheumatoid arthritis—males of present series with onset between 15 and 75 compared with male population of Massachusetts in 1930

Age group*	Census population No. (thousands)	Per cent	Present series No.	Per cent
15–19	181.0	12.3	11	11.1
20–24	163.1	11.1	14	14.1
25–29	153.3	10.4	16	16.2
30–34	154.0	10.5	15	15.2
35–39	163.5	11.1	10	10.1
40–44	147.5	10.0	8	8.1
45–49	130.7	8.9	11	11.1
50–54	114.0	7.8	5	5.0
55–59	95.7	6.6	1	1.0
60–64	76.0	5.2	4	4.0
65–69	54.6	3.7	2	2.0
70–74	35.5	2.4	2	2.0
Total	1,468.9	100.0	99	99.9

$\chi^2 = 13.61; p > 0.1$

* Patients with onset before age 15 were not tabulated because so few of them were available for inclusion in the study.

Table 6.2

Age at onset of rheumatoid arthritis—females of present series with onset between 15 and 75 compared with female population of Massachusetts in 1930

Age group*	Census population No. (thousands)	Per cent	Present series No.	Per cent
15–19	185.2	11.8	16	9.1
20–24	182.5	11.6	21	11.9
25–29	170.8	10.9	19	10.8
30–34	167.5	10.6	18	10.2
35–39	172.0	10.9	19	10.8
40–44	148.5	9.4	15	8.5
45–49	134.8	8.6	16	9.1
50–54	120.3	7.6	28	15.9
55–59	101.6	6.5	15	8.5
60–64	83.3	5.3	4	2.3
65–69	63.0	4.0	3	1.7
70–74	43.4	2.8	2	1.1
Total	1,572.9	100.1	176	99.9

$\chi^2 = 26.72; p < .01$

* See note on Table 6.1.

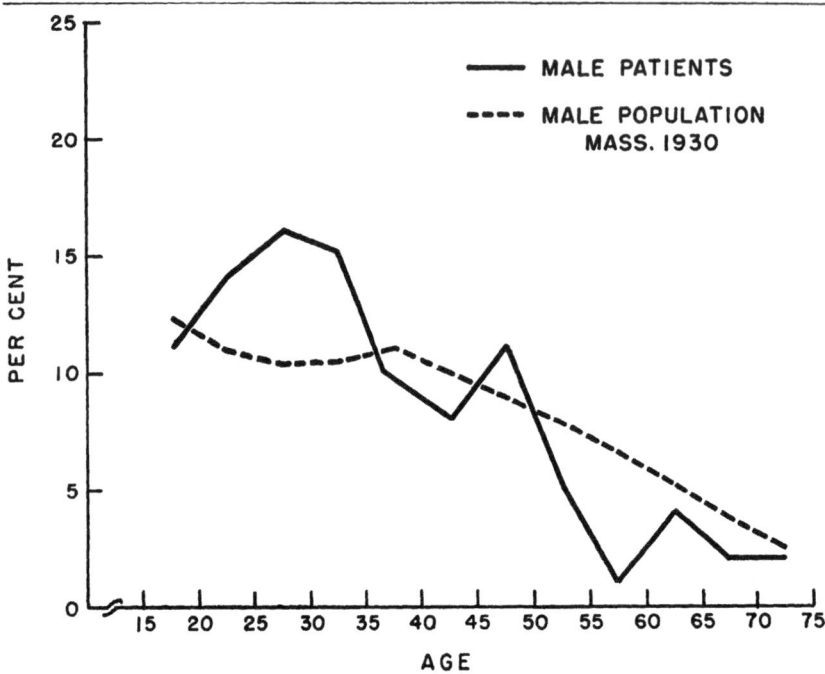

Figure 6.1 Percentage distribution of ages of disease onset of 99 male patients with rheumatoid arthritis compared with expected frequencies based on the 1930 Massachusetts Census figures. (Although the chart shows an excess of onsets between the ages of 20 and 35 and a decline from the population percentages after the age of 50, these variations lack significance, as shown in Table 6.1)

tion figures after age 49, there was no significant departure from the age distribution of the Massachusetts male population (see Table 6.1). In females, on the other hand, a significant difference was obtained owing to the increased frequency of onset between the ages of 50 and 55 and the decreased frequency after age 59. More women gave a history of onset at the age of 54 than during any other single year of life.

6.3   Computed by decades, the sex ratio is found to be nearly constant at approximately 3 to 2, with females predominating, up to the age of 50. In the next decade it rises to 7 to 1, and after 59 the numbers are equal. As noted before (par. 2.16), the present series differs from others in the literature with respect to the inclusion of patients with spondylitis, whether or not peripheral joints were also involved. If those

Age at Onset

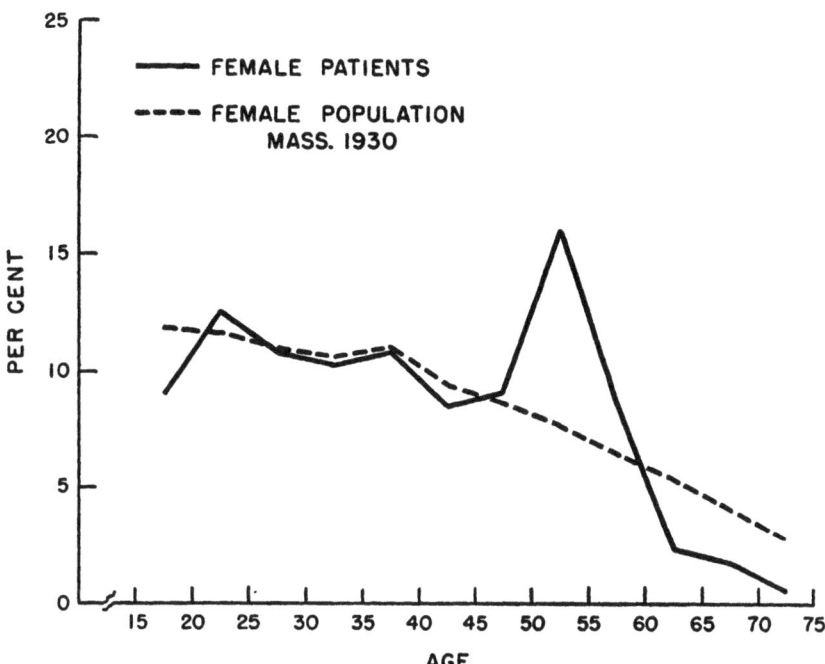

Figure 6.2 Percentage distribution of ages of disease onset of 176 female patients with rheumatoid arthritis compared with expected frequencies based on the 1930 Massachusetts Census figures

with spinal arthritis are deducted, the results in Tables 6.1 and 6.2 remain unchanged.*

6.4 A similar study of the age at onset in rheumatoid arthritis in respect to the age distribution of the population of Scotland was made by Sclater [454] in 1943. In comparing his results with ours, the reader should note, in addition to the difference in geographical location, that involvement of interphalangeal or wrist joints was necessary for inclusion in the Scottish series. Furthermore, ten-year rather than five-year groups were used, and spondylitics were excluded from the series. On this basis, Sclater found that distribution in females by age at onset dif-

* In the analysis of clinical and laboratory data to follow, the presence or absence of association will be noted between certain factors and age at onset. To avoid repetition, such results will not be listed in this chapter, but they may be found under the appropriate heading in Appendix Table 47.

fered significantly from that of the Scottish population, chiefly because of the excess of cases starting between the ages of 35 and 45. He also found a higher incidence in males of the same age group. These findings were not duplicated in our patients, even when they were selected and grouped like Sclater's. In females, for example, the excess occurred in the next decade, from 45 to 55.

6.5   Lewis-Faning [320] recently compared the age distribution of 540 patients with rheumatoid arthritis and that of a general population —in this case, of Great Britain. The patients were divided not only by sex, but also by marital state. The series was limited to patients with arthritis of five years' duration or less, and ten-year age groups were made up according to age on admission to the study rather than age at the onset of the disease. Again patients with spondylitis were excluded. A direct comparison with our results as expressed in Tables 6.1 and 6.2 is therefore not possible, but in an attempt to verify the British figures we retabulated our data, after excluding the spondylitics and the patients with onset of more than five years' duration. Although we were unable to confirm Lewis-Faning's inference that the risk of incurring the disease increases between the ages of 15 and 55 in males and single females, when our data were reassembled it appeared that this risk is practically the same in all groups of married women. The high incidence of onset in women in the 50–54 age group, shown in Table 6.2, was thus obscured.

6.6   In a third study, published in 1952 by Clemmesen and Arnsø [91], the age-at-onset distribution of 849 patients with rheumatoid arthritis was compared with the age distribution of the population of Copenhagen in 1945—the results being presented graphically rather than numerically. In this study the patients were divided into those with insidious and those with acute onset. Furthermore, the criteria for the selection of patients differed from those employed in the present series, notably in respect to the exclusion of patients with spondylitis or psoriasis. While it is therefore impossible to make a direct comparison with the results obtained in our study, certain points should be mentioned. The first is that, in females, two peaks are evident in the authors' graphs, one showing onset between the ages of 35 and 40 and the other showing onset between the ages of 45 and 55. This later peak corresponds to the

Age at Onset

high frequency of onset in our females aged 50 to 55. A second point is that a decline in liability to acquire the disease in females after the age of 60 can be computed from the authors' data; this agrees with the findings in the present series and in the two British series [320, 454]. In males, however, the Danish report differs from the three others in demonstrating a distinct rise in onset between the ages of 65 and 75.

6.7 It is our impression and that of others [133, 199, 333] that rheumatoid arthritis occurs much less frequently in children than in adults. From childhood on, according to our data, males of all ages would appear equally liable. Of the three other reports in which comparisons have been made with the population at risk, none is in agreement with this finding. The results are more consistent with regard to females in that all four report a decline in liability to acquire the disease after the age of 60 and, in the majority of the groups considered, the onset occurred with greater than expected frequency between the ages of 50 and 55. The latter finding immediately suggests an influence of the menopause, a possible relationship which will be considered in a subsequent chapter. The points of disagreement among the four studies may be related to differences in geographical location or in criteria for selection of patients and for determining disease onset. All, however, are limited by the assumption, which cannot be subjected to direct validation, that the series under consideration is representative of rheumatoid arthritis occurring in the population. Major difficulties in interpretation are thus presented by the type of approach used in the present series and comparable studies. Better information can be obtained only by epidemiologic field studies of suitable populations. If such become available, hints in regard to the causation or pathogenesis of rheumatoid arthritis may be gathered by comparison with the age distribution of other diseases. Those occurring more frequently in childhood include infections to which immunity is acquired (exanthemata, anterior poliomyelitis), conditions associated with streptococcal infections (scarlet fever, rheumatic fever) and dietary deficiencies such as rickets and scurvy. On the other hand, individuals from middle life on are more liable to familial metabolic diseases such as diabetes mellitus and gout and to degenerative vascular disease prone to involve the heart and kidneys. Finally, many diverse conditions, including infections not conferring immunity, diseases of known allergic origin (asthma, hay fever), an endocrinopathy (thyrotoxicosis), and a deficiency disease (pellagra) show no predilection for any age group.

SUMMARY

6.8   In the present study of the age at onset in rheumatoid arthritis an attempt has been made to take into consideration the age distribution of the population at risk. Actual frequencies have thus been compared with expected frequencies based on census figures. The results suggest that males of all ages above 15 are equally susceptible, while in females a marked increase in disease frequency occurs between the ages of 50 and 55, along with a decrease at 60 and over. Two similar studies from Great Britain [320, 454] and one from Denmark [91] are in general agreement in regard to females, but the results are inconsistent in regard to males. While the differences may depend somewhat on variations in method, studies of this type are seriously limited by the unconfirmed assumption that the patients chosen are representative of rheumatoid arthritis occurring in the population. Better information should be obtainable from epidemiologic studies of suitable population groups.

6.9   Objectives for further study:

1.   The age at onset of rheumatoid arthritis in the general population in different localities.

2.   A more exact definition of a relationship between the menopause and the age at onset in women.

7

National Origin

7.1   No attempt was made to subdivide the patients of the present series according to anthropological criteria in regard to racial stock. In Tables 7.1 and 7.2 an estimate of national origins has been made and compared with the U.S. Census figures for the population of Massachusetts in 1930. The higher proportion of patients classified as of United States origin in each table may be accounted for by a difference in definition of this group. In our analysis a native-born patient was placed in this category if only one parent was a native. Even so, about half our patients were tabulated as being of foreign extraction, although two-thirds were actually born in the United States. Figures for the hospital population for the eight years 1928–1935 furnished by Richardson [432] in a racial study of liver disease show only 32 per cent of this population to have been native-born. This difference may be of only apparent significance, since patients admitted for injuries and surgical emergencies may well have been drawn to a great extent from areas neighboring the hospital and containing a large proportion of foreign-born.

7.2   The foreign countries of origin of our patients represent those from which immigration to New England in the last fifty or more years has been common. No differences in regard to sex have been observed. That only two Negroes (both females) were included in the series merely reflects the relatively low Negro population in the area served

Table 7.1

White males of present series compared with male population of Massachusetts in 1930 by country of origin

Country of origin	Census Per cent	Present series No.	Present series Per cent
United States	34.4	57	53.3
Foreign	65.6	50	46.7
Total	100.0	107	100.0
Canada	25.2	11	22.0
Ireland	19.0	9	18.0
Russia, Poland, Latvia, Lithuania, Finland	16.0	10	20.0
Italy	12.7	4	8.0
England, Scotland, Wales	9.9	7	14.0
Norway, Sweden, Denmark	3.8	6	12.0
All others	13.1	3	6.0
Total (foreign)	99.7	50	100.0

$\chi^2 = 13.14; p < .05$

Table 7.2

White females of present series compared with female population of Massachusetts in 1930 by country of origin

Country of origin	Census Per cent	Present series No.	Present series Per cent
United States	33.8	89	48.4
Foreign	66.2	95	51.6
Total	100.0	184*	100.0
Canada	27.0	29	30.5
Ireland	21.6	18	18.9
Russia, Poland, Latvia, Lithuania, Finland	14.6	13	13.7
Italy	10.7	6	6.3
England, Scotland, Wales	10.4	8	8.4
Norway, Sweden, Denmark	3.6	10	10.5
All others	11.6	11	11.6
Total (foreign)	99.5	95	99.9

$\chi^2 = 15.48; p < .02$

* 2 Negroes not included in this table.

National Origin

by the Massachusetts General Hospital, since rheumatoid arthritis is not infrequently encountered in the Negro race [*133*]. As shown in Tables 7.1 and 7.2, the distribution of our patients of foreign extraction differs significantly from the Census distribution, owing almost entirely to a greater frequency of patients with national origin in the Scandinavian countries. Although we are not aware of any unusual concentration of patients of Scandinavian origin in the hospital population, no data are available to exclude such a possibility. These figures thus hardly establish an association between the Scandinavian origin and the development of rheumatoid arthritis severe enough to require hospitalization. Nor is information yet obtainable in regard to the prevalence of rheumatoid arthritis as influenced by regional and racial factors.

SUMMARY

7.3 Over two-thirds of the patients in the present series were born in the United States. The country-of-origin distribution of those who were considered to be of foreign extraction approximated that of the population of Massachusetts in 1930, except that the series showed a higher proportion of individuals of Scandinavian origin.

7.4 Objective for further study:

The prevalence of rheumatoid arthritis as influenced by geographic and racial differences.

8

Family History

8.1 The data pertaining to family history in rheumatoid arthritis were obtained by questioning the patients of the series in regard to disease in blood relatives, including grandparents, parents, uncles, aunts, cousins, siblings, and children. Information acquired in this way is, of course, subject to error and should not be relied upon to furnish absolute rates of the occurrence of disease in the families of our patients. Moreover, no attempt was made to record family size. However, this would not appear to be a serious omission, since a similarity in family size between rheumatoid arthritics and controls matched for age, sex, and civil state has been established by a recent British study [320]. A more valuable point in any such comparison is the possibility that arthritics would tend to be more aware than would controls of articular disease in the family.

8.2 Ordinary difficulties encountered in obtaining an accurate family history are enhanced by the confusion in both medical and lay nomenclature of the arthritides. In addition, the diagnosis of joint disease, which may be uncertain even when the patient is available for examination, becomes doubly so when the evidence must be obtained by questioning another person. For these reasons, we have been unwilling to classify family histories of rheumatic disease into types, unless the de-

Family History

scription given was reasonably characteristic. In this way, by far the largest subdivision in Table 8.2 is entitled "Undetermined and other forms of rheumatism," the latter referring to a few cases of what seemed to be arthritis due to specific infections and gout. Early or mild cases of rheumatoid arthritis, atypical rheumatic fever, and degenerative joint disease not sufficiently characteristic for recognition have undoubtedly been labeled "undetermined," but again it should be stressed that the same standards were applied to the data obtained from controls.

8.3   In the study of family background in rheumatoid arthritis, we were interested in other conditions which have been considered familial, in an attempt to determine whether or not the rheumatoid stock was generally vulnerable. As shown in Table 8.1, no significant differences in frequency were observed in diseases of the heart, blood vessels, and kidneys; cancer; diabetes mellitus; migraine; and allergic diseases. The last are listed here, although a more detailed discussion of their relationship to rheumatoid arthritis will be found in a subsequent chapter. Degenerative joint disease showed an unusually low frequency in the families of both arthritics and controls, one undoubtedly far below the real prevalence of this condition, which is present, although often asymptomatic, in most of the population from middle life on [34]. If the "Undetermined and other forms of rheumatism" in Table 8.2 could be broken down, this seeming discrepancy might be remedied.

Table 8.1

Diseases occurring with about the same frequency in families of 293 rheumatoid arthritics and 293 controls

Type of disease	Distribution of diseases in families with 1 or more cases (exclusive of patient or control)	
	Percentage of patients' families	Percentage of controls' families
Cardio-vascular-renal disease	41.0	43.7
Cancer	17.8	21.5
Diabetes mellitus	9.6	9.6
Migraine	3.4	4.1
Allergy (asthma, hay fever, urticaria)	16.0	16.0
Degenerative joint disease	5.8	5.1

8.4   As shown in Table 8.2, rheumatoid arthritis occurred more often in the families of arthritics than in the families of controls. Somewhat higher frequencies were recorded in comparable series in the literature (Table 8.3); in all but one the results were obtained, as far as we can tell, largely by questioning the patient rather than by examination of members of the family. The study forming the one exception was carried out by Talkov [520], who examined family members as far as possible and in addition obtained information from their physicians or from hospital records. Controls were utilized only in the present study and by Stecher et al. [496]. The latter found that relatives of patients were affected with rheumatoid arthritis five times as frequently as relatives of controls.

8.5   Of the patients in our series, 26 reported single additional cases of rheumatoid arthritis in their families, 4 reported two additional cases, and 5 reported three. Of the 14 patients with familial histories studied by Dawson [133], 6 patients reported two cases in the family, and 2 patients reported three cases. As a matter of fact, individual instances of more than four cases of rheumatoid arthritis in the same family have been reported not infrequently in the literature. Examples include: 4 siblings and the paternal grandmother [510]; 4 brothers and their mother with rheumatoid spondylitis [21]; 4 siblings and both

Table 8.2

Diseases occurring with significantly greater frequency in families of 293 rheumatoid arthritics than in families of 293 controls

	Patients' families		Controls' families		Difference in percentages
	No.	Per cent	No.	Per cent	
With 1 or more cases of disease, exclusive of patient or control (total)	124	42.3	71	24.2	18.1 ± 3.9
Type of disease	*Distribution of cases (exclusive of patients or controls)*				
Rheumatoid arthritis	35	11.9	15	5.1	6.8 ± 2.3
Rheumatic fever	34	11.6	10	3.4	8.2 ± 2.2
"Undetermined and other forms of rheumatism"	68	23.2	37	12.6	10.6 ± 3.2

Family History

Table 8.3
Rheumatic diseases in families of rheumatoid arthritics—present series compared with representative series from the literature

Source	No. of patients in series	Percentage of families with 1 or more cases of disease (exclusive of patient or control)				Difference in percentages
		Rheumatoid arthritis	Rheumatic fever	Rheumatic disease		
				Patients' families	Controls' families	
Garrod [199]	500	16.8	12.8	43.2	20.0	23.2 ± 2.9
Strangeways and Burt [510]	200	30.0	12.5	56.5		
Coates [96]	50		32.0			
Dawson and Tyson [138]	100	15.0	14.0			
Edström [165]	504			52.0		
Talkov [520]	50	32.0	18.0	48.0		
Stecher et al. [496]	224	21.0				
Present series	293	11.9	11.6	42.3	24.2	18.1 ± 3.9

parents [199]; and 3 brothers, 3 sisters, and their father [199]. In the last family only 1 child, a girl, escaped the disease. Cecil [73] also mentions a family with rheumatoid arthritis in four generations.

8.6 We are in agreement with others [13, 199] that patients with positive familial histories of rheumatoid arthritis do not tend to develop the disease at an earlier age than those without such histories. For patients with 1 or more arthritic relatives the mean age at onset was 38.9 years, as compared with 35.2 years for the remaining members of the series. In addition, an association was found between family history of rheumatoid arthritis and onset after the age of forty (Table 8.4). The

Table 8.4
Family history of rheumatoid arthritis in relation to age at onset among patients of present series

Age at onset	No. of patients	Family history of rheumatoid arthritis	
		No.	Per cent
Total	293	35	11.9
Under 40	177	15	8.5
40 or more	116	20	17.2
		Difference in percentages:	8.7 ± 3.8

opinion that an acute, severe onset is more likely to occur when other members of the family are affected [13] has not been substantiated by our data (Table 8.5). Other factors found unrelated to the presence or absence of a family history of rheumatoid arthritis include sex; constitutional, vasomotor, or neurologic symptoms; joints first involved; total severity on admission; and course, both before and after hospitalization. Thus, family history of rheumatoid arthritis does not appear to influence the nature of the arthritis present, nor to be of prognostic importance. On the other hand, as pointed out by Barter [19], a positive family history lends weight to the diagnosis of rheumatoid arthritis when a patient is suspected of being in a prodromal or early stage of this disorder.

8.7 The clinical impression that multiple cases of rheumatoid spondylitis are frequently encountered in the same family has been subjected to careful analysis in two recent publications. Rogoff and Freyberg [435] discovered additional cases in the families of 10 out of the 114 spondylitics of their series, while Stecher *et al.* [497] summarized their findings by the statement that rheumatoid spondylitis occurred 70 times as often in relatives of 50 patients as in relatives of 394 controls. In both investigations inquiries were made into the presence of peripheral rheumatoid arthritis among other members of the family. The findings agreed with those reported by Talkov [520] in suggesting a familial pattern for arthritis in general and also a familial pattern for spinal localization as compared with peripheral localization. No special search for spondylitis was made among the relatives of our patients, but the data available do not suggest a familial pattern. It can at least be said that a positive family history of rheumatoid arthritis, with or without spinal involvement, was elicited in approximately the same frequency from patients with spondylitis (12.2 per cent) as from those with only peripheral joints affected (11.9 per cent).

8.8 A highly interesting finding, in view of the relationship often postulated between rheumatoid arthritis and rheumatic fever, is the significant difference between patients and controls with respect to family history of rheumatic fever (Table 8.2). The validity of this finding is supported by the familial frequency discovered by other workers —Coates [96] having reported that nearly a third of a rather small series of patients with rheumatoid arthritis gave familial histories of

Family History

Table 8.5

Family history of rheumatoid arthritis in relation to type of onset in patients of present series

Type of onset	No. of patients	Family history of rheumatoid arthritis	
		No.	Per cent
Total	293	35	11.9
Acute	64	7	10.9
Gradual	229	28	12.2
	Difference in percentages:		1.3 ± 5.0

rheumatic fever. More detailed description of the familial relationship of the two diseases awaits further investigation.

8.9 As shown in Table 8.2, a higher frequency of rheumatic disease in general, whether or not classified into types, was recorded in the families of the patients than in the families of the controls. This finding confirms an observation by Garrod [199], who studied 500 patients with rheumatoid arthritis and an equal number of non-rheumatic controls.* Strangeways and Burt [510] and Talkov [520] obtained even higher percentages than we did for any form of rheumatic disease in the family (Table 8.3), but neither of these studies used controls. In two other studies [19, 165] striking frequencies of rheumatic disease were encountered in the patients' families. In both, rheumatoid arthritis and rheumatic fever were lumped together in tabulating the results, and in one, a control group showed a significantly lower proportion of relatives with positive histories. Comments have also been made [21] on the frequent occurrence of different forms of arthritis, as well as of psoriasis, in the same family, with the suggestion that there may be hereditary transmission of a susceptibility of the joints to various forms of disease. Thus far data are lacking either in the present study or in the literature to confirm this hypothesis, except for the apparent familial association between rheumatoid arthritis and rheumatic fever.

8.10 Although it would seem reasonable to assume that a familial tendency exists in rheumatoid arthritis, no conclusions can yet be drawn as to the relative influence of environment, contagion, or heredity. A

---

* For his controls Garrod recorded the frequency of a family history of rheumatic disease (Table 8.3) but not of rheumatoid arthritis (par. **8.4**).

recent study of 302 patients [*320*] and an equal number of controls reveals no significant difference in the home conditions of the two groups which could be related in point of time to the onset of disease. Occurrences of the disease in both marital partners have been noted in our clinic, raising the possibility of contagion or of a common environmental factor. If heredity plays an important part, no generally accepted genetic mechanism has been proposed which would account for its familial nature. Edström [*165*] has expressed the belief that an irregularly dominant gene is operative in the production of a susceptibility to either rheumatoid arthritis or rheumatic fever, while Stecher *et al.* [*496*] are of the opinion that the hereditary factor in rheumatoid arthritis is probably autosomal and dominant, with incomplete "penetrance." Further work is clearly indicated in the direction of sifting out the etiologic importance of heredity, environment, and contagion. The collection and study of rheumatoid arthritics who are twins, in which a beginning has been made [*53, 165*], should do much toward solving the problem, as should a long-term, detailed investigation of the occurrence of rheumatoid arthritis in members of a suitable community.

SUMMARY

8.11   Information in regard to disease in blood relatives was obtained by questioning patients and controls. No differences were evident in certain conditions usually considered familial, including diabetes mellitus, migraine, and allergic diseases, but both rheumatoid arthritis and rheumatic fever were present more frequently in the families of patients than in the families of controls. A family history of rheumatoid arthritis was not associated with onset of the disease at an earlier age, nor was it of prognostic assistance. While the familial nature of rheumatoid arthritis appears to have been demonstrated in the present series and in previous studies, the available data are not sufficient to establish the existence of an hereditary factor or to define a genetic mechanism.

8.12   Objectives for further study:

1. The familial occurrence of rheumatoid arthritis in relation to environment and opportunity for transmission as well as to heredity.

2. The familial association of rheumatoid arthritis and rheumatic fever as seen in a selected population.

9

Allergic Diseases

9.1 As an outgrowth of the failure to demonstrate an infectious etiology for rheumatoid arthritis by the isolation of a pathogenic agent, an allergic hypothesis has been proposed. Since direct evidence is lacking, this hypothesis must depend for the present on relevant clinical data. If rheumatoid arthritis is of allergic origin, we should expect by analogy with known allergic disease: (1) an increased familial occurrence of asthma, hay fever, or other definitely allergic manifestations and (2) co-existence of these same manifestations in a greater number of patients than of controls.

9.2 As demonstrated in Table 9.1, asthma, hay fever, and urticaria occurred with essentially the same frequency in the families of patients and controls. In a similar study [320], no real difference was found between 532 patients and an equal number of controls as regards the proportion of parents, grandparents, and siblings with allergic disease. Table 9.2 shows that the patients were not more subject than the controls to these three allergic diseases. Two other studies tend to corroborate these findings: one [320] dealt with various allergic diseases, including migraine and eczema; and the other [276] with bronchial asthma.

9.3 It is estimated [537] that from 2 to 4 per cent of the general population of the United States are affected by asthma or hay fever or both. The corresponding figures for our patients and controls were 3.8

Table 9.1

Frequency of allergic diseases in families of 293 rheumatoid arthritics and 293 controls

	Patients' families		Controls' families	
	No.	Per cent	No.	Per cent
With 1 or more cases of disease, exclusive of patient or control (total)	47	16.0	47	16.0
Type of disease	Distribution of cases (exclusive of patient or control)			
Asthma	21	7.2	29	9.9
Hay fever	16	5.5	9	3.1
Urticaria	17	5.8	19	6.5

and 6.8 per cent, respectively. In regard to bronchial asthma alone, a recent survey [541] indicated fairly general agreement that the frequency of this condition in the populations of Western Europe and the United States is about 0.5 per cent. This percentage, while confirmed by Järvinen [276] in studies conducted in Finland on nearly 2,000 patients with rheumatoid arthritis, is distinctly less than that obtained for our patients and controls, especially the latter. The explanation for this discrepancy may be simply the relatively small number of individuals studied or, more likely, the age distribution of patients and controls, whose mean age at the time of examination was forty-two. It should also be noted that the majority of the controls were hospital employees, a group likely to include individuals with chronic disease. Two smaller series should also be mentioned in which the frequency of allergic disease found in patients was compared with that found in a smaller number of unmatched controls. Except for increased proportions of patients with hay fever in one series [535] and with "allergic dermatitis" in the other [572], no significant differences were observed. Eaton [157] also encountered a significantly higher percentage of urticaria in 173 patients with rheumatoid arthritis than in 120 patients with degenerative joint disease serving as controls. This result was unchanged when patients and controls were divided according to sex, but the control group was made up of much older individuals. In the present study a tendency toward a higher frequency of urticaria was observed in patients (Table 9.2). Further study of the association between urticaria

Allergic Diseases

Table 9.2

Frequency of past or present allergic diseases among 293 rheumatoid arthritics and 293 controls

	Patients		Controls		Difference in percentages
	No.	Per cent	No.	Per cent	
With 1 or more allergies (total)	39	13.3	40	13.7	
Type of allergy		Distribution of cases			
Asthma	5	1.7	9	3.1	1.4 ± 1.3
Hay fever	10	3.4	13	4.4	1.0 ± 1.6
Urticaria	31	10.6	20	6.8	3.8 ± 2.4

and rheumatoid arthritis seems indicated, in view especially of the occurrence of purpura [23, 132] and of decreased capillary resistance [532] in rheumatoid subjects.

9.4 Other authors [131, 362, 422] have expressed the opinion, without furnishing numerical evidence, that the finding of allergic disease in a rheumatoid arthritic constitutes no more than a chance observation. From the opposite point of view, it has been stated that rheumatoid arthritis affects individuals with allergic disease in no more than the expected frequency [131, 422]. Among 400 asthmatics Harkavy and Hebald [239] encountered 9 patients with a migratory form of joint disease which was consistent with an atypical form of rheumatoid arthritis. The most convincing and careful study on this subject that has thus far come to our attention was conducted by Järvinen [276] on 563 patients with bronchial asthma and 748 controls. In the former the proportion with rheumatoid arthritis was 1.2 per cent and in the latter 0.94 per cent. Reference will be made in a subsequent chapter (par. 20.9) to the same author's interesting observations on an alternation between the symptoms of arthritis and asthma in the 7 patients in whom both diseases were present.

SUMMARY

9.5 From our observations and those of others, no analogy can be drawn between rheumatoid arthritis and diseases of recognized allergic origin on the basis of an increased frequency of asthma, hay fever, or urticaria in rheumatoid subjects or their families.

9.6 Objective for further study:
The association between urticaria and rheumatoid arthritis.

10

Illnesses, Operations, and Injuries

10.1 The present chapter is concerned with the total number of illnesses, operations, or injuries recorded in the lifetime of each patient up to the time of hospitalization for arthritis, rather than with possible precipitating factors in close proximity to the onset. A comparison can thus be made with the control group, since the controls were chosen to correspond in age distribution to the patients on hospital admission. In this area of our investigation the main object has been to determine whether certain diseases, groups of diseases, operations, or injuries may be associated with the development of rheumatoid arthritis of sufficient severity to warrant hospital study and treatment, although not immediately preceding the onset. We have also been concerned with the possibility of uncovering hitherto unrecognized systemic manifestations of rheumatoid arthritis in the form of disease conditions more prevalent in the patients of the present series than in the controls, whether preceding or accompanying the development of articular involvement. Finally, we have tried to discover some evidence as to whether or not the rheumatoid stock is more vulnerable to illness or injury than the general population.

10.2 One objection may be raised at the outset against many of the data presented in this section, which were obtained entirely by questioning the patients and controls. It can be stated with some justifi-

Illnesses, Operations, and Injuries

cation that a group of patients with a potentially serious disease may search their memories more diligently for previous illnesses or injuries in an effort to uncover factors relevant to their present complaint. Although the controls were questioned carefully by the same observers who gathered information from the patients, the tendency of patients to give more complete and accurate information cannot be dismissed as a possibility, nor, if present, can the magnitude of its effect on the tabulation be estimated. For this reason, findings which may be weighted will be kept to a minimum in the following paragraphs, and impressions rather than conclusions should be derived from the figures to be presented.

10.3   The frequency of serious illnesses in patients and controls is shown in Table 10.1. (Examples of illness considered "serious" are found in Tables 10.2 and 10.3, which omit many of the upper respiratory infections, including tonsillitis, sinusitis, and otitis media, and most of the contagious diseases of childhood.) As may be seen in Table 10.1, the percentage of serious illnesses reported by patients was significantly higher than that reported by the controls. However, when the two groups were broken down according to sex and age, the differences were significant only for males and for females over forty. Male patients showed a consistently higher frequency than female patients, but the reverse was true of the controls. Male and female patients over forty

Table 10.1

Frequency of serious illnesses among patients of present series and corresponding controls divided according to sex and age

	No. in each group	History of 1 or more serious illnesses				Difference in percentages
		Patients		Controls		
		No.	Per cent	No.	Per cent	
Total	293	170	58.0	126	43.0	15.0 ± 4.1
Males	107	68	63.0	41	37.3	25.7 ± 6.8
Females	186	102	54.8	85	45.7	9.1 ± 5.2
Under 40	144	72	50.0	59	41.0	9.0 ± 5.9
40 or over	149	98	65.8	67	45.0	20.8 ± 5.8
Males under 40	64	37	57.8	23	35.9	21.9 ± 8.8
Males 40 or over	43	31	72.1	18	41.9	30.2 ± 10.7
Females under 40	80	35	43.8	36	45.0	1.2 ± 7.7
Females 40 or over	106	67	63.2	49	46.2	17.0 ± 6.9

showed higher frequencies than those who had not reached this age, and the controls reflected this tendency although the differences were not significant. In one other study [320] in which patients and controls were compared as regards their general resistance to disease in the past, no differences of any importance could be demonstrated between the two groups. However, the results are hardly comparable with those obtained in the present study in that the illnesses considered were of all degrees of severity and were limited to those occurring before the onset of the arthritis. Ailments arising subsequent to onset were separately tabulated, with the excess among rheumatoid subjects accounted for by tonsillitis, sore throat, and coryza.

10.4 No significant differences between patients and controls were discovered with respect to the individual illnesses listed in Table 10.2, although several, including cholecystitis, nervous breakdown, pleurisy, rheumatic fever, and thyrotoxicosis occurred with somewhat greater frequency among the patients, and the total for the controls is smaller. Cases of jaundice have been lumped together, whatever the possible cause, but the large majority presumably represented infectious hepatitis. In most instances the jaundice occurred long before the onset of the arthritis. (In the 4 patients who had jaundice during their arthritis, amelioration of symptoms was noted twice.) In view of the equal occurrence of jaundice among patients and controls, previous liver disease cannot reasonably be assigned the responsibility for the alterations in liver function encountered in rheumatoid arthritis [327, 358, 426, 438, 560], nor is there even suggestive evidence from these data that hepatitis may be one of the systemic manifestations of this disease. On the other hand, pleurisy has been frequently described [179, 227, 249] as an extraarticular localization of rheumatoid arthritis, but Table 10.2 shows no significant difference between patients and controls. While 9 patients in comparison with 5 controls gave a history of previous attacks, and 5 new cases were diagnosed among the patients as opposed to 3 among the controls, the figures at hand lend no real support to the possibility that rheumatoid arthritis may appear in the pleura before it appears in the joints. As already mentioned, attacks of rheumatic fever or chorea were reported by more patients than controls, but it is possible, of course, that some of the illnesses regarded as rheumatic fever may actu-

Illnesses, Operations, and Injuries

Table 10.2

Serious illnesses reported with about the same frequency by 293 rheumatoid arthritics and 293 controls (see Table 10.1)

Type of illness	Distribution of illnesses	
	No. of patients	No. of controls
Bronchiectasis, lung abscess	2	0
Cerebrovascular accident	1	1
Cholecystitis	10	5
Colitis	5	2
Diabetes	0	1
Diphtheria	10	13
Eclampsia	1	0
Influenza	22	19
Jaundice	22	22
Malignant tumor	3	1
Nervous breakdown	5	1
Neurologic disease	3	1
Peptic ulcer	0	1
Pernicious anemia	3	0
Pleurisy	9	5
Renal calculus	3	0
Rheumatic fever or chorea	14*	7
Scarlet fever	26	30
Syphilis	2	5
Thyrotoxicosis	5	1
Tuberculosis, pulmonary	5	4
Typhoid fever	17	14
Miscellaneous infections	11	6
Total	179†	139†

* 4 patients with history of chorea alone.
† These totals are larger than those in Table 10.1 because certain patients gave a history of more than 1 serious illness.

ally have been atypical attacks of rheumatoid arthritis. A more than coincidental association between thyroid disorders and rheumatoid arthritis has been frequently cited in the literature [6, 97, 150, 286, 421, 528]. On this point our figures suggest a relationship, but the apparently increased frequency of thyrotoxicosis among the patients is not statistically significant. In Chapter 41 further evidence will be presented in regard to an association between rheumatoid arthritis and thyroid disorders.

10.5   Gonorrhea and pneumonia were the only illnesses found with significantly greater frequency among the patients than among the controls (Table 10.3). In the case of gonorrhea, it is reasonable to surmise that patients with arthritis might be more willing to admit to histories of venereal disease than a control group largely made up of hospital employees and that the former group may have been questioned more searchingly in this regard. In partial answer to these objections, it may be pointed out that slightly more controls than patients gave histories of syphilis (Table 10.2). While about 80 per cent of the attacks of gonorrhea in the patients occurred before the onset of the arthritis, none were in close proximity to the development of joint involvement. In the controlled study previously cited [320], histories of gonorrhea were not obtained in excess among the patients. It is also fair to state that, if the figures for gonorrhea are discarded as unreliable, the differences shown in Table 10.1 cease to exist as far as males are concerned.

10.6 The higher frequency of pneumonia found in our patients has not been confirmed by Lewis-Faning [320]. Most of the attacks reported by our patients took place well before the onset of the arthritis, and, as shown in Table 10.3, the older age group was the only one significantly affected. An explanation of the latter finding is not immediately apparent. Examination of the age distribution of the attacks fails to show that the patients incurred the disease at a more advanced age than the controls. Recent reports [5, 38, 41, 170, 322, 353] of pulmonary infiltration occurring in the course of rheumatoid arthritis raise the possibility that the lungs may share in the systemic involvement of this condition and add interest to the finding of an increased frequency of pneumonia in the patients of the present series.

10.7 Figures for the prevalence of certain illnesses among patients with rheumatoid arthritis are available in the literature and are presented in Table 10.4. Diabetes was not found in our patients or in a similar series composed of 254 rheumatoid arthritics [187], but the combination of these two conditions has been encountered by Cecil [73] as well as in our own more recent experience. In a study by Järvinen [277] of 1,008 patients with rheumatoid arthritis and 766 diabetics, along with suitable control groups, the two diseases were found together in approximately the frequency expected by chance. The absence of myxedema in the present series and in one other [187] contrasts with

Table 10.3

Illnesses reported with significantly greater frequency by 293 rheumatoid arthritics than by 293 controls divided according to sex and age (see Table 10.2)

	Distribution of illnesses				Difference in percentages
	Patients		Controls		
Type of illness	No.	Per cent	No.	Per cent	
Gonorrhea					
Total	24	8.2	7	2.4	5.8 ± 1.8
Males	23	21.5	4	3.7	17.8 ± 4.8
Pneumonia					
Total	44	15.0	22	7.5	7.5 ± 2.6
Males under 40	11	17.2	6	9.4	7.8 ± 6.3
Males 40 or more	8	18.6	1	2.3	16.3 ± 6.9
Females under 40	8	10.0	9	11.2	1.2 ± 5.6
Females 40 or more	17	16.0	6	5.7	10.3 ± 4.4

Table 10.4

Frequency of certain illnesses among rheumatoid arthritics—present series (293 patients) compared with representative series from the literature

	Percentage of		
Type of illness	Present series	Other series	
Diabetes	0.0	0.0	Fletcher and Lewis-Faning [187]
Diabetes		1.3	Järvinen [277]
Diphtheria	3.4	3.8	Jones [286]
Gonorrhea	8.2	3.7	Ibid.
Myxedema	0.0	0.0	Fletcher and Lewis-Faning, op. cit.
Nephritis	0.3	0.4	Jones
Peptic ulcer	0.0	2.9	Ibid.
Peptic ulcer		0.0	Fletcher and Lewis-Faning, op. cit.
Pleurisy	3.1	3.3	Jones
Pneumonia	15.0	2.1	Ibid.
Rheumatic fever or chorea	4.8	2.4	Fletcher and Lewis-Faning, op. cit.
Scarlet fever	8.9	4.6	Jones
Scarlet fever		1.6	Fletcher and Lewis-Faning, op. cit.
Syphilis	0.7	0.4	Ibid.
Thyrotoxicosis	1.7	1.2	Ibid.
Thyrotoxicosis		2.0	Douthwaite [150]
Thyrotoxicosis		1.0	Smith [479]
Tuberculosis	1.7	4.3	Fletcher and Lewis-Faning, op. cit.
Tuberculosis		4.0	Douthwaite, op. cit.
Tuberculosis		1.0	Brabazon [52]

the relative frequency with which thyrotoxicosis is associated with rheumatoid arthritis. However, Macalister [337] described in detail a striking instance of myxedema in a patient with rheumatoid arthritis, and Monroe [361] found 3 patients with this form of arthritis in a series of 98 cases of spontaneous or acquired myxedema. We have since encountered 2 patients with this combination, in one of whom the myxedema was postoperative and, in the other, spontaneous. In both instances, the myxedema appeared well in advance of the arthritis. While none of the patients in the present series gave histories of peptic ulcer up to the time of hospitalization, subsequent studies in our clinic have shown this condition to be at least as common in rheumatoid arthritics as in the general population (par. 25.4). The discrepancies between our findings and those in the literature regarding gonorrhea and pneumonia are not readily explainable and may depend on the methods used in questioning the patients or in the clinical material studied.

10.8 As shown in Table 10.5, the frequency of severe injuries, chiefly fractures, was essentially the same in both groups. This was also true in regard to serious surgical operations. Orthopedic operations in treatment of the patients' arthritis were excluded, as were minor operations on the nose and throat, since the latter were often performed in order to remove foci of infection. When the patients and controls were broken down according to sex and age, as was done in Table 10.1 in the study of the frequency of serious illnesses, the only significant difference obtained was the higher frequency of operations in females. The patients and controls were also compared in respect to certain types of surgical operations commonly performed in both groups. Although more breast, thyroid, and mastoid operations were performed on patients and more hernia repairs on controls, the differences in frequency were not significant. An approximately equal number of appendectomies and of operations on bones and joints (excluding those done in treatment of the arthritis) took place in both groups. As may be seen in Table 10.6, the female patients had more operations than the controls on their genital organs. While the frequency of hysterectomies was about the same in the two groups, more of the patients had one or both ovaries removed. Non-mutilating operations, chiefly curettage, suspension of the uterus, and perineal repair, occurred only slightly more

Illnesses, Operations, and Injuries

Table 10.5
Frequency of severe injuries and serious surgical operations among 293 rheumatoid arthritics and 293 controls

	Patients		Controls	
History of 1 or more	No.	Per cent	No.	Per cent
Severe injuries	42	14.3	37	12.6
Serious operations	115	39.2	101	34.5

Table 10.6
Frequency of gynecological operations among females of present series (186 patients) and 186 controls and distribution of types of operation performed

	Patients		Controls		Difference in percentages
	No.	Per cent	No.	Per cent	
With 1 or more operations (total)	48	25.8	28	15.1	10.7 ± 4.2
Type of operation	Distribution of operations				
Hysterectomy	12	6.5	10	5.4	1.1 ± 2.5
Ovariectomy	17	9.1	3	1.6	7.5 ± 2.3
Uterus and/or ovary removed	23	12.4	11	5.9	6.5 ± 3.0
Other types	25	13.4	17	9.1	4.3 ± 3.8

often among the arthritics. In the majority of instances (about 70 per cent in each category), the operations were performed before the onset of arthritis. Some basis at least for speculation as to the influence of ovariectomy on the development of rheumatoid arthritis in women is provided by the foregoing data.

10.9 As might be expected, a significantly greater number of controls (106) than patients (78) gave no histories of serious illnesses, operations, or injuries. From the figures already presented, this difference may be ascribed chiefly to the findings in regard to histories of serious illnesses. When the patients with spondylitis were compared with the remainder, a somewhat higher frequency of illnesses, operations, and injuries was found in those with peripheral involvement alone, but to a significant degree only in respect to operations. Arthritis of marked severity* on admission was distributed approximately equally

* For definition, see par. 4.26.

between those patients with positive histories of serious illnesses, injuries, or operations and those whose past had been relatively uneventful.

SUMMARY

10.10   The patients of the present series have been compared with matched controls in respect to a history of serious illness, injury, or operation before admission to the hospital but not necessarily antedating the onset of their arthritis. More illness in general was found among the patients, but only two diseases, gonorrhea and pneumonia, were elicited with significantly greater frequency. With the exception of these two infections and of thyroid disorders, ulcerative colitis, and psoriasis, no evidence was encountered either in the present study or in the literature of association or antagonism* between rheumatoid arthritis and another disease.

10.11   No differences were obtained in respect to injuries and surgical operations, but more patients than controls had had one or more of their ovaries removed. Since the frequency of jaundice, presumably due to hepatitis, was the same in patients and controls, our data fail to furnish evidence either that liver disease is an additional systemic manifestation of rheumatoid arthritis or predisposes to its development in a form severe enough to warrant hospitalization. The results reported in this chapter must be interpreted with caution in view of the likelihood that patients gave more complete histories than controls.

10.12   Objective for further study:

More exact definition of a relationship between castration in women and the development of rheumatoid arthritis.

* See par. 28.5 in regard to a possible antagonism between severe hypertension and rheumatoid arthritis.

11

Occupation

11.1 This chapter will deal with the distribution of the patients of the present series by occupation, in an effort to ascertain whether or not any particular type of occupation may predispose to the development of rheumatoid arthritis severe enough to require hospitalization. A review of the literature reveals no direct studies of either the attack rate or the prevalence of rheumatoid arthritis in workers divided according to occupation. However, figures are available on the occupations stated at the time of hospital or clinic admission by patients in whom diagnoses of rheumatoid arthritis had been made. In a study of 102 patients Smith [*479*] concluded that specific occupations did not "play much role in the etiology of the disease," since his patients gave histories of widely diversified occupations, without showing any predilection toward jobs involving unusual strain or exposure. In a later study of 573 patients with rheumatoid arthritis admitted to a Copenhagen hospital, Snorrason [*483*] similarly concluded that rheumatoid arthritis attacked "all social classes without regard to economic circumstances" and that relatively light indoor work "almost appeared" more predisposing than heavy outdoor work. In several British studies [*98, 263, 480*], published about fifteen years ago, patients consecutively admitted to hospitals largely devoted to rheumatic diseases were divided according to diagnosis and to the type of occupation followed at the time of admission. In this way various occupations can be compared in regard to the relative frequency of rheumatoid arthritis and other diseases involving the skeletal system, including osteoarthritis, fibrositis, and sciatica. In two out of three such studies [98, 263] a higher proportion of patients with diagnoses of rheumatoid arthritis were found among males with indoor rather than outdoor occupations, while the reverse finding was obtained in the third [480]. In interpreting these results, it must be remembered that the patients listed the occupations they were pursuing at the time of admission to the hospital and that some may have changed to indoor occupations consequent to their disease. One interesting finding agreed to by three authors [60, 263, 480] and warranting further investigation was the relatively low frequency of rheumatoid arthritis among miners. This group, although undergoing severe and often hazardous physical labor, was exposed to a constant temperature between 70° and 80° F. and a high humidity. (On the other hand, in a recent epidemiologic survey of a Welsh mining community [352], the frequency of rheumatoid arthritis in miners and ex-miners approximated that in males engaged in other occupations.) The patients studied by Coates and Delicati [98] were divided according to whether the outdoor occupation involved marked or "less" exposure to damp and whether or not a combination of mental and physical stress was probably operative. The last group included policemen, engine and train drivers, and chauffeurs. No difference was found in the frequency of rheumatoid arthritis in those with marked or "less" exposure to damp, but a diagnosis of this disease was made in a significantly greater proportion of those working under stress than in the remainder of the outdoor workers.

11.2   The most recent investigation of the relation between occupation and rheumatic diseases appeared in 1947 as part of a statistical study by Lewis-Faning [319] of 1,000 patients attending rheumatism clinics in the London area. Relatively more rheumatoid arthritis than other forms of rheumatism was found among indoor workers, with the possibility remaining that the arthritis had altered the patients' occupations in some instances. A comparison between the patients in our series and those studied in London is set forth in Table 11.1, which utilizes the classification adopted by the British workers (except that patients with rheumatoid arthritis and those with ankylosing spondyli-

Occupation

Table 11.1

Occupations of rheumatoid arthritics—males and females of present series compared with a series of patients admitted to London clinics [319]

Occupation group		Males			
		British series		Present series	
		No.	Per cent	No.	Per cent
I	Outdoor workers (heavy)	12	17.1	21	19.8
II	Outdoor workers (other)	6	8.6	11	10.4
III	Indoor workers on materials	17	24.3	36	34.0
IV	Indoor workers (other) and persons not gainfully employed	35	50.0	38	35.8
Total		70	100.0	106*	100.0
		Females			
I	Housewives and persons not gainfully employed	192	81.0	149	81.0
II	Office and shop workers	31	13.1	23	12.5
III	Factory workers and cleaners	14	5.9	12	6.5
Total		237	100.0	184†	100.0

* Occupation undetermined for 1 patient.
† Occupation undetermined for 1 patient; 1 patient 5 years old at onset.

tis are combined). The results are in remarkable agreement, although the occupations noted for our patients were those pursued at the time of disease onset rather than at the time of hospital admission. The percentages are almost identical among females. Among males, outdoor workers made up 25.8 per cent of the total in the British series compared with 30.3 per cent in our series, with indoor workers amounting to 74.2 per cent and 69.7 per cent, respectively.

11.3 In none of the British series was it possible to compare the distribution of patients by occupation with that of the population from which they were drawn. In Table 11.2, we have attempted to make this comparison by utilizing the Census figures for the occupations of the population of Massachusetts in 1930. Such a comparison can be only approximate, of course, since the arthritis began before 1930 in a number of our patients. In order to avoid the formation of subgroups too small for statistical evaluation, three arbitrary combinations for each sex were made from occupational classifications employed in the Census. The first group of males was composed of manual laborers, whether engaged in agriculture or industry; the second group, of men engaged in less strenuous activity; and the third group, of students and unem-

Table 11.2

Occupations of rheumatoid arthritics—males and females of present series compared with population of Massachusetts in 1930 (see par. 11.3 for definition of groups)

Occupation group	Males				
	Census population		Present series		
	No.	Per cent	No.	Per cent	Expected no.
I	704,648	42.4	49	46.2	44.9
II	570,654	34.3	40	37.7	36.4
III	387,914	23.3	17	16.0	24.7
Total	1,663,216	100.0	106*	99.9	106.0
	Females				
I	219,771	12.4	25	13.6	22.8
II	307,095	17.4	41	22.3	32.0
III	1,238,439	70.2	118	64.1	129.2
Total	1,765,305	100.0	184†	100.0	184.0

* Occupation undetermined for 1 patient.
† Occupation undetermined for 1 patient; 1 patient five years old at onset.

ployed persons. The first group of females was composed of factory workers and others whose jobs made special demands on the physique; the second, of clerical workers and those performing domestic and personal services; and the third, of housewives, students, and others not gainfully employed. When these classifications were adopted, as may be seen in the table, no significant departure was found from the occupational distribution of the population. In order to allow for variations between the age distribution of the population and the age-at-onset distribution of the patients, a comparison was made similar to that expressed in Table 11.2 with both males and females divided into the two age groups, 10 to 45 years and 45 to 75 years. Again no significant differences were obtained among the females or the younger males. In the older males, differences were evident, as shown in Table 11.3. However, the groups of patients were very small, and the differences would not be significant if Groups II and III were recombined. It seems fair, then, to state in summary that, with the occupational classifications employed, there is no apparent association between the type of occupation at the time of onset and the development of rheumatoid arthritis severe enough to require hospitalization.

11.4 As shown in Table 11.4, males were divided according to

Occupation

Table 11.3

Males of present series with onset of arthritis between the ages of 45 and 75 compared by occupation group with males aged 45 to 75 in 1930 Massachusetts population

Occupation group	Census population		Present series		Expected no.
	No.	Per cent	No.	Per cent	
I	264,334	52.2	10	41.7	12.5
II	187,378	37.0	14	58.3	8.9
III	54,611	10.8	0	0.0	2.6
Total	506,323	100.0	24	100.0	24.0

$\chi^2 = 6.02; p < .05$

Table 11.4

Frequency of spondylitis among males of present series—patients having outdoor occupations at onset of rheumatoid arthritis compared with those having indoor occupations (see Table 11.1)

Occupation	No. of males	Spondylitis present	
		No.	Per cent
Total	106*	32	30.2
Outdoor	32	9	28.1
Indoor	74	23	31.1
	Difference in percentages:		3.0 ± 9.5

* Occupation undetermined for 1 patient

whether they were following an outdoor or an indoor occupation at the time disease became manifest. No difference is evident in the frequency of spondylitis in the two groups, a result confirmed by the distribution in Lewis-Faning's series [319]. Our group of 8 females with spinal arthritis alone (1 case) or both spinal and peripheral arthritis was too small for comparison with the group having peripheral arthritis alone. It is interesting to note, however, that in the British series the women of Group I showed no difference in this respect. Whether there was any relationship between the type of occupation and the total severity* of the arthritis was the next point to be investigated. As shown in Table 11.5, the proportions with disease of mild, moderate, and marked severity remained essentially the same irrespective of the type of occupation pursued at the time of onset.

* See definition, par. **4.26**.

Table 11.5

Total severity of rheumatoid arthritis on hospital admission among males and females of present series divided according to occupation group (see Table 11.1)

Occupation	No. of patients	Total severity among males					
		Mild		Moderate		Marked	
		No.	Per cent	No.	Per cent	No.	Per cent
Total	106*	27	25.4	64	60.3	15	14.2
Outdoor	32	9	28.1	18	56.2	5	15.6
Indoor	74	18	24.3	46	62.2	10	13.5
		Total severity among females					
Total	184†	45	24.4	105	57.0	34	18.5
Group I	149	35	23.5	85	57.0	29	19.5
Groups II and III	35	10	28.6	20	57.1	5	14.3

* Occupation undetermined for 1 patient.
† Occupation undetermined for 1 patient; 1 patient five years old at onset.

SUMMARY

11.5 Most preceding studies have shown an excess of rheumatoid arthritis in indoor workers in comparison with other rheumatic diseases. Since the occupations listed were those followed by the patients on admission to clinic or hospital, the possibility exists that the type of occupation was in some instances determined by the disease. When a simple classification into broad occupational groups was employed, we found no significant departure from the Census figures for Massachusetts in 1930 regarding occupation at the onset of the disease. The evidence at hand is thus insufficient to demonstrate a relationship between types of occupation and the onset or development of rheumatoid arthritis.

11.6 Objective for further study:

The attack rate or prevalence of rheumatoid arthritis in workers in various occupations, with special reference to environmental conditions and liability to stress.

12

The Menopause

12.1   As indicated in paragraph 6.7, the increased frequency of onset of rheumatoid arthritis in women between the ages of 50 and 55 immediately suggests an influence of the menopause. Such a relationship was postulated by Garrod [*199*] over sixty years ago and more recently by Clemmesen and Arnsø [*91*]. This chapter will therefore be devoted to a detailed review of the time of menopause in females of the series in relation to the onset and development of their disease. With respect to patients in whom the menopause had been artificially produced by surgical castration or irradiation, the cessation of ovarian activity could be fixed with some certainty. When the menopause occurred naturally, we used the date of the last menses as the reference point, although realizing that ovarian function sometimes begins to wane before this time and sometimes persists after it. Table 12.1 demonstrates little difference between patients and controls in regard to the age or type of menopause. Almost half the women in both groups had experienced the menopause at the time of questioning, and the frequency of artificial menopause was approximately the same in patients as in controls, a finding confirmed in the patients and controls studied by Lewis-Faning [*320*]. As an additional check, a comparison was also made with a representative series of American women [*448*]. As shown

Table 12.1

Females of present series (186 patients) compared with 186 controls in regard to type of menopause and average age at menopause

	Patients		Controls	
Menopausal group	No.	Per cent	No.	Per cent
Artificial	15	8.1	11	5.9
Natural	73	39.2	70	37.6
Total	88	47.3	81	43.5
Average age				
Artificial	38.1 years		40.5 years	
Natural	46.6 years		47.2 years	
Whole group	45.2 years		46.2 years	

by Table 12.2, we were not able to confirm the suggestions of Bauer [20] and Fox [189] that rheumatoid arthritis is related to an early menopause or to discover any evidence to the effect that rheumatoid arthritis, like breast cancer [392], is associated with a late menopause.

12.2   The scatter diagram presented in Figure 12.1 does not show any temporal association between the onset of rheumatoid arthritis and natural menopause, but that in Figure 12.2 suggests an apparent linear relationship between onset and artificial menopause in 15 patients. In 2 patients, the arthritis even began within six months of the sterilization. The relationship seems less close, however, when we note that in 5 patients the arthritis preceded the menopause and, in another 5, from eight to sixteen years elapsed between the menopause and the onset of arthritis. It may also be seen in Table 12.3 that about two-thirds of the women in the natural menopause group stopped menstruating at least two years before or after the onset of the disease—the median interval being seven years. Of the women with artificial menopause, although the median interval was two years, only a third experienced the onset within two years *after* sterilization. The relatively large number with onset between the ages of 50 and 55 is presented in the last column of this table. Again no close relationship apparently existed between the last menstrual period and the start of the arthritis.

12.3   Seven studies of the relationship of age at menopause to age at the onset of rheumatoid arthritis have been found in the literature.

Table 12.2

Age at natural menopause—73 patients of present series compared with 70 controls and with a series of 567 American women [448]

	Percentage reaching natural menopause		
Age group	Patients	Controls	American women
Under 35	1	1	3
35–39	7	3	5
40–44	19	21	17
45–49	40	36	40
50–54	33	35	31
55 or more	0	4	4
Total	100	100	100
Average age at natural menopause	46.6	47.2	47.1

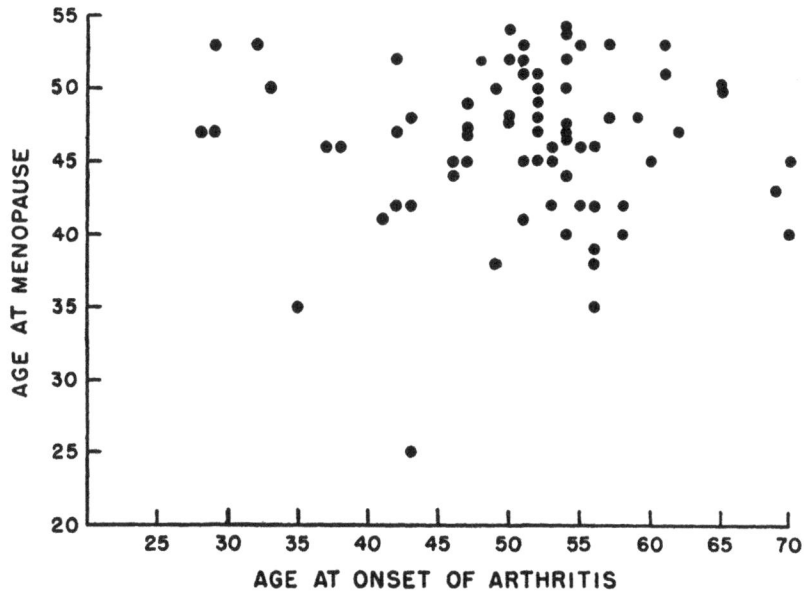

Figure 12.1 Scatter diagram showing relationship between age at natural menopause and age at onset of rheumatoid arthritis in group of 73 women

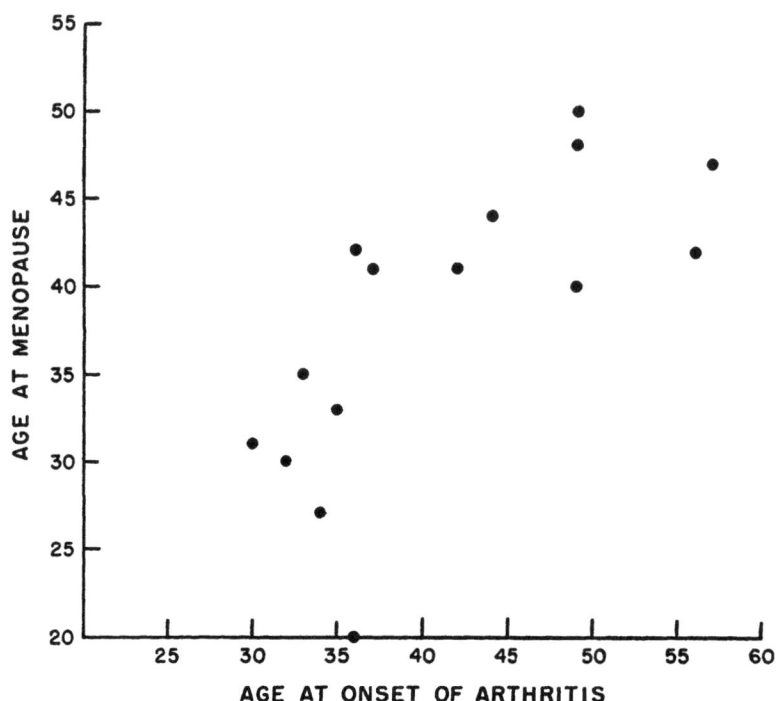

Figure 12.2 Scatter diagram showing relationship between age at artificial menopause and age at onset of rheumatoid arthritis in group of 15 women

In Table 12.4 the data have been grouped according to the proportion of all females utilized and the interval chosen to denote proximity of the two events. When the data are arranged in this fashion, a general agreement is evident among the several studies, as well as with the figures obtained from the present series, that no close temporal relationship has been demonstrated between onset of rheumatoid arthritis and cessation of menses. However, in spite of the failure by numerical means to implicate the menopause as an important factor in the onset of rheumatoid arthritis, the possibility that loss of ovarian function is concerned with its development should not be discarded. As pointed out above, the actual cessation of menses is the only readily available reference point for a study of this type, although the climacteric, or period of diminishing ovarian activity, may extend over months and years [475].

Table 12.3 Postmenopausal group and females aged 50–54 of present series divided according to interval between menopause and onset of rheumatoid arthritis

Onset of arthritis	Whole group		Natural menopause		Artificial menopause		Aged 50–54	
	No.	Per cent	No.	Per cent	No.	Per cent	No.	Per cent
Within 2 years before or after menopause	31	35.2	23	31.5	8*	53.3	11	40.7
More than 2 years before	22	25.0	20	27.4	2	13.3	2	7.4
More than 2 years after	35	39.8	30	41.1	5	33.3	14	51.7
Total	88	100.0	73	100.0	15	99.9	27	99.8
In the same year	10	11.4	8	11.0	2	13.3	3	11.1
Median interval between onset and menopause:	7 years		7 years		2 years		4 years	

* 3 patients before menopause; 5 after menopause.

Table 12.4 Relationship of menopause and age of onset in rheumatoid arthritis—females of present series compared with representative series from the literature

Source	No. of females	Proportion utilized	Onset related to menopause		
			Interval	No.	Per cent
Jones [286]	201	All		5	2.5
Vrtiak and Jordan [546]	43	All		4	9.3
Fletcher and Lewis-Faning [187]	254	All		25	9.8
Present series	186	All	Onset in same year	10	5.4
Smith [479]	60	All	1 year before or after	6	10.0
Present series	186	All	1 year before or after	18	9.7
Garrod [199]	411	All	2 years before or after	64	15.6
Present series	186	All	2 years before or after	31	16.7
Clemmesen and Arnsø [91]	292	Age of onset 35–59	1 year before or after	60	20.5
Present series	93	Age of onset 35–59	1 year before or after	18	19.4
Lewis-Faning [320]	115	Postmenopausal	1 year before or after	28	26.3
Present series	88	Postmenopausal	1 year before or after	18	20.5

12.4   It has been stated in the literature [150, 189] that cases of rheumatoid arthritis arising at the menopause are generally milder and progress more slowly. No evidence to this effect is shown in Table 12.5, in which the three groups of females, divided according to degree of total disease severity on admission, contain approximately equal proportions of women experiencing the onset of arthritis within two years of the menopause. Similarly no association has been found between proximity of disease onset to menopause and either (1) a progressive compared with an intermittent course before admission or (2) improvement or failure to improve in follow-up studies. From the data just presented, the suggestion is drawn that neither a favorable nor an unfavorable influence is exerted upon the severity or course of rheumatoid arthritis when it starts near the menopause. It must be remembered, however, that other factors may have been operative, such as age at onset and age on admission—in nearly all of this group after the age of forty. When the women who were post-menopausal on admission are compared with those still menstruating, no difference in respect to degree of total severity was found, but an association emerged between the post-menopausal state and failure of subsequent improvement. In this instance the age factor may have been responsible, since those admitted after forty were also less likely to do well after leaving the hospital.

Table 12.5

Onset of rheumatoid arthritis within 2 years of menopause in relation to total disease severity on hospital admission among females of present series

Total disease severity*	No. of females	Onset within 2 years of menopause	
		No.	Per cent
Total	186	31	16.7†
Mild	45	6	13.3†
Moderate	107	19	17.8†
Marked	34	6	17.6†
$\chi^2 = .48; p > 0.7$			

* See definition, par. **4.26**.

† Approximately the same results were obtained when women of the 35–59 age group and post-menopausal women were considered separately.

The Menopause

SUMMARY

12.5 In women with rheumatoid arthritis the age and type of menopause corresponds closely with information in this regard obtained from controls. No close temporal relationship between time of menopause and disease onset was found either in our series or in others. Onset of arthritis within two years of menopause had no detectable influence on the severity or subsequent course of the disease. In the interpretation of the data in this chapter, it must be remembered that the cessation of menses was necessarily used as a reference point, while the climacteric, or period of diminishing ovarian function, may precede and follow this event for months or years.

12.6 Objectives for further study:

1. Hormonal determinations on women with rheumatoid arthritis arising soon after cessation of menses or at the usual time of menopause.

2. The prevalence of rheumatoid arthritis in women with artificial menopause compared with the prevalence in women in the same age groups.

13

Prodromal Symptoms

13.1   In the earliest descriptions of rheumatoid arthritis, it has been noted that symptoms not necessarily related to the joints may precede the actual development of arthritis. As far back as 1868, Trousseau [536] alluded to muscle spasm and pains in the limbs, while Homolle [264], in 1882, stated that sensory disturbances especially related to weather changes and fatigue, neuralgic pains, and muscle stiffness might be present for several weeks or even a few months before the onset of joint involvement. Various designations have been applied to this period in the development of rheumatoid arthritis, including "premonitory symptoms" (Garrod [199], 1890), "period of invasion" (Teissier and Roque [525], 1897), "prodromata" (Jones [286], 1909), and "the pre-arthritic stage" (Copeman [117], 1938). In recognition of Jones' inclusive and vivid description of this group of symptoms, we shall also employ the terms "prodromata" or "prodromal symptoms."

13.2   The symptoms attributed to the prodromal stage of the disease involve nearly all bodily systems, and number at least thirty-five in the studies that we have reviewed.* It seems reasonable to agree with

---

* Arranged roughly according to frequency of mention, they include: sensory disturbances, pains in skeletal structures, fatigue, vasomotor instability, weight loss, nervousness, muscle atrophy, appetite loss, sweating, muscle weakness, muscle spasm, muscle twitching, crepitus, association of symptoms with weather changes, tachycardia, dyspnea, palpitation, increased reflexes, fever, headaches, migraine, asthma, pallor, sensitivity to

Prodromal Symptoms

Jones [286] that there is nothing distinctive about most of them and that they may occur often in patients who never develop rheumatoid arthritis. To make a diagnosis of the disease at this stage is hazardous and the interpretation of therapeutic results impossible. In fact, the existence of a prodromal period can be established only if the patient later develops unmistakable signs of rheumatoid arthritis and, except in rare instances, a history of these symptoms can be elicited from the patient only after an appreciable interval has elapsed. For this reason, perhaps, reports on the actual frequency of prodromata are lacking except for Smith's [478] analysis of about 50 patients in respect to the duration and nature of the symptoms and for a study by Lewis-Faning [320] to be referred to later. Furthermore, it may be difficult to determine the point when prodromata are interrupted by actual arthritis, often accompanied by similar symptoms. It has been stated with some reason that the prodromal period must mark the real onset of this constitutional disease [133] or, as Jones [286] puts it, the "primary manifestations of a chronic toxemia." This seems plausible until we read clinical histories of patients whose first symptoms, especially vasomotor instability, appeared in early childhood, even thirty or forty years before the articular disease developed. Perhaps, in some instances, the prodromal period represents rather a constitutional background favorable to the development of rheumatoid arthritis. Such questions cannot be elucidated at present, and in our discussion this interesting period must be delimited by arbitrary clinical criteria.

13.3 In the data to follow, prodromal symptoms are those noted by the patient before the actual onset of the first attack of arthritis. Symptoms preceding exacerbations or secondary attacks of the disease are thus excluded. The actual onset of the arthritis may be difficult to ascertain in some patients. We have held it to be the first appearance of persistent pain, inflammation, or limitation of motion of one or more joints. Since many of our patients have been studied five, ten, or more years after the onset, it is obvious that the patients' memory of the sequence of events cannot be relied upon with confidence. For this reason, the group with disease duration of one year or less has been

---

cold, urinary frequency, intermittent exophthalmos, intermittent thyroid swelling, scleroderma, atrophy of skin, hair or nails, ecchymoses, soreness under heels, insomnia.

compared with the remaining members of the series. The next question is which of the thirty-five or more symptoms we have listed should be chosen for study. On the basis of clinical descriptions in the literature, the previously mentioned series of 51 patients analyzed by Smith [478], and our own experience, we settled upon three of the admittedly most common symptoms: fatigue, pain, and sensory disturbances, and, in addition, chose appetite loss and crepitus. Finally, if the patient or control had had one or more of these symptoms, he was asked whether or not it had been intensified by changes in the weather. The word "fatigue" was used in a broad sense to cover lack of energy and unaccustomed tiring of muscles or of the body as a whole. Pain might be localized in bones, joints, or muscles and included so-called "neuralgic pains" and muscle cramps and stiffness. Sensory disturbances were usually perceived in the extremities and variously described by the patients as numbness, pins and needles, stinging, or burning. Crepitus referred to cracking sounds heard or felt in the vicinity of joints. Nervousness, weight loss, and vasomotor disturbances are frequently mentioned in the literature as common prodromal symptoms. Since the beginning of our study we have also found such to be the case, but unfortunately did not include them in our questionnaire.

13.4 We have mentioned that these prodromal symptoms are not distinctive and may occur in patients with other diseases and even in apparently normal individuals. To examine the relationship of all five symptoms* to the onset of rheumatoid arthritis, we compared the frequencies found in the arthritic group prior to the onset of joint disease with the frequencies found in the control group at or preceding the time of examination. Table 13.1 demonstrates that, while controls were more likely to be free of all the symptoms investigated, fatigue and appetite loss were the only symptoms which occurred with significantly greater frequency in the arthritic group. In other words, pain of the type described, sensory disturbances, and intensification of any of these symptoms by weather cannot necessarily be regarded as true prodromal symptoms, since they occurred with nearly equal frequency in the control group. This control group was not strictly comparable to the arthritic group in regard to the ages at which the symptoms oc-

---

* The controls were not questioned in regard to crepitus.

Prodromal Symptoms

Table 13.1
Frequency of prodromal symptoms among 293 rheumatoid arthritics and 293 controls

	Patients		Controls		Difference in percentages
	No.	Per cent	No.	Per cent	
With 1 or more symptoms (total)	174	59.4	142	48.5	10.9 ± 4.1
Type of symptom	Distribution of symptoms				
Fatigue	137	46.8	62	21.2	25.6 ± 3.9
Pain	86	29.4	82	28.0	1.4 ± 3.8
Appetite loss	50	17.1	28	9.6	7.5 ± 2.8
Crepitus	49	16.7	Not questioned		
Sensory	37	12.6	27	9.2	3.4 ± 2.6
Intensified by weather	32	10.9	27	9.2	1.7 ± 2.5

curred. Since by definition the prodromata appeared before the onset of joint disease in the patients and since the controls were examined at ages corresponding to the ages at which the patients were admitted to the hospital, the controls were somewhat older than the patients with respect to the occurrence of prodromal symptoms. In order to check this discrepancy the patients and controls were divided by sex and by age (above and below forty) and compared with respect to the frequency of fatigue and appetite loss. No significant difference was found except for a higher frequency of fatigue in female controls aged forty or over. Since this last finding would tend to make the results even more significant, the age differences between the patients and controls can probably be disregarded. It seems safe to state then, that, of the symptoms used for our study, only fatigue and appetite loss preceded the onset of arthritis in our series of patients more frequently than they affected the comparable group of normal controls. In the results to be presented, we shall confine our analysis to these two symptoms and refer to them alone as "prodromal symptoms."

13.5 In Lewis-Faning's [320] study of 302 patients and controls, inquiries concerning prodromal symptoms were made in the case of controls relative to a reference point in time comparable to the date of disease onset in the patient with whom the control was paired. Under this method, prodromal symptoms were present to a much greater degree in the patients than in the controls—none being recorded for 34 per cent of patients compared with 88 per cent of the controls. In addition to fatigue, pains in joints and muscles, weight loss, sweating, and paresthesias were found with significantly greater frequency in the patients.* Appetite loss occurred as frequently in controls as in patients. While in general agreement, Lewis-Faning's results thus differ somewhat from ours, perhaps because in his study the controls as well as the patients were questioned about the occurrence of symptoms preceding the date of inquiry by as long as five years. In the present study, on the other hand, the patients were asked to recall more distant episodes than were the controls. It should also be pointed out that, although three prodromata were found in approximately equal frequency in the patients and the controls (Table 13.1), in a given patient these symptoms may still constitute manifestations of the disease.

13.6 As stated above, data pertinent to symptoms occurring in the relatively distant past are open to serious criticism. For this reason we divided the arthritics into two groups—the first composed of patients hospitalized one year or less after onset and the second of patients hospitalized more than one year after onset. Controls of corresponding sex and age were selected for each group according to chance. In the 84 patients with more recent onset fatigue and appetite loss were again the only prodromal symptoms elicited with significantly greater frequency from patients than from controls (Table 13.2). In the group with longer duration of disease, fatigue alone among the prodromata studied was found more often in patients than in controls (Table 13.3). In Table 13.4 direct comparison of the two groups shows that a history of prodromal symptoms (fatigue and appetite loss) was obtained with significantly greater frequency from patients whose arthritis had lasted one year or less. Now, while the mean age at onset of the females in the two groups is not significantly different, in the males with disease of recent onset the mean age of onset was forty years compared with thirty years in the remainder. Although this gives a significant difference of 10 ± 3.7, the conclusions are not affected, since the frequency of prodromata is not increased in older males with arthritis present one year or less. It seems reasonable that the higher frequency of prodromal

* Inquiries were not made about intensification of symptoms by weather.

Table 13.2

Frequency of prodromal symptoms among 84 patients with shorter duration of rheumatoid arthritis on hospital admission (1 year or less) and among corresponding controls

	Patients with shorter duration		Controls		Difference in percentages
	No.	Per cent	No.	Per cent	
With 1 or more symptoms (total)	62	73.8	41	48.8	25.0 ± 7.5
Type of symptom	Distribution of symptoms				
Fatigue	53	63.1	17	20.2	42.9 ± 7.6
Pain	22	26.2	25	29.8	3.6 ± 7.0
Appetite loss	22	26.2	6	7.1	19.1 ± 5.8
Crepitus	15	17.9	Not questioned		
Sensory	11	13.1	5	6.0	7.1 ± 4.5
Intensified by weather	4	4.8	4	4.8	0.0

Table 13.3

Frequency of prodromal symptoms among 209 patients with longer duration of rheumatoid arthritis on hospital admission (more than 1 year) and among corresponding controls

	Patients with longer duration		Controls		Difference in percentages
	No.	Per cent	No.	Per cent	
With 1 or more symptoms (total)	112	53.6	101	48.3	5.3 ± 4.9
Type of symptom	Distribution of symptoms				
Fatigue	84	40.2	45	21.5	18.7 ± 4.5
Pain	64	30.6	57	27.3	3.3 ± 4.4
Appetite loss	28	13.4	22	10.5	2.9 ± 3.2
Crepitus	34	16.3	Not questioned		
Sensory	26	12.4	22	10.5	1.9 ± 3.1
Intensified by weather	28	13.4	23	11.0	2.4 ± 3.2

Table 13.4

Prodromal symptoms (fatigue and appetite loss) in relation to disease duration before hospital admission among patients of present series

Disease duration	No. of patients	History of prodromata	
		No.	Per cent
Total	293	139	47.3
Shorter (1 year or less)	84	56	66.7
Longer (more than 1 year)	209	83	39.7
	Difference in percentages: 27.0 ± 6.4		

symptoms in the group with shorter duration of disease depended largely upon the more exact memory of these patients for more recent events.

13.7 Fatigue and appetite loss were reported less frequently as prodromal symptoms by male members of the series than by females, as shown in Table 13.5. Since there was no such difference in the controls, it would be unwise to assume that this finding was due to a greater degree of stoicism in men. Lewis-Faning's [320] findings agree with ours in respect to a higher frequency of prodromal fatigue in females and in patients more than forty years of age; he also found a slightly higher frequency in older controls, but the difference between

Table 13.5

Sex distribution of prodromal symptoms (fatigue and appetite loss)—patients of present series compared with controls

Sex	No. in each group	Patients			
		History of fatigue*		History of appetite loss†	
		No.	Per cent	No.	Per cent
Total	293	137	46.8	50	17.1
Males	107	32	29.9	9	8.4
Females	186	105	56.5	41	22.0
		Controls			
Total	293	62	21.2	28	9.6
Males	107	17	15.9	12	11.2
Females	186	45	24.2	16	8.6

*Difference in percentages:
Patients—26.6 ± 6.1
Controls—8.3 ± 5.0

†Difference in percentages:
Patients—13.6 ± 4.7
Controls—2.6 ± 3.5

Prodromal Symptoms

the two age groups was not significant. Fatigue and appetite loss were also reported more commonly by those of our patients whose disease began after the age of forty (Table 13.6). That this age difference is peculiar to rheumatoid arthritis is suggested by the fact that a similar situation was not found among the controls. The conclusion may thus be drawn that fatigue and appetite loss as prodromal symptoms in rheumatoid arthritis are more frequent in females and in older patients for reasons that as yet remain unexplained.

13.8 Although the reasons have been set forth for including patients with rheumatoid spondylitis in the present series, we thought it would be of interest to compare the patients with and without spinal involvement in respect to prodromal symptoms. Table 13.7 shows a distinctly lower frequency in the patients with spondylitis. This finding can be explained by the well-known reversal in sex distribution in the spinal type of rheumatoid arthritis, exemplified in the present series by a distribution of 32 males and 9 females. In fact, if the comparison is limited to males with and without spondylitis, the difference disappears.

13.9 In a study of psychic factors in rheumatoid arthritis, Thomas [527] pointed out that what are commonly regarded as prodromal

Table 13.6

Prodromal symptoms (fatigue and appetite loss) in relation to age at onset of rheumatoid arthritis—patients of present series compared with corresponding controls

Age at onset	No. in each group	Patients* History of prodromata No.	Per cent
Total	293	139	47.5
Under 40	177	75	42.4
40 or more	116	64	55.2
On admission to study		Controls†	
Total	293	83	28.3
Under 40	144	35	24.3
40 or more	149	48	32.2

* Difference in percentages: 12.8 ± 6.0
† Difference in percentages: 7.9 ± 5.8

Table 13.7

Prodromal symptoms (fatigue and appetite loss) in relation to presence or absence of spondylitis on hospital admission among patients of present series

Spondylitis	No. of patients	History of 1 or more prodromata	
		No.	Per cent
Total	293	139	47.5
Present	41	13	31.8
Absent	252	126	50.0
	Difference in percentages:	18.2 ± 8.5	

symptoms are "readily recognized as often due to emotional disturbances." It thus seemed worth while to examine the relationship of prodromal symptoms to mental or physical strain. (See the discussion of precipitating factors in the next chapter.) Table 13.8 indicates that those with prodromal symptoms had been exposed to stresses in the pre-arthritic period with greater frequency than those without, but not that such stresses were necessarily productive of symptoms by a psychosomatic mechanism. Furthermore, as shown in Table 13.9, no significant association was found between prodromal symptoms and a history of nervousness or emotional upsets. More detailed psychiatric study, and especially long-term follow-up of patients with symptomatology suggesting the prodromal phase of rheumatoid arthritis, are obviously indicated. Until this is accomplished, no conclusions can be drawn in regard to Thomas' [527] interpretation of prodromal symptoms, one which would certainly lend support to the importance of psychogenic factors in the onset and development of this disease.

13.10   The ability of the physician to prognosticate the ultimate outcome is less certain in rheumatoid arthritis than in many chronic diseases. In this chapter we have therefore attempted to ascertain whether the presence or absence of prodromal symptoms may be related to the future course. In Table 13.10 the proportion of patients whose course* progressed between onset and hospital admission is essentially the same in the groups with and without prodromata. In Table 13.11 the patients' status on admission has been considered in respect to a history of prodromal symptoms. Again no differences are apparent

---

* See definition, par. **4.13**.

Table 13.8

Strain as a precipitating factor in relation to presence or absence of prodromal symptoms among patients of present series

Prodromata	No. of patients	Strain as a precipitant	
		No.	Per cent
Total	293	80	27.3
Present	139	60	43.2
Absent	154	20	13.0
Difference in percentages: 30.2 ± 5.2			

Table 13.9

History of nervousness and/or emotional upsets in relation to presence or absence of prodromal symptoms among patients of present series

Prodromata	No. of patients	History of nervousness and/or emotional upsets	
		No.	Per cent
Total	293	177	60.4
Present	139	90	64.7
Absent	154	87	56.5
Difference in percentages: 8.2 ± 5.7			

Table 13.10

Progressive course before hospital admission in relation to presence or absence of prodromal symptoms (fatigue and appetite loss) among patients of present series

Prodromata	No. of patients	Progressive course	
		No.	Per cent
Total	293	214	73.0
Present	139	104	74.8
Absent	154	110	71.4
Difference in percentages: 3.4 ± 5.2			

Table 13.11

Total severity of disease on hospital admission in relation to presence or absence of prodromal symptoms (fatigue and appetite loss) among patients of present series

Prodromata	No. of patients	Total severity of disease					
		Mild		Moderate		Marked	
		No.	Per cent	No.	Per cent	No.	Per cent
Total	293	73	24.9	172	58.7	48	16.4
Present	139	34	24.5	82	59.0	23	16.5
Absent	154	39	25.3	90	58.4	25	16.2

160   *Rheumatoid Arthritis*

in the degree of "total severity"* between the two groups. Finally, follow-up study of the patients after they had left the hospital suggests that a history of prodromal symptoms was not an important factor in the ultimate outcome. The observations reported in this paragraph, which were obtained from consideration of the series as a whole, were duplicated in the group with disease duration of one year or less. Whether or not fatigue or appetite loss or both precede the development of arthritis would thus seem to be of no value in prognosis.†

13.11   In the next chapter we shall enumerate and attempt to evaluate the influence of what might be called precipitating factors. These include disturbing events or situations in close proximity to the onset of the arthritis—i.e., acute infections, usually of the upper respiratory tract; mental or physical strain; surgical operations; acute trauma; and unusual exposure to cold and dampness. It would seem pertinent at this point to determine their relationship to the prodromal symptoms which may also precede the beginning of definite joint disease. The 84 patients whose onset antedated hospital admission by one year or less were chosen as the most likely to have unimpaired recollection of the pertinent information. In 13 of the patients composing this group the onset appeared out of an entirely clear sky with neither antecedent prodromata nor precipitating factors. In 21 cases the onset was preceded by prodromal symptoms but not by other disturbances, while in 17 cases the onset was preceded by some of the events or situations listed above but not by constitutional symptoms. In 21 of the 33 patients whose histories contained both precipitants and prodromata, the sequence of events leading up to the onset could be reasonably well outlined. A summary of the pre-arthritic histories of these patients is presented in Table 13.12. In every case in Group I prodromal symptoms were present for periods of four weeks to two years before either an infection (upper respiratory, 9 cases; phlebitis, 1 case), strain (5 cases), trauma (1 case), or exposure (1 case) preceded the development of arthritis. In Group II strain in the form of overwork preceded the onset of fatigue, which in turn was followed by infection or exposure and then by involvement

---

* See definition, par. **4.26**.

† The degree of association between prodromal symptoms and other factors will be mentioned in subsequent chapters and, to avoid repetition, omitted here. A complete list is also available in Appendix Table 47.

Table 13.12

Relationship of prodromal symptoms and precipitating factors in 21 patients of present series giving a history of both (see par. 13.11 for explanation of groups)

Age at onset	Sex	Sequence of events before onset
		GROUP I
44	F	Fatigue 8 months; fracture 1 week before onset
58	F	Fatigue and appetite loss for 1½ years; emotional stress associated with onset
20	M	Fatigue 6 weeks; cold 1 week before onset
45	F	Fatigue 2 years; emotional stress associated with onset
38	F	Fatigue 4 weeks; quinsy a few weeks before onset
28	F	Fatigue 1 year; sore throat 3 months before onset
15	M	Fatigue 6 months; sore throat just preceding onset
54	F	Fatigue and appetite loss for 20 months; phlebitis 1 month before onset
34	F	Fatigue and appetite loss for 14 months; head cold just preceding onset
53	F	Fatigue 1 year; strain (caring for sick relative) before onset
50	F	Fatigue 7 months; strain (overwork) preceding onset
35	F	Fatigue 8 months; strain (overwork) preceding onset
30	M	Fatigue and appetite loss for 3 months; exposure (cold-water swimming preceding onset)
22	F	Fatigue 3 months; sore throat just preceding onset
43	F	Fatigue 5 months; quinsy 10 days before onset
32	F	Fatigue and appetite loss for 6 months; sore throat just preceding onset
47	F	Fatigue 9 months; grippe just preceding onset
		GROUP II
25	F	Strain (overwork) for 1 year; fatigue for 2 months; laryngitis 1 month before onset
27	M	Strain (overwork) for 4 years; fatigue for 6 months; exposure to cold for 1 week before onset
		GROUP III
53	F	Intestinal grippe followed by fatigue for 2 months; sore throat just before onset
27	F	Grippe followed by fatigue for 4 months; tonsillectomy performed 1 week before onset

of the joints. In Group III the sequence was infection, fatigue, another infection or operation, and finally arthritis. Thus, in 80 per cent of the 21 cases, what may have been constitutional features of the disease were already present when the acute infection or other disturbance apparently initiated a clinically recognizable stage of arthritis. No formal conclusions can be drawn from these observations. The situation in Groups II and III, where strain or infection occurred even before the prodromal period, might not turn out to be less common if a greater number of patients were studied. The cases cited do illustrate, however, the difficulty in fixing upon the exact onset of the disease and the fallacy in a given case of assigning a causative role to an upper respiratory infection, for example, without attempting to trace back and record the earliest non-articular manifestations of the disease.

SUMMARY

13.12   In the literature on rheumatoid arthritis, references have frequently been made to a prodromal period preceding the onset of arthritis. Of five prodromal symptoms studied, only fatigue and appetite loss occurred with significantly greater frequency in patients than in controls. These two symptoms were less common in males than in females and in younger than in older patients, but no prognostic value could be attached to the presence or absence of prodromal fatigue or appetite loss. Analysis of the group experiencing the onset of arthritis one year or less before hospital admission corroborated the findings in the whole series.

13.13   The onset of rheumatoid arthritis may be entirely unheralded or may be preceded by constitutional symptoms or precipitating factors or both. In the last situation the precipitating factor was preceded by prodromal symptoms in a majority of the small group of patients from whom accurate data could be obtained. These findings suggest that, if we assume the disease to be already begun when constitutional manifestations are evident, apparent precipitants (infection, strain, operation, trauma, or exposure) then merely determine a more disabling phase with articular localization of the morbid process.

13.14   Objectives for further study:

1. Clinical, laboratory, and psychiatric observation and follow-up of

Prodromal Symptoms

patients without definite arthritis whose presenting symptoms resemble those of the prodromal stage of rheumatoid arthritis. Such individuals might be encountered in general medical practice, in a medical outpatient clinic, or in a population study.

2. Detailed recording of the sequence of events in patients with rheumatoid arthritis of recent origin whose histories include both a prodromal stage and precipitating factors.

3. The occurrence of "prodromal" symptoms in relatives of patients with rheumatoid arthritis.

4. Observations on the persistence of or changes in prodromal symptoms following the onset of joint involvement, especially in relation to exacerbations and remissions.

14

Precipitating Factors

14.1 As pointed out in the previous chapter, it is often difficult to fix upon the exact time of onset in rheumatoid arthritis. The prodromal constitutional symptoms which frequently come first may rightly mark the beginning of the disease, with so-called "precipitating factors" preceding the more easily recognizable phase of actual arthritis. In spite of this uncertainty, it seemed worth while to record some of the more common potentially disturbing events and conditions which have been found in association with the earliest evidence of arthritis in our patients. Such events and conditions have been frequently mentioned as predisposing causes or precipitating factors in descriptions of rheumatoid arthritis and have been cited in support of theories of the etiology or pathogenesis of the disease.

14.2 A list of the precipitating factors most commonly mentioned in the literature, together with their frequency in the present series, is given in Table 14.1. The latter may be seen to vary from 5.1 to 27.3 per cent—the highest frequency being found in the case of mental or physical strain. An additional factor, not listed in the table, is childbirth, since 4 women in the series dated the onset of their disease to the post-partum period. A detailed consideration of each precipitating factor will be found below, along with a review of the pertinent literature. Table 14.1 also demonstrates that a history of one or more precipitating fac-

Precipitating Factors

Table 14.1
Frequency of certain precipitating factors which antedated onset of rheumatoid arthritis among 293 patients

	Patients	
	No.	Per cent
With 1 or more precipitants (total)	144	49.1
Type of precipitant	*Distribution of precipitants*	
Strain: mental, physical, or both	80	27.3
Infection	49	16.7
Exposure to cold or dampness	31	10.6
Surgical operation	16	5.5
Trauma	15	5.1
Total	191	65.2

tors was given by about half the patients, a proportion approximating that obtained in two other series [13, 180]. Since a number of patients reported more than one, the sum of the percentage frequency of individual factors is well over 50 per cent. Reference will be made in later paragraphs to combinations of precipitating factors recorded for individual patients, and their significance will be discussed.

14.3 An attempt was made to check the accuracy of the figures obtained for the frequency of precipitating factors (Table 14.2). To

Table 14.2
Precipitating factors in relation to disease duration before hospital admission—84 patients having shorter duration (1 year or less) compared with 209 patients having longer duration (more than 1 year)

	Disease duration				Difference in percentages
	Shorter		Longer		
	No.	Per cent	No.	Per cent	
Patients with 1 or more precipitants (total)	52	61.9	92	44.0	17.9 ± 6.5
Type of precipitant	*Distribution of precipitants*				
Strain	27	32.1	53	25.4	6.7 ± 6.0
Infection	22	26.2	27	12.9	13.3 ± 4.4
Exposure	10	11.9	21	10.0	1.9 ± 4.1
Operation	7	8.3	9	4.3	4.0 ± 2.9
Trauma	2	2.4	13	6.2	3.8 ± 2.8

this end, the patients were divided into two groups. The first, 84 in number, included those admitted to the hospital with disease duration of one year or less, and the second comprised 209 patients with disease of longer duration. A significant difference was found only in the case of infection (probably due to reasons outlined in par. 14.10), but histories of one or more precipitating factors were elicited from a greater number of patients with shorter duration than from the remainder. This suggested that the patients seen later in the course of their disease forgot or minimized possible predisposing causes.

STRAIN

14.4 Strain was found to be the most common precipitating factor, with over one-fourth of the patients admitting to a period of unusual anxiety, excessive physical exertion, or both associated with the onset of arthritis. Although an attempt might be made to divide these patients according to whether the strain experienced was mental or physical, it seemed likely in most cases that both types had been present. For example, work demanding long hours or of a fatiguing nature was usually accompanied by anxiety and tension, while illness in the family, histories of which were obtained from 20 patients, as a rule involved excessive physical labor as well as worry.

14.5 It should be noted at this point that data in regard to the frequency and type of strain were gathered in this series by superficial questioning. No attempt was made to obtain a detailed analysis of the emotional state of the patient preceding the start of his arthritis nor, by means of a social history, to determine whether or not there was a temporal relationship between environmental stress and the first signs of joint disease. The results of such studies, performed on smaller groups of patients with rheumatoid arthritis [67, 100, 171, 236, 400, 527], indicate that more searching investigation would undoubtedly have yielded an even higher frequency of strain as a precipitating factor.

14.6 The types of strain encountered are listed in Table 14.3, with the patients divided according to sex. Although the frequency of strain as a precipitating factor was not significantly different in males and females, the strain was of an occupational nature in nearly all of the males compared with slightly over half of the females. Table 14.4

Table 14.3

Types of mental or physical strain associated with onset of rheumatoid arthritis by male and female patients with history of strain

Type of strain	No. of patients	
Males		24
Occupational	21	
Sick relative	1	
Occupational and sick relative	1	
Unemployment	1	
Females		56
Occupational (own housework, outside occupation, or both)	30	
Sick relative	16	
Death of near relative	4	
Occupational and sick relative	2	
Marital discord	2	
Own health	1	
"Nervous breakdown"; causes undetermined	1	
Total		80

Table 14.4

Strain as a precipitating factor in relation to age at onset of rheumatoid arthritis among females of present series—those having shorter duration before hospital admission (1 year or less) compared with entire group

	All females*		
	No. of patients	With strain before onset	
Age at onset		No.	Per cent
Total	186	57	30.6
Under 40	103	21	20.4
40 or more	83	36	43.4
	Females with shorter duration†		
Total	56	20	35.7
Under 40	29	8	27.6
40 or more	27	12	44.4

* Difference in percentages: 23.0 ± 6.8
† Difference in percentages: 16.8 ± 12.5

shows that strain was a more common precipitating factor in women whose disease began after the age of forty than in the group with earlier onset. When cases of shorter duration are considered, in which the data are probably more accurate, a similar difference was found but not to a significant degree. In males the frequency of strain as a precipitant was not related to age at onset of the arthritis. As might be expected, an association was obtained between patients with histories of strain antecedent to onset and of nervousness and emotional upsets (Table 14.5). No difference was noted in regard to the type of onset, whether or not strain preceded, but this was not true of infection (par. 14.10). In patients with spondylitis (with or without peripheral arthritis) strain preceded the onset with about the same frequency as in patients with peripheral arthritis alone. Finally, the presence or absence of strain as a precipitating factor was not found to be of prognostic value concerning the course of the disease before hospital admission,* total severity on admission,† and subsequent course.**

14.7 One or more additional precipitating factors were mentioned by 34 of the 80 patients who gave histories of strain preceding the onset of arthritis.†† The most common combination was infection and strain, which was present in 16 cases. This number is no more than would be expected by chance, as shown in Table 14.6. (The independence of these two factors is also brought out by their failure to share in the same associations. See par. 14.11.) Most of the 16 patients had been under strain for some time preceding the development of an infection in close proximity to the first definite signs of joint disease. A similar situation prevailed in two groups of three each, respectively reporting operation and trauma as the second precipitant. Both strain and exposure were reported as precipitating factors by 10 patients, the majority of whom held occupation to be responsible for each factor.

14.8 In 1860 Fuller [195] expressed the opinion that ". . . when

* See definition, par. 4.13.
† See definition, par. 4.26.
** The degree of association between antecedent strain and other factors will be mentioned in subsequent chapters, and, to avoid repetition, omitted here. A complete list is also available in Appendix Table 47.

†† Patients mentioned in this paragraph total more than 34 because some patients are included in more than one group.

Precipitating Factors

Table 14.5

History of nervousness and/or emotional upsets in relation to presence or absence of strain before onset of rheumatoid arthritis among patients of present series

Onset of arthritis	No. of patients	History of nervousness and/or emotional upsets	
		No.	Per cent
Total	292*	177	60.6
Preceded by strain	80	60	75.0
Not preceded by strain	212	117	55.2
		Difference in percentages:	19.8 ± 6.4

* 1 patient not questioned in regard to a history of nervousness and/or emotional upsets.

Table 14.6

Infection as a precipitating factor in relation to presence or absence of strain before onset of rheumatoid arthritis among patients of present series

Onset of arthritis	No. of patients	Infection as a precipitant	
		No.	Per cent
Total	293	49	16.7
Strain present	80	16	20.0
Strain absent	213	33	15.5
		Difference in percentages:	4.5 ± 5.0

the rheumatic poison is present in the system, any disturbing circumstance, even of temporary duration, such as overfatigue, anxiety, grief or anger, by rendering the system more susceptible of its influence, may prove the accidental or exciting cause of the disease. . . ." Thus, nearly a hundred years ago, strain was recognized as a common precipitating factor of the articular phase of rheumatoid arthritis, which does not necessarily mark the real onset of the disease. Since then nearly every treatise on rheumatoid arthritis has mentioned mental or physical strain or both in association with the beginning of joint involvement [*133, 183, 205, 271, 286, 427, 514, 564*]. Representative papers in which the frequency of strain has been expressed numerically are listed in Table 14.7. In some instances [*67, 199, 236, 400, 502*] mental strain was studied exclusively, but as in the present series, in all probability many of the patients were also subject to unusual physical exertion. It is not surprising that the frequency of strain has been higher in the more modern tabulations, in view of recently increasing awareness of the importance of

Table 14.7

Strain as a precipitating factor in rheumatoid arthritis—present series compared with representative series from the literature

Source	No. of patients	Strain as a precipitant	
		No.	Per cent
Earlier authors (total)	1,033	95	9.2
Garrod [199], 1890*	500	34	6.8
Stewart [502], 1897*	40	4	10.0
Bannatyne [13], 1898	293	4	1.4
Strangeways and Burt [510], 1907	200	53	26.5
Later authors (total)	437	124	28.4
Smith [479], 1932	102	23	22.5
Ellman and Mitchell [171], 1936	40	15	37.5
Burt et al. [67], 1938*	50	11	22.0
Halliday [236], 1942*	20	9	45.0
Patterson et al. [400], 1943*	25	12	48.0
Fletcher [186], 1947	200	54	27.0
Present series	293	80	27.3

* Series in which only mental strain was considered.

emotional and environmental factors in the development of rheumatoid arthritis. The highest figures, approaching 50 per cent, were obtained in two small series [236, 400] compiled by physicians especially interested in the psychosomatic aspects of the disease.

14.9 References should also be made to other papers in which the data given were not adapted for inclusion in Table 14.7. Thomas [527] presented evidence that significant emotional disturbances were present before the onset of arthritis in 31 patients whom he interviewed; in 9 of these the disease developed weeks or months after the beginning of a depression. In another study [283] impressive similarities were found in the conflict situations and psychodynamic backgrounds of 33 patients. A control series was utilized by Lewis-Faning [320] to evaluate the psychological precipitants in rheumatoid arthritis. The 292 patients in his series were directly questioned as to whether any one of a list of potentially disturbing circumstances had arisen either within two years or within two months previous to onset. Controls matched in age, sex, and civil state were similarly questioned in regard to a reference point in time fixed to correspond with disease onsets in the patients. When the results were tabulated, no differences were observed between the

Precipitating Factors

two groups, and Lewis-Faning concluded "that such mental stresses as may be engendered by the circumstances studied are likely to occur as frequently among nonsufferers as sufferers." However, he pointed out that the study had not excluded the possibility that such factors may play a role in the onset of the disease, with the difference in reaction of patients and controls perhaps residing "in some feature of the sufferer himself rather than in any difference of stress experience." Controls were also employed in a study [*100*] conducted in 1939 on 50 members of the present series. Data in regard to potentially upsetting emotional and environmental factors, obtained by questioning each patient, were recorded in one column of his life chart [*351*]. At a subsequent time, medical data were entered in a parallel column without reference to the social information previously listed. The medical data included past illnesses, prodromal symptoms, onset of the arthritis, and course of the disease to date. In 31 of the 50 patients a close temporal relationship appeared to exist between life stress and the course of the arthritis. As controls, 25 patients comparable in age, sex, and social status, entering the hospital because of varicose ulcers, were interviewed in exactly the same way. In only 3 cases was there a coincidence of onset of ulceration and social stress. The conclusion was drawn that environmental stresses "seem to bear more than a chance relationship to the onset and exacerbations of rheumatoid arthritis." Thus far only a beginning has been made in assessing the relative importance of psychological factors in rheumatoid arthritis. Much more detailed studies will be necessary to establish the relationship of such factors to the onset and course of the disease.

INFECTION

14.10 The prevalence of recognizable infections in association with the onset of joint involvement, has been cited as an argument in favor of the theory that rheumatoid arthritis has an infectious etiology. In the present series, about one-sixth of the patients gave such histories (Table 14.1). As mentioned above (par. **14.3**, Table 14.2), the frequency of this precipitating factor was significantly higher in the group with disease duration of one year or less before hospital admission. While the difference may be due, as pointed out by Sclater [*454*], to an increased likelihood that such persons remember events connected with the beginning of their illness, it is also possible that the nature of the ensuing arthritis was responsible for earlier hospital admission. Table 14.8 demonstrates the higher proportion of antecedent infections in those with acute rather than gradual onset,* an association also noted by Sury [513] in children. Associations were also found (1) between acute onset and admission to the hospital within one year (Table 15.3) and (2) between early admission and antecedent infection (Table 14.2). Further analysis of the mutually operative factors suggests that the association between early admission and antecedent infections was probably not due to the patients' failure to remember such infections, but rather to the association of antecedent infections with acute onset, which in turn led to early hospitalization.

14.11 No significant difference in the frequency of antecedent infections was evident in respect to sex or to onset before or after age forty—findings which have been confirmed in two other series [454, 479]. Likewise the groups with and without spinal involvement contained approximately equal numbers of patients with infections in association with the beginning of their arthritis. In regard to prognosis, the presence or absence of antecedent infection was found to bear no relation to the patient's course either before admission or after leaving the hospital. The absence of an association between the precipitating factors, strain and infection, has already been mentioned. In line with this finding was the almost complete lack of similar relationships between strain or infection and other factors. For example, infection, but not strain, was associated with an acute onset and with early admission, while strain, but not infection, was associated with prodromal symptoms, with a history of fatigability and weakness, with a history of nervousness, and with a family history of rheumatoid arthritis. A first suggestion thus emerges of the possibility of verification by numerical methods of the oft-cited clinical concept of an "infectious" type of rheumatoid arthritis. The evidence derived from the present study for and against this concept is summarized in a later chapter (pars. **16.14** and **16.15**).†

14.12 Table 14.9 lists the types of infection preceding the onset in our series. Almost nine-tenths of them involved the upper respira-

---

* See definition of acute onset, par. **4.8**.

† The degree of association between antecedent infection and other factors will be mentioned in subsequent chapters, and, to avoid repetition, omitted here. A complete list is also available in Appendix Table 47.

Precipitating Factors

Table 14.8

Infection as a precipitating factor in relation to type of onset of rheumatoid arthritis among patients of present series

Type of onset	No. of patients	Infection as a precipitant	
		No.	Per cent
Total	293	49	16.7
Acute	64	24	37.5
Gradual	229	25	10.9
Difference in percentages: 26.6 ± 5.3			

tory tract and nearly half of these were located in the throat. In four other series, the respiratory tract was also the most common site, with frequencies of 94 per cent [320], 92 per cent [13], 70 per cent [479], and 54 per cent [502]. The absence of gonorrhea or of a nonspecific urethritis as precipitating factors in our patients may seem unusual in view of the findings in a series of 100 soldiers studied in World War II [180] and recent reference [10, 254] in the literature to "post-gonorrheal" rheumatoid arthritis. The most likely explanation is that, at the time the series was selected, we were reluctant to include such patients in a group with undoubted rheumatoid arthritis.

14.13   The interval between infection and onset was two months

Table 14.9

Types of infection preceding onset of rheumatoid arthritis among patients with history of infection

Type of infection	No. of patients
Upper respiratory tract infections	43
Sore throat or tonsillitis	18
Upper respiratory infection, not localized	11
Grippe or influenza	9
Sinusitis	3
Laryngitis	1
Scarlet fever	1
Miscellaneous infections	6
Phlebitis	2
Ulcerative colitis	1
Pulmonary tuberculosis	1
Carbuncle	1
Mumps	1
Total	49

or less, except in 1 patient whose severe sore throat antedated his arthritis by three months. In certain cases the infection was still present when the joints became affected. In nearly all instances the infection was of relatively short duration, but the single patient with ulcerative colitis had had colitis for six months before developing arthritis and another patient had had pulmonary tuberculosis for three years.

14.14 Infection was reported as the sole precipitant by 28 of 49 patients, while the remaining 21 mentioned additional factors.* Reference has been made in the preceding section on strain to the combination of this precipitant with infection in 16 patients, most of whom recalled that the infection was preceded by a long period of strain. Of the 4 patients reporting both exposure and infection, the exposure was twice regarded by the patient as responsible for the development of an upper respiratory infection which antedated his arthritis. For 5 patients, the combination of infection and operation was recorded. In 3 instances, the tonsils were removed because of frequent upper respiratory infections, in 1 a carbuncle was incised, and in another sinus drainage performed, with the operation directly preceding the onset in each case. For the other patients with one or more additional precipitants, no regular sequence of events was observed.

14.15 The reports in the literature pertaining to infection as a precipitant in rheumatoid arthritis are listed in Table 14.10. Although the frequency varies from 8.9 to 32.5 per cent, the figure obtained from the whole group is very close to the percentage in the present series. Lewis-Faning's study [320] is of especial interest in that, by a method referred to above (par. 14.9) and similar to that employed in his study of psychological precipitants, comparison was made with a control series. A significant difference was found with frequencies of 18.5 per cent for the patients and 10.6 per cent for the controls—the excess in the patients being chiefly due to tonsillitis. The author also rightly pointed out that persons with rheumatoid arthritis, in seeking to find an explanation for their disease, might remember such infections more readily than would controls. In a paper not listed in Table 14.10, Dawson [134] stated, without giving actual figures, that from 20 to 25 per cent

---

* Patients referred to in this paragraph total more than 21, because some patients were included in more than one group.

Precipitating Factors

Table 14.10

Infection as a precipitating factor in rheumatoid arthritis—present series combined and compared with representative series from the literature

Source	No. of patients	Infection as a precipitant		Remarks
		No.	Per cent	
Total	1,718	306	17.8	
Stewart [502], 1897	40	13	32.5	URI,* 54 per cent; Gonorrhea, 15.4 per cent
Bannatyne [13], 1898	293	26	8.9	URI,* 92.4 per cent
Strangeways and Burt [510], 1907	200	40	20.0	
Smith [479], 1932	102	30	29.4	URI,* 70 per cent; Gonorrhea, 3.9 per cent
Sclater [454], 1943	388	71	18.3	
Finney et al. [180], 1947	100	21	21.0	Gonorrhea or non-specific urethritis, 52.2 per cent
Lewis-Faning [320], 1950	302	56	18.5	URI,* 94 per cent
Present series	293	49	16.7	URI,* 88 per cent
Not considered in above total				
Cecil and Angevine [76], 1938	200	19	9.5	URI,* alone considered
Boots and McCollom [48], 1942	180	37	20.6	URI,* alone considered

* Upper respiratory infection.

of the rheumatoid arthritics interviewed by him gave "clinical histories" of antecedent streptococcal infections. The highest frequency encountered in the literature for any type of antecedent infection was 40 per cent, mentioned by Davidson and Goldie [131] but again without reference to basic figures. We may conclude then, from our own findings and those of others, that infection has been shown to precede the onset of rheumatoid arthritis in about one-sixth of the cases studied.

EXPOSURE

14.16 The third most common precipitating factor reported by the patients in the present series was exposure to cold or dampness, which was mentioned by 10.6 per cent (Table 14.1). We have included in this category the patients who had lived or worked under unusually cold or wet conditions for some time before the onset of arthritis and those who had been chilled or wet through in a single episode closely connected with the start of their disease. These two groups are set off in Table 14.11, in which types of exposure are classified. Slightly over one-third had been subjected to sudden exposure, while the remainder had worked or lived under cold or damp conditions for some time. As may be seen in the table, chronic exposure was usually associated with the patient's occupation. In some cases damp or cold factory conditions were cited; in others, the workers had been exposed to the weather in occupations such as truck-driving. Two female patients had had their hands in and out of water over long periods of time while washing clothes or dishes. Two other patients had lived in cold and damp environments, and one believed that repeated swimming in cold water was contributory to the development of his arthritis.

14.17 Exposure was recorded more frequently as a precipitating factor for males than for females in a tabulation of the entire series (Table 14.12)—a finding which was confirmed by similar analysis of the group of patients who had been hospitalized one year or less after the onset of disease. The difference was apparently related to chronic occupational exposure, since the latter group was made up of 10 males and 6 females. In a series of cases reported by Smith [479] no significant difference was found between the sexes in the frequency of exposure as a precipitant. Table 14.13 demonstrates the tendency (without statistical significance) toward a higher frequency of antecedent exposure in patients with increasing total severity of disease on admission to the hospital. A ready interpretation of this finding is not available at present. No differences regarding the proportion with exposure before onset were found in patients with onset after or before the age of forty, with or without spinal involvement, or with acute as compared with gradual onset. Similarly, the course pursued before admission or after discharge did not appear to be related to a history of exposure preceding the appearance of arthritis.

14.18 Exposure was reported as the sole precipitating factor by only 13 of the 31 patients. Of the remaining 18 patients, 14 reported that strain was present in combination with exposure. In most of these cases, both factors were associated with the patients' occupations. Exposure

Table 14.11

Types of exposure preceding onset of rheumatoid arthritis among patients with history of exposure

Type of exposure	No. of patients	
Acute		12
To cold	7	
Caught in rain or wet feet	3	
Working one week in damp cellar	1	
Type undetermined	1	
Chronic		19
Industrial, in cold and damp environment	8	
Outdoor work, exposed to weather	6	
Dishwashing	1	
Laundry work	1	
Lived over flooded cellar	1	
Lived near sea	1	
Frequent cold-water swimming	1	
Total		31

Table 14.12

Exposure as a precipitating factor in rheumatoid arthritis among males and females of present series

Sex	No. of patients	Exposure present	
		No.	Per cent
Total	293	31	10.6
Males	107	17	15.9
Females	186	14	7.5
	Difference in percentages: 8.4 ± 3.7*		

* See text for a possible explanation of this difference.

Table 14.13

Exposure as a precipitating factor in relation to total severity of rheumatoid arthritis on hospital admission among patients of present series

Degree of severity	No. of patients	Exposure present	
		No.	Per cent
Total	293	31	10.6
Mild	72	5	6.9
Moderate	172	17	9.9
Marked	49	9	18.4

Difference in percentages between mild and marked severity: 11.5 ± 6.0
$\chi^2 = 4.19; p > 0.1$

Table 14.14

Exposure as a precipitating factor in rheumatoid arthritis—present series compared with representative series from the literature

Source	No. of patients	Exposure present	
		No.	Per cent
Literature (total)	1,507	201	13.3
Stewart [502], 1897	40	5	12.5
Bannatyne [13], 1898	293	26	8.9
Strangeways and Burt [510], 1907	200	48	24.0
Jones [286], 1909	240	2	0.8
Smith [479], 1932	102	10	9.8
Finney [180], 1947	100	12	12.0
Lewis-Faning [320], 1950	532	98	18.4
Present series (total)	293	31	10.6

and infection were recalled as precipitants by 4 patients. In 2 of these cases the sequence was sudden exposure followed by an upper respiratory infection in close proximity to the onset of arthritis.

14.19 Exposure to cold and dampness has long been thought to exert an adverse effect upon the symptomatology of rheumatoid arthritis, and attempts have been made to correlate meteorological conditions with subjective manifestations of the disease [362, 430]. In addition, various authors [183, 190, 199, 205, 271] since the time of Charcot [81] have considered exposure to be an important precipitating factor. The results from the seven papers in which numerical data were presented are listed in Table 14.14. In spite of some variation in the frequencies reported, the percentage obtained by combining the data is reasonably close to that found in the present series.*

OPERATION

14.20 Only 16 patients reported surgical operations antecedent to the onset of their arthritis—a frequency of 5.5 per cent. Table 14.15

---

* Two pieces of indirect evidence against there being a relationship between exposure and the development of rheumatoid arthritis are available. As outlined in Chapter 11, in our series an outdoor occupation did not appear to be associated with the development of rheumatoid arthritis any more than an indoor, while Finney et al. [180] were unable to discover a single case of rheumatoid arthritis among 1,200 American soldiers who had developed trench foot under combat conditions.

Precipitating Factors

Table 14.15
Types of operation preceding onset of rheumatoid arthritis among patients with history of surgery

Type of operation	No. of patients
Ear, nose, or throat	6
Pelvic	2
Bone or joint	2
Testicular tumor	1
Fistula in ano	1
Cataract	1
Thyroidectomy	1
Dental extractions	1
Drainage of carbuncle	1
Total	16

lists the types of operation with the largest number performed on the ears, sinuses, or tonsils. The interval between operation and the first evidence of arthritis was usually brief, but in 3 cases three, four, and six months had elapsed. No differences in the frequency of operation were found in respect to the age or sex of the patients, the presence or absence of spinal involvement, the type of onset, the total severity of the arthritis on admission, or the subsequent course both before and after admission. From 10 of the 16 patients, histories of one or more additional precipitating factors were elicited. The combination of infection and operation has been mentioned above, with the operation performed immediately before the onset and in treatment of the infectious process in all 5 instances. In 3 cases the patient had been under strain for some time before the operation, which took place shortly before the first signs of joint disease.

14.21 Ghrist and Hench [205] included surgical operation among the precipitating factors in rheumatoid arthritis, while Jones [286] referred to the onset of the disease following surgical procedures on the thyroid or ovaries. Only 1 of a series of 100 soldiers gave a history of an antecedent operation [180], but Smith [479] recorded a frequency of 5.9 per cent in 102 civilian patients—a figure closely corresponding to the one obtained in the present series. In line with Jones' [286] observations, 2 of Smith's [479] patients had thyroidectomies and 1 had a testicle removed. As shown in Table 14.15, only 1 of our patients had a thyroidectomy, but operations were performed on parts of the male or female genital system in 3 cases.

TRAUMA

14.22 Histories of trauma in association with the onset of arthritis were given by 15 patients—a frequency of 5.1 per cent. In 11 instances injuries to joints or neighboring skeletal structures were sustained from a fall, sprain, or direct blow. In the remainder, the injuries consisted in unusual strain to the back or arms from unaccustomed work, such as heavy lifting or wood-chopping. The injuries occurred within two months of the development of arthritis in all cases, and, in at least half, symptoms due to trauma merged without perceptible interval into those of arthritis. While coincidence cannot be entirely excluded in a given case when assessing the significance of trauma as a precipitating factor, in all but 1 of our patients the injury involved at least one of the joints first affected by arthritis. For this reason, trauma may be considered as at least operative in the localization of the arthritis in a particular joint [30, 199, 287, 295, 447, 483, 498].

14.23 No differences in the frequency of trauma were found in respect to the age or sex of the patients, the presence or absence of spinal involvement, the type of onset, the severity of the disease on admission, or the subsequent course before or after admission. In distinction to other precipitating factors, trauma was found less often in combination than alone. In 3 cases, however, a long period of occupational strain, with or without simultaneous exposure, had been present before the injury which occurred immediately before the onset.

14.24 A number of reports [30, 81, 133, 180, 190, 199, 498] have mentioned trauma as an infrequent precipitating factor in rheumatoid arthritis, and seven series [13, 167, 287, 295, 320, 447, 479] reported in the literature lend themselves to comparison with the present one (Table 14.16). As in the case of exposure, the percentage obtained by combining the data is fairly close to that found in our patients. In respect to antecedent trauma, the frequency of 8 per cent obtained by Buckley [59] in a series made up entirely of spondylitics is approximately the same as that (10.2 per cent) obtained by us for the patients with spondylitis in the present series. While no association between

Precipitating Factors

Table 14.16

Trauma as a precipitating factor in rheumatoid arthritis—present series compared with representative series from the literature

		Trauma present	
Source	No. of patients	No.	Per cent
Literature (total)	5,135	199	3.9
Bannatyne [*13*], 1898	293	7	2.4
Smith [*479*], 1932	102	8	7.8
Rydén [*447*], 1943	905	19	2.1
Jonsson and Berglund [*287*], 1949	1,669	12	0.7
Lewis-Faning [*320*], 1950	532	31	5.8
Kelly [*295*], 1951	600	50	8.3
Edström [*167*], 1952	1,034	72	7.0
Present series (total)	293	15	5.1

trauma and the onset of arthritis was found in one study of 200 patients [*510*], and in two others was believed to be purely coincidental [*271, 287*], analysis of our data and those shown in Table 14.16 lends support to the opinion that trauma is occasionally a precipitating or localizing factor in rheumatoid arthritis.

PREGNANCY

14.25 Of the 186 women in our series 4 experienced the onset of arthritis within four weeks after childbirth. The frequency of this precipitating factor was thus 2.1 per cent among all the women in the series and 7.4 per cent among the women whose arthritis began before the age of forty-five and who were known to be fertile. Although a certain amount of mental and physical strain is necessarily present after childbirth, 1 of the 4 women in the series gave a story of an unusual degree of mental strain at the time of and following her delivery. In 1 case joint involvement began after a miscarriage and in 1 case during the third month of pregnancy. In the latter instance acute exposure to cold was also cited as a precipitating factor.

14.26 Previous reports in the literature concerning the frequency of the onset of rheumatoid arthritis after childbirth [*13, 187, 199, 307, 510*] are in general agreement with our findings, and several authors have commented on the occurrence of the first manifestation of this disease after childbirth or miscarriage [*81, 205, 454, 514*] and on the relative rarity of onset during pregnancy [*81, 454*]. Data are presented in regard to the latter by four authors [*13, 199, 286, 479*], all of whom agree essentially with the frequency of 1.9 per cent obtained in fertile women in our series with arthritis starting before the age of forty-five. Lewis-Faning's [*320*] studies on the relationship of pregnancy to the disease are of particular interest, in that paired controls were used (see par. **14.9**). Of the 52 women who had borne children and whose arthritis began in the child-bearing age, the onset occurred less than one year after delivery in 19.2 per cent, while the comparable figure for 55 controls was 10.9 per cent. The difference is not significant, but Lewis-Faning stressed the advisability of collecting data on a larger series. Another important point brought out in his study was the lack of evidence that women with rheumatoid arthritis as a group had more children than did the general population of married women as represented by the controls.

14.27 That relapses in rheumatoid arthritis are common after delivery has also been noted in the literature [*454, 514*] and the strong likelihood of remissions during pregnancy is generally accepted [*255*]. In the cases apparently starting after delivery, it is possible, of course, that the disease was already present with its manifestations masked by the as yet unknown mechanism which is responsible for remissions in pregnancy. At any rate, the conclusion may be expressed that signs of rheumatoid arthritis occasionally arise after delivery or miscarriage, but less frequently appear during the pregnant state.

SUMMARY

14.28 About half the patients in the present series gave histories of one or more potentially disturbing events (so-called "precipitating factors") preceding the onset of a persistent arthritis. Strain was noted most commonly, with infection, exposure, operation, trauma, and childbirth, following in this order. Some gave histories of two or more; information concerning a total of 198 precipitating factors was elicited from 144 patients. The most common combination was strain of long duration before an onset immediately preceded by an infection, operation, or injury. When strain and exposure were both present, each factor was usually considered to be of occupational origin. In several

Precipitating Factors

instances, operation in treatment of an antecedent infection had been performed shortly before the arthritis began.

14.29 Of the five precipitating factors studied, infection alone was noted more frequently by patients with disease duration of one year or less than by the remainder. Analysis of the data indicates that this difference was not primarily due to the influence of memory but rather to the association between an antecedent infection and early severity of disease leading to a more rapid hospitalization. On the other hand, we found no evidence that the presence or absence of infection or any one of the other factors studied lends assistance in predicting the subsequent course.

14.30 Under the heading of strain, both mental and physical types were included. In most of the males but in only half of the females, the strain was believed to be of occupational origin. Of the patients whose arthritis was preceded by infection, the upper respiratory tract was the site in about 90 per cent. While exposure was usually of a chronic nature and often associated with occupation, certain patients gave histories of sudden exposure to severe cold or dampness shortly before the arthritis began. That trauma exercised at least a localizing function in certain instances was suggested by the finding in nearly all such cases that the injured joint was one of the first to be involved in the arthritic process. The arthritis began directly after delivery in 4 cases and after a miscarriage in 1, but during pregnancy in only 1.

14.31 Previous reports in the literature are largely in agreement with the results obtained in the present study in regard to the frequency of precipitating factors, except that several recent studies assign increasing importance to psychologic factors. More extensive studies are needed to determine the relationship of these as well as other factors to the onset and course of rheumatoid arthritis.

14.32 Objectives for further study:

1. Forward rather than retrospective observations on the so-called "precipitating factors," based on their relationship to alterations in the course of the disease following the actual onset.

2. Objective 2, par. 13.14.

15

Type of Onset

15.1 The type of onset in the patients of the present series showed wide variation, ranging from the insidious to the explosive. For the purpose of analysis, only two groups were recognized, the first termed "acute" and the second "gradual." In the group listed as having acute onset, the disease not only began suddenly, but also was so incapacitating that the patients were forced to bed, and, in a number of instances, fever and marked joint inflammation were present. In other words, the deciding criterion was the severity rather than the abruptness with which the disease began. In the remainder, the disease reached a stage sufficiently incapacitating to warrant hospitalization over a much longer period. In each patient, the final classification of type of onset was agreed upon by two observers.

15.2 In a minority of the patients, 21.8 per cent, the onset was classified as acute. Statements encountered in the literature [*133, 199, 251, 286, 356, 427*] are in general agreement that the disease more often starts gradually or insidiously. In one paper [*510*] which presents the actual figures on a series of 200 patients the proportion (17.5 per cent) with acute onset is very close to ours. Five other authors [*78, 307, 320, 333, 546*], however, have recorded a distinctly higher percentage of patients with an acute onset—42.3 per cent in a combined series of 1,464 cases of rheumatoid arthritis. Since the term "acute" as applied to the

Type of Onset

onset of arthritis in these patients was not defined, the reason for this disparity is not evident, but it may be inferred that acuteness connoted abruptness more often than severity.

15.3 As may be seen in Table 15.1, no significant difference in type of onset was encountered in male as compared with female patients, a finding confirmed by Lambert [307]. That an acute onset was more common in patients whose disease started before the age of forty is demonstrated in Table 15.2. No explanation is apparent for this finding, which was not confirmed by one of the studies mentioned above [320], either in regard to a febrile onset or to an acute as compared with an insidious onset. Since the author fails to define "acute," the discrepancy may actually lie in a difference in the meanings assigned to this word in the two series. As shown in Table 15.3, the frequency of an acute onset was higher in patients admitted to the hospital with disease duration of one year or less than in those with longer duration, and the same association was found when the patients were divided according to sex. It seems reasonable to assume that the relationship between early admission and an acute type of onset rests upon a disease of great initial severity leading to early hospitalization. Age at onset was not a factor, since the patients with arthritis of one year's duration or less and the patients with disease of longer duration were about equally divided with respect to onset before and after the age of forty. Nor, as brought out in the preceding chapter (par. **14.10**) can responsibility be assigned to the co-association of acute onset and shorter disease duration with antecedent infection. The last chapter also stressed the finding that infection was the only precipitating factor occurring in a larger proportion of patients with an acute as compared with a gradual onset of articular symptoms (Table 14.8). For example, strain, the precipitant most commonly reported by our patients, contrasted with infection in this as well as other associations.

15.4 As pointed out before, it seems likely that the actual onset of rheumatoid arthritis may coincide with the start of prodromal constitutional symptoms. Such symptoms may even precede abrupt and severe articular manifestations, as mentioned by Jones [286], and in fact were present in nearly half of our patients classified as having an acute onset. No association was found, however, between the type of

Table 15.1
Acute onset of rheumatoid arthritis among males and females of present series

Sex	No. of patients	Acute onset	
		No.	Per cent
Total	293	64	21.8
Males	107	23	21.5
Females	186	41	22.0

Table 15.2
Acute onset of rheumatoid arthritis in relation to age at onset among patients of present series

Age at onset	No. of patients	Acute onset	
		No.	Per cent
Total	293	64	21.8
Under 40	177	46	26.0
40 or more	116	18	15.5

Difference in percentages: 10.5 ± 4.9

Table 15.3
Acute onset in relation to duration of rheumatoid arthritis before hospital admission among patients of present series

Disease duration	No. of patients	Acute onset	
		No.	Per cent
Total	293	64	21.8
Shorter (1 year or less)	84	33	39.3
Longer (more than 1 year)	209	31	14.8

Difference in percentages: 24.5 ± 5.3

onset and the presence or absence of prodromal symptoms, since acute onset was found with approximately equal frequency in each group. A similar absence of association was recorded by Lewis-Faning [320] in respect to either an acute (undefined) or a febrile disease onset. In the next chapter (par. **16.12**) reference will be made to the absence of an essential difference in the distribution of primary joint involvement in patients with acute onset as compared with gradual onset. It is also interesting to note that the disease began acutely almost as often in patients with spinal involvement (with or without peripheral involvement) as in those with peripheral arthritis alone (Table 15.4). Other

Type of Onset

Table 15.4

Acute onset of rheumatoid arthritis in relation to presence or absence of spondylitis on hospital admission among patients of present series

Spondylitis	No. of patients	Acute onset No.	Per cent
Total	293	64	21.8
Present	41	7	17.1
Absent	252	57	22.6
		Difference in percentages:	5.5 ± 6.8

associations, which will be referred to in subsequent chapters, include those between acute onset and (1) fever while the patient was under hospital observation (par. 26.5), (2) the finding of subcutaneous nodules (par. 33.3), and (3) weakness or anorexia following onset (par. 21.4). It is not surprising that the last two constitutional symptoms should frequently follow an onset of acute type as herein defined. In women an association was also found between an onset of the gradual type and an onset occurring within two years of the menopause. This association is not found if only postmenopausal women, or women admitted between the ages of thirty-five and fifty-nine are considered. Lewis-Faning [320] found no difference in respect to the frequency of acute (undefined) or febrile onsets in women whose disease began within one year of the menopause and in the remaining postmenopausal females. Finally, the absence of association should be mentioned between acute onset and certain factors to be taken up in later chapters. These include a unilateral distribution of joint involvement at onset (par. 17.3) and the findings on admission of lymphadenopathy (par. 30.4), splenomegaly (par. 30.6), and anemia (par. 38.3).*

15.5 A question which might be asked is whether an abrupt, severe onset foretells a less favorable course, progressing eventually to a severe form of disease, or the reverse. Table 15.5 shows that an acute type of onset was more common in patients who experienced remissions before hospitalization than in those without remissions. However, both an acute onset and an intermittent course before hospitalization were found to be more common in patients with onset before the age of forty. Further analysis does not permit a decision in regard to the rela-

---

* For a complete list of associations, see Appendix Table 47.

Table 15.5

Acute onset of rheumatoid arthritis in relation to type of course before hospital admission among patients of present series, divided according to sex

Course before admission	No. of patients	Acute onset No.	Acute onset Per cent
*Total series**			
Total	293	64	21.8
Intermittent	80	25	31.2
Progressive	213	39	18.3
Males†			
Total	107	23	21.5
Intermittent	29	8	27.6
Progressive	78	15	19.2
*Females***			
Total	186	41	22.0
Intermittent	51	17	33.3
Progressive	135	24	17.8

* Difference in percentages: 12.9 ± 5.5
† Difference in percentages: 8.4 ± 8.8
** Difference in percentages: 15.5 ± 6.7

tive influence of any one of these three factors. When the patients were divided according to the total severity of their disease on admission, as shown in Table 15.6, mild, moderate, and marked severity occurred with approximately equal frequencies in patients with acute onset and patients with gradual onset. Similarly, in a study (Chapter 44) of the course of rheumatoid arthritis in 250 members of the series who received

Table 15.6

Total severity of rheumatoid arthritis in relation to type of onset among patients of present series

Type of onset	No. of patients	Total severity of arthritis*					
		Mild No.	Mild Per cent	Moderate No.	Moderate Per cent	Marked No.	Marked Per cent
Total	293	72	24.6	172	58.7	49	16.7
Acute	64	19	29.7	33	51.6	12	18.8
Gradual	229	53	23.2	139	60.7	37	16.2

$\chi^2 = 1.81; p > .3$

* See definition, par. **4.26**.

Type of Onset

only simple medical and orthopedic therapy, the type of onset apparently made no difference in the proportion considered improved at the time of last examination.

SUMMARY

15.6 An abrupt, severe onset was much less common than a gradual one in our series of patients. Acute onset occurred with equal frequency in males and females but more often in those whose disease began before the age of forty. Prodromal symptoms, which may mark the real beginning of the disease, were reported as frequently by those with an acute onset as by the remainder. Antecedent infection and early admission to the hospital were both associated to a significant degree with an acute type of onset. As far as could be ascertained from our data, the type of onset, whether acute or gradual, was of prognostic assistance only because of the association between an acute onset and an intermittent course before hospital admission.

15.7 Objective for further study:

Additional information in regard to the course pursued by patients with acute onset compared with those whose disease began gradually.

16

Joints First Involved

16.1 Enumeration of the primary sites of articular involvement has formed an integral part of the majority of clinical descriptions of rheumatoid arthritis. In some [183, 251, 252, 286, 427], only general statements have been set down as to the joints most commonly involved at the onset of disease; but, in others [199, 307, 321, 333, 454, 510], careful tabulations have been based on studies of patients comparable in number to the present series. While such information furnishes a certain amount of assistance in the early diagnosis of rheumatoid arthritis, the data which follow will point out that no joint or group of joints is uniformly the first to be attacked. More useful diagnostically is the tendency of the disease to exhibit a symmetrical pattern with involvement of corresponding joints on both sides of the body. The spine was primarily affected in 31 patients of the present series, while bilateral involvement, not necessarily of corresponding joints, was apparent from the beginning in 70 per cent of the 262 patients with onset in the peripheral joints. This important characteristic of the disease will be treated in detail in the next chapter, while the joints first involved will be considered here, irrespective of whether the involvement was unilateral or bilateral.

16.2 To permit statistical analysis and comparison with other series our data on initial joint involvement were arbitrarily arranged in

Joints First Involved

Table 16.1. The joints of the hands, feet, and wrists and the temporomandibular joints were grouped under the heading "Small joints," and the joints of the shoulders, elbows, hips, knees, and ankles under "Large joints." The disease process was considered to be "Monarticular" when no other joints were affected for a period of at least a week. Primary involvement of the neck was included under the heading "Spine," while the last heading, "Large and small," allowed for a rather uncommon combination. As may be seen in the table, small joints were initially involved more often than large joints by a rather narrow margin. However, the reverse is found if those with monarticular onset are not considered separately.

16.3 In view of the long interval frequently existing between the beginning of the arthritis and the time of questioning, in many instances from ten to twenty years, Table 16.2 was set up as a check upon the accuracy of the preceding table. But no essential differences emerged in regard to the distribution of primary joint involvement between the patients with disease dating back one year or less, whose memory should be relatively accurate, and the remainder.

16.4 Our finding that large and small joints were first involved with almost equal frequency runs counter to a long-prevailing clinical impression, supported by the authority of certain older writers [81, 183, 199, 286, 427], that the onset of rheumatoid arthritis is predominantly in the smaller articulations. Of six pertinent studies reported in the literature (Table 16.3), three are in agreement with our findings, while

Table 16.1

Frequency of initial involvement of groups of joints, single joints, and spine among patients of present series

Joint involvement	Patients No.	Per cent	Remarks
Small joints	109	37.2	(39.3 per cent if monarticular included)
Large joints	84	28.7	(42.3 per cent if monarticular included)
Monarticular	46	15.7	
Spine	31	10.6	
Large and small joints	23	7.8	
Total	293	100.0	

Table 16.2

Initial involvement of groups of joints, single joints, and spine in relation to duration of rheumatoid arthritis before hospital admission among patients of present series

Joint involvement	Shorter duration (1 year or less)		Longer duration (more than 1 year)	
	No.	Per cent	No.	Per cent
Small joints	33	39.3	76	36.4
Large joints	25	29.8	59	28.2
Monarticular	13	15.5	33	15.8
Spine	8	9.5	23	11.0
Large and small joints	5	6.0	18	8.6
Total	84	100.1	209	100.0

the remainder support the belief that initial involvement of small joints is distinctly more common. This difference in opinion may be partly explained by variations in the selection of patients and in the criteria for division of joints into "large" and "small," which are listed in the table under "Remarks." (In our series, large joints were more often involved in patients who had developed spondylitis at the time of admission but whose symptoms had begun in peripheral joints.) At any rate, the physician should not hesitate to entertain the diagnosis of rheumatoid arthritis in a patient with one or more large joints initially affected or in a patient with involvement only in the large joints. It might also be mentioned in passing that there are many more small joints in the body than large, with the spinal joints intermediate in number. If we think of rheumatoid arthritis in terms of exposure of synovial tissue to a noxious agent, the larger number of small joints might be balanced by the greater amount of this tissue in the larger articulations.

16.5   In Table 16.4 the individual joints first involved are listed in order of frequency. For this purpose the hands and feet, although each comprising multiple joints, are counted as units and initial spinal involvement and simultaneous involvement of different joints are classified separately. As shown in the table, the knees, feet, and hands head the list—50 per cent of the patients considered having been affected in one of these sites. A sex difference, to be referred to later, was also brought out in respect to primary involvement of the hands and of the spine. In other series of comparable size [*307, 454, 510*] the same three

Table 16.3

Initial involvement of small and large joints in rheumatoid arthritis—present series compared with representative series from the literature

		Involvement in				
		Small joints		Large joints		
Source	No. of patients	No.	Per cent	No.	Per cent	Remarks
Strangeways and Burt [510], 1907	168	83	49.4	85	50.6	
Lambert [307], 1908	150	74	49.3	76	50.7	
McCrae [333], 1915			43.0		57.0	Percentages only given; spondylitis excluded.
Sclater [454], 1943	288	167	58.3	121	41.7	Spondylitis excluded; involvement of finger or wrist joints required for inclusion in series.
Lewis-Faning and Fletcher [321], 1945	254	160	63.0	94	37.0	Spondylitis excluded.
Lewis-Faning [320], 1950	510	357	69.4	153	30.6	Spondylitis excluded; ankles included among small joints.
Present series	239	115	48.0	124	52.0	Initial involvement in spine (31 patients) and in both large and small joints (23 patients) excluded.

Table 16.4

Frequency of initial involvement of individual joints among males and females of present series

Joints initially involved	Total series		Males		Females		Difference in percentages
	No.	Per cent	No.	Per cent	No.	Per cent	
Knees	57	19.5	18	16.8	39	21.0	
Feet	46	15.7	17	15.9	29	15.6	
Hands	43	14.7	7	6.5	36	19.4	12.9 ± 4.3
Shoulders	15	5.1	5	4.7	10	5.4	
Ankles	13	4.4	3	2.8	10	5.4	
Wrists	8	2.7	1	0.9	7	3.8	
Hips	6	2.0	5	4.7	1	0.5	
Elbows	3	1.0	1	0.9	2	1.1	
Temporo-mandibular	1	0.3	1	0.9	0	0.0	
Spine	31	10.6	23	21.5	8	4.3	17.2 ± 3.7
Onset in 2 or more different locations	70	23.9	26	24.3	44	23.7	
Total	293	99.9	107	99.9	186	100.2	

joints made up the majority of those first affected, with the wrists, shoulders, and ankles next in line. In Table 16.5 the present series is compared with a combined series from the literature [307, 454, 510] in regard to the three articulations most commonly first affected. No striking differences emerged, except that in our series the hands and feet were first involved with about equal frequency, while in the combined series onset occurred more often in the hands. In each case initial involvement of the hands was more common in females than in males. This table may also serve to counteract statements in the literature to the effect that in the majority of patients rheumatoid arthritis is first apparent in the hands or in either the hands or the feet [81, 183, 251, 252, 286, 427, 510].

16.6 The pronouncement that the upper limbs are almost always the first to be attacked in rheumatoid arthritis has been ascribed to Charcot [82]. Evidence to the contrary was presented by McCrae [333], who concluded that many more patients have their first symptoms in a leg joint than in an arm joint. The data in Table 16.6 show that the lower extremities of our patients were more frequently involved at the onset of the disease. This difference was apparently greater in males than in females, and was accompanied by a higher frequency in spinal

Table 16.5

Frequency of initial involvement of knees, hands, and feet—males and females of present series compared with a combined series from the literature [307, 454, 510]

Source	No. of patients	No. of Males	No. of Females
Combined series (total)	668	187	481
Present series (total)	293	107	186

Joints	Series	Total No.	Total Per cent	Males No.	Males Per cent	Females No.	Females Per cent	Difference in percentages between males and females
Knees	combined	148	22.2	35	18.7	113	23.5	
	present	57	19.5	18	16.8	39	21.0	
Feet	combined	66	9.9	26	13.9	40	8.3	
	present	46	15.7	17	15.9	29	15.6	
Hands*	combined	191	28.6	30	16.0	161	33.4	17.4 ± 3.9
	present	43	14.7	7	6.5	36	19.4	12.9 ± 4.3
Hands and/or feet	combined	257	38.4	56	30.0	201	41.7	11.7 ± 4.2
	present	89	30.4	24	22.4	65	35.0	12.6 ± 6.2

* Difference in percentages between combined series and present series: 13.9 ± 3.0

Table 16.6

Frequency of initial joint involvement of upper and lower extremities and of spine among males and females of present series

Site of primary involvement*	Total series No.	Total series Per cent	Males No.	Males Per cent	Females No.	Females Per cent
Upper extremities	89	30.4	21	19.6	68	36.6
Lower extremities	140	47.8	51	47.7	89	47.8
Upper and lower extremities	33	11.3	12	11.2	21	11.3
Spine	31	10.6	23	21.5	8	4.3
Total	293	100.1	107	100.0	186	100.0

* Difference in percentages between primary involvement of upper and lower extremities: total series—17.4 ± 4.0; males—28.1 ± 6.5; females—11.2 ± 5.1

involvement. In two other series [454, 510] the disease started with approximately equal frequency in arm and leg joints, but Lambert's [307] and McCrae's [333] figures are in essential agreement with those in Table 16.6. The conclusion may be drawn from the combined data that rheumatoid arthritis is at least as likely to start in the legs as in the arms, and the possibility should be kept in mind that onset in the feet may be overlooked and the symptoms there assigned to foot strain.

16.7 That the distribution of joint involvement in rheumatoid arthritis is usually bilateral and often symmetrical has already been mentioned. A further characteristic is the tendency of the disease process to be polyarticular from the beginning. Atypical forms, however, involving one or a few joints, have been recognized [113, 225, 251, 325, 463, 474]. The disease began in single joints in 46 patients of the present series, or nearly one-sixth of the total number. Although monarticular onset was found to vary in frequency from 32 to 42 per cent in three other series [307, 320, 510], the authors do not state whether the process had been monarticular for at least a week—the period used as the criterion for monarticular onset in our patients. Table 16.7 shows the joints affected among the patients with monarticular onset. In both the present series and a combined series from the literature [307, 510] the knee joint was by far the most frequently involved; the others, chiefly large joints, were involved with about the same frequency. As noted in the table, no definite predilection was shown for either side of the body in the two series. Among our 46 patients the arthritis remained monarticular for periods ranging from one week to eighteen years. In 22 patients other joints were involved within a month; in 17, within one year; and in the remaining 7, the disease was confined to a single joint for over a year. In only 3 patients, however, was the process monarticular on admission. The occasional persistence of rheumatoid arthritis in one joint is exemplified in Smith's [474] series of 24 patients by duration of monarticular involvement ranging from a few months to ten years. In each of these patients tuberculosis or infectious arthritis due to some other agent was effectively excluded by biopsy. In some of those with initial involvement in a single joint, the arthritis subsided for a time before other joints were attacked. This was the case in 13 of our 46 patients, in about half of whom the remission lasted a year or more before

Joints First Involved

Table 16.7
Frequency of individual joints involved and lateral distribution in monarticular onset—present series compared with a combined series from the literature [307, 510]

	Patients with monarticular onset			
	Combined series		Present series	
Joint involvement	No.	Per cent	No.	Per cent
Knee	48	39.0	25	54.3
Shoulder	17	13.8	7	15.2
Wrist	21	17.1	4	8.7
Hip	16	13.0	3	6.5
Ankle	14	11.4	3	6.5
Elbow	7	5.7	2	4.3
Metatarso-phalangeal	0	0.0	1	2.2
Temporo-mandibular	0	0.0	1	2.2
Total	123	100.0	46	99.9
Right side of body	58	47.2	27	58.7
Left side of body	65	52.9	19	41.3

joint symptoms reappeared. These were located in the joints originally involved with slightly less frequency than in new ones. Rheumatoid arthritis, then, should occupy a high place in the differential diagnosis of a persistent or remittent monarticular arthritis, unless there is specific evidence of an infectious or gouty etiology. One author [225], in fact, found that persistent arthritis involving one or a few joints in children is more commonly "nonspecific" (presumably rheumatoid) than due to tuberculosis or syphilis.

16.8   The arthritis first attacked the spine in 31 patients of the present series, or about 10 per cent. The frequency was higher than in four other series [307, 320, 333, 510], probably because the patients eventually developing rheumatoid spondylitis were excluded from these series. Two-thirds of our patients whose arthritis first appeared in the spine were classified on admission in the group with spondylitis and had typical roentgenographic changes in the sacro-iliac joints. On the other hand, in about half the group with spondylitis, the process began in one or more peripheral joints. The joints first involved in the 41 patients with spondylitis on admission are summarized in Table 16.8. It may be noted that the disease began only once in the upper extremities

Table 16.8

Frequency of initial involvement of individual joints among patients having spondylitis at time of hospital admission

Joint involvement	Patients	
	No.	Per cent
Spine	22	53.7
Feet	5	12.2
Hip(s)	4*	9.8
Knees	4*	9.8
Hips and knees	2	4.9
Ankles, hips, and knees	1	2.4
Temporo-mandibular	1*	2.4
Shoulders	1	2.4
Ankles	1	2.4
Total	41	100.0

* Indicates 3 patients who had initial monarticular involvement in hip, knee, and temporo-mandibular joints, respectively.

and then in the shoulders rather than in the elbows, wrists, or hands. These findings have been confirmed in a series of 1,035 patients with rheumatoid spondylitis studied at the Mayo Clinic [413], except that in the latter series a smaller proportion, 23.4 per cent, experienced onset in the peripheral joints. In 13 per cent of these the process was monarticular in the beginning. A marked predilection for involvement of the lower extremities was also found in the prespondylitic phase, with the initial arthritis confined to upper extremity articulations in only 4 per cent of these patients.

16.9   Table 16.9 shows the frequency of onset in groups of joints in respect to sex. Significant differences may be seen only under "Small joints" and "Spine." Regarding the former, some predilection is also shown for females in four other series [307, 321, 454, 510], but to a significant degree in only one [454]. This increased frequency of small joint involvement in females evidently depends upon a similar finding in regard to primary hand involvement (Tables 16.4 and 16.5). Furthermore, the greater tendency in other series for arthritis to start in the feet of males (Table 16.5) may account for the lack of significant findings in the sex frequency of primary small joint involvement. That males should far outnumber females among patients with arthritis origi-

Joints First Involved

Table 16.9
Frequency of initial involvement of groups of joints, single joints, and spine among males and females of present series

Joint involvement	Males		Females		Difference in percentages
	No.	Per cent	No.	Per cent	
Small joints	28	26.2	81	43.5	17.3 ± 5.9
Large joints	30	28.0	54	29.0	
Monarticular	19	17.8	27	14.5	
Spine	23	21.5	8	4.3	17.2 ± 3.7
Large and small joints	7	6.5	16	8.6	
Total	107	100.0	186	100.0	

$\chi^2 = 25.42; p < .001$

nating in the spine is not surprising in view of the large proportion of males who were found to have spondylitis on admission.

16.10 Patients with onset before and after the age of forty were compared with respect to initial involvement of various groups of joints (Table 16.10). No significant difference was observed between the older and younger groups. Except that a monarticular onset was more common in females whose disease began before rather than after the age of forty, no information of statistical significance was obtained from tabulating the distribution of primary joint involvement in males and females divided according to age at onset.

Table 16.10
Initial involvement of groups of joints, single joints, and spine in relation to age at onset of rheumatoid arthritis among patients of present series

Joint involvement	Age at onset			
	Under 40		40 or more	
	No.	Per cent	No.	Per cent
Small joints	60	33.9	49	42.2
Large joints	49	27.7	35	30.2
Monarticular	33	18.6*	13	11.2
Spine	21	11.9	10	8.6
Large and small	14	7.9	9	7.8
Total	177	100.0	116	100.0

$\chi^2 = 4.6; 0.5 > p > 0.3$

* Monarticular onset was significantly more frequent in females whose disease began before the age of 40 than in those with later onset.

Table 16.11

Initial involvement of groups of joints, single joints, and spine in relation to type of course before hospital admission among patients of present series

	Type of course				Difference in percentages
	Intermittent		Progressive		
Joint involvement	No.	Per cent	No.	Per cent	
Small joints	22	27.8	87	40.7	12.9 ± 6.4
Large joints	26	32.9	58	27.1	
Monarticular	19	24.1	27	12.6	11.5 ± 4.7
Spine	5	6.3	26	12.1	
Large and small joints	7	8.9	16	7.5	
Total	79	100.0	214	100.0	

$\chi^2 = 10.08; .05 > p > .02$

16.11 The patients in the present series were also divided according to whether the course of the disease was intermittent* or progressive before hospital admission. Table 16.11 sets forth the groups of joints primarily affected in each division. A significant association was found between initial joint involvement and type of course before admission, due largely to a relationship between small joints and a progressive course (irrespective of whether joints of the hands or feet were the ones primarily attacked) and between monarticular onset and a course marked by remissions. Reference has already been made (par. **16.7**) to the long remissions taking place in a certain number of patients while the arthritis was still in a monarticular phase. Otherwise, the distribution of primary joint involvement afforded no assistance in prognosis, as far as total severity† on admission and the subsequent course were concerned.

16.12 In Table 16.12 the distribution of initial joint involvement is tabulated in patients whose arthritis was immediately preceded by so-called "precipitating factors," an aspect of the course of rheumatoid arthritis discussed in Chapter 14. No significant differences from the distribution of joints first involved in the whole series were evident in patients with either strain or infection before onset. In patients with the remaining three precipitating factors, some striking deviations were found, but the groups were so small that chance variation cannot be

---

* See definition, par. **4.13**.

† See definition, par. **4.26**.

Table 16.12

Initial involvement of groups of joints, single joints, and spine in relation to various precipitating factors among patients of present series

	No. of patients	Groups of joints								Monarticular		Spine	
		Small		Large		Large and small							
		No.	Per cent	No.	Per cent	No.	Per cent			No.	Per cent	No.	Per cent
Total	293	109	37.2	84	28.7	23	7.8			46	15.7	31	10.6
Type of precipitant					Distribution of precipitants								
Strain	80	30	37.5	21	26.2	7	8.8			11	13.7	11	13.7
Infection	49	18	36.7	16	32.7	5	10.2			7	14.3	3	6.1
Exposure	31	9	29.0	7	22.6	0	0.0			9	29.0	6	19.4
Surgery	16	9	56.2	1	6.2	0	0.0			2	12.5	4	25.0
Trauma	15	5	33.3	1	6.7	0	0.0			5	33.3	4	26.7

excluded as the explanation. The distribution of joints first involved was also essentially the same irrespective of the type of onset, whether acute or gradual. We were unable to confirm Lewis-Faning's [320] finding that a polyarticular onset is related to a history of prodromal symptoms, but we agree that onset near the menopause is not related to initial involvement of a single joint or of more than one. Finally, the type of primary joint involvement was apparently not associated in our series with the development of fever (par. 26.3), lymphadenopathy (par. 30.4), or subcutaneous nodules (par. 33.3).*

16.13   In the introductory section of the monograph, devoted chiefly to a definition of rheumatoid arthritis as a disease entity, the pertinent literature was summarized in regard to the place of an atypical form of rheumatoid arthritis variously termed "infectious," "secondary," or "focal" (par. 2.101). The criteria for the recognition of this type of arthritis may be listed as follows: an antecedent infection; an abrupt, febrile onset; unilateral involvement of one or a few large joints; a tendency to remission; and the absence of constitutional symptoms. Two of these criteria have already been taken up in the series analysis (par. 14.11 and Chapter 15), and the remainder will be discussed in subsequent chapters (Chapters 17, 19, and 21). At this point, however, their inter-relationships will be outlined and an attempt made to determine whether or not an atypical form of rheumatoid arthritis emerges, which, from a study of the literature, seemingly constitutes merely a stage in the development of a more typical form of the disease.

16.14   Table 16.13 shows the positive and negative associations* among these criteria, and a brief discussion of each factor may be found below.

1. ANTECEDENT INFECTION (Chapter 14). Reference has already been made (par. 14.11) to a suggestive difference between onset preceded by strain and that preceded by infection, due to the absence of similar associations with other factors. In Table 16.13 antecedent infection is associated only with acute onset.

2. ONSET ACUTE (Chapter 15). In addition to antecedent infection, this factor is associated with an intermittent course before admission and also with weakness and anorexia. As pointed out before (par. 15.4),

* For a complete list of associations, see Appendix Table 47.

Joints First Involved

Table 16.13
Associations among commonly applied criteria for the "infectious" type of rheumatoid arthritis

Criterion	Associations
Infection preceding onset	Onset acute
Onset acute	Infection preceding onset Intermittent course before admission Weakness Anorexia
Onset unilateral	Absence of anorexia
Onset monarticular	Intermittent course before admission Absence of anorexia
Onset in large joints	None
Course intermittent before admission	Onset acute Onset monarticular Absence of tremor

it seems likely that these constitutional symptoms would accompany a severe type of onset.

3. ONSET UNILATERAL (Chapter 17), MONARTICULAR, OR IN LARGE JOINTS. No study was made in the present series of primary involvement of a few as compared with many joints, but onset in one joint is considered in the table along with unilateral onset and onset in large joints. Positive associations were found only between monarticular onset and intermittent course, but negative associations were found between anorexia and both monarticular and unilateral onset.

4. INTERMITTENT COURSE (Chapter 19). Associations between this factor and both acute and monarticular onset have already been mentioned. There was also a negative association with one neurological symptom, tremor.

16.15 Although there are a certain number of pertinent positive and negative associations among the criteria listed in Table 16.13, this evidence seems insufficient to identify an atypical "infectious" stage of rheumatoid arthritis. From the data presented, at least, no support is given to the rigid subdivision of the disease into primary and secondary, typical and atypical, or atrophic and "infectious" forms. As Jones

[286] pointed out, endless transitional forms exist between the "infectious" and the more typical cases. Follow-up observations in this clinic [550] and elsewhere [74, 251] have demonstrated that many patients whose disease begins in an atypical form may eventually go on to a typical progressive polyarthritis. As concluded from the survey of the literature (par. 2.103), the "infectious" type probably represents a stage of rheumatoid arthritis that is seen relatively early in its course and one in which the prognosis is more favorable for at least temporary remission. Nevertheless, the recognition of an "infectious" stage can at times serve a useful purpose, both in diagnosis and prognosis.

SUMMARY

16.16 According to the evidence of the present study, rheumatoid arthritis does not invariably or even usually begin in the small articulations of the hands and feet. The patients of the present series experienced initial involvement of the large and small joints with about equal frequency (40 per cent in each instance). The rest (20 per cent) experienced onset in both types of joints or in the spine. Small joints were first attacked more commonly in females than in males, a finding associated with the greater proportion of females whose disease began in the joints of the hands. No difference was observed in the distribution of primary joint involvement among patients with onset before or after the age of forty. A higher frequency of small joint onset was found in patients who ran a progressive course before hospital admission than in those with exacerbations and remissions, but monarticular onset was more common in the latter group. Otherwise the type of initial articular involvement was not of prognostic assistance. There were no significant differences in the distribution of primary joint involvement in respect to the presence or absence of prodromal symptoms or to an acute as opposed to a gradual onset. The precipitating factors studied in Chapter 14 were distributed according to chance in regard to the groups of joints first involved.

16.17 The knee joints were most commonly involved, with the joints of the hands and feet next in order. About half the patients of the series experienced onset in one of these three locations, but less than a third had primary involvement of hands or feet. In the present series,

Joints First Involved

contrary to the majority opinion expressed in the literature, onset was more common in the joints of the legs than in those of the upper extremities. In about one-sixth of our patients, the disease first appeared in a single joint, most often the knee, and did not involve other sites for at least a week. As noted by others, this monarticular stage may persist and occasion difficulty in formulating the final diagnosis. The spine was first affected in 10 per cent of the patients, the majority of whom developed obvious spondylitis. On the other hand, in about half of those with spondylitis at the time of admission, the disease had begun in peripheral joints, almost invariably the joints of the lower extremities. This finding, which was independently arrived at in another series [413], furnishes a valuable addition to the clinical description of rheumatoid arthritis involving the spine.

16.18 The concept of an atypical, "infectious" form of rheumatoid arthritis has not been definitely established by testing for associations among the criteria usually assigned to this stage of the disease. Follow-up observations have proved more useful in its recognition and in defining its relationship to the more typical, progressive forms.

16.19 Objectives for further study:

1. Additional observations of the subsequent course of patients who are apparently in an atypical, "infectious" stage of rheumatoid arthritis.

2. Explanation of differences in the initial localization of the arthritis, with special attention to the role of trauma, over-use, and psychological factors.

17

Unilateral and Bilateral Joint Involvement

17.1 "In 1836, when attending the medical practice of the Middlesex Hospital, my attention was arrested by several cases of rheumatism, in which, as the disease passed into a chronic state, corresponding parts of the limbs became affected in pairs, in perfectly symmetrical order." Thus Budd [62] recorded one of the early observations of the marked tendency of rheumatoid arthritis to involve corresponding joints on opposite sides of the body. Later authors [199, 286, 427] have confirmed this observation and extended the symmetry to nodules and tenosynovitis [564].

17.2 The patients in the present series were questioned in regard to whether the disease was bilateral at the time of onset, was unilateral for at least a week only to become bilateral, or remained unilateral until admission. (Whether or not exactly corresponding joints were simultaneously affected at the start of the arthritis could not be determined reliably in many instances.) The findings are shown in Table 17.1 in regard to the patients without spinal involvement. Those with spondylitis on admission were excluded, although in half of these 41 patients peripheral joints were affected, usually bilaterally, before the spine. It is evident from the table that in nearly 30 per cent the arthritis was limited to one side at onset and therefore could hardly involve corresponding opposite joints, but, by the time of admission,

Unilateral and Bilateral Joint Involvement

Table 17.1

Lateral distribution of joint involvement among patients of present series without spondylitis on hospital admission (see par. 17.2 for explanation of groups)

Type of onset		Patients No.	Per cent
Group I	Bilateral at onset	178	70.6
Group II	Unilateral becoming bilateral	60*	23.8
Group III	Unilateral on admission	14	5.6
Total		252	100.0

* Includes 1 patient with onset in spine and right shoulder and 1 patient with unilateral peripheral joint involvement following onset in the spine.

joints on both sides of the body showed involvement in all but a very few cases. We have also tried to answer from our data the question as to how long the arthritis remained unilateral. The findings show a wide variation, from one week to eighteen years, with the majority becoming bilateral within six months (Table 17.2). Among the 14 patients with unilateral disease on admission (Table 17.1), the duration before hospital admission varied between a few days and five years, with the median figure 5.5 months. One of the present authors [463], in a study of 132 American soldiers with rheumatoid arthritis, found 13.2 per cent with arthritis confined to one side of the body. In half of these, the arthritis was of long duration, averaging ten years. It may thus be concluded that, although rheumatoid arthritis is typically a bilateral disease,

Table 17.2

Duration of unilateral joint involvement before bilateral arthritis became apparent among patients of Group II (see Table 17.1)

Duration	Patients No.	Per cent
6 months or less	34	56.7
1 year to 6 months	10	16.7
2 years to 1 year	9	15.0
5 years to 2 years	4	6.7
10 years to 5 years	2	3.3
Over 10 years	1	1.7
Total	60	100.1
Mean: 1.4 years		
Median: 6 months		

it may remain strictly unilateral over long periods in a small proportion of patients.

17.3   For the purposes of statistical analysis, Groups II and III in Table 17.1 were joined together and compared with Group I. For convenience, the latter will henceforth be designated the Bilateral Group and the remainder the Unilateral. A higher proportion of males was found in the Unilateral Group than in the Bilateral Group (Table 17.3), whereas the reverse was true of females. As explained below, the strength of this association is open to question. Although no differences were observed in respect to age on admission, onset of the disease under the age of forty was observed more often in the Unilateral Group (Table 17.4). Another distinction between the two groups was found in regard to a history of prodromal symptoms. Table 17.5 shows a higher frequency of patients with prodromata among those with bilateral onset. It must be remembered, however, that the patients with prodromal symptoms and those with bilateral arthritis from the beginning showed significantly higher proportions of females. Further analysis of the data revealed that only the association between prodromata and female sex distribution remained valid when the three variables were considered simultaneously. Comparison of the two groups in regard to the total severity* of the arthritis on admission brought out one further difference between the two groups (Table 17.6). The Unilateral Group included a significantly higher proportion of patients with mild severity and a lower proportion with moderate severity, while those with marked severity appeared in both groups in about equal frequency. No differences were noted between the two groups in respect to other factors tested. These included: course (both before and after admission), type of onset, duration of arthritis before admission, primary involvement of large or small joints, and strain or infection as precipitating factors.† From our data, then, we may characterize the patient with unilateral onset as more likely to be a male with arthritis starting before the age of forty and with a relatively milder disease process on admission.

17.4   Numerical data on the proportion of patients with bilateral arthritis at the onset of disease are few, and there are no precise state-

---

* See definition, par. **4.26**.

† For a complete list of associations, see Appendix Table 47.

Table 17.3
Proportion of males among patients with bilateral and with unilateral joint involvement (see Table 17.1)

Type of involvement	No. of patients	No. of males	Percentage of males
Total	252	75	29.8
Bilateral (Group I)	178	46	25.8
Unilateral (Groups II and III)	74	29	39.2

Difference in percentages: 13.4 ± 6.3

Table 17.4
Age at onset in relation to lateral distribution of joint involvement among patients of present series (see Table 17.1)

Type of involvement	No. of patients	Onset before age 40 No.	Onset before age 40 Per cent
Total	252	147	58.0
Bilateral (Group I)	178	96	53.9
Unilateral (Groups II and III)	74	51	68.9

Difference in percentages: 15.0 ± 6.8

Table 17.5
History of prodromal symptoms in relation to lateral distribution of joint involvement among patients of present series (see Table 17.1)

Type of involvement	No. of patients	History of prodromata No.	History of prodromata Per cent
Total	252	126	50.0
Bilateral (Group I)	178	97	54.5
Unilateral (Groups II and III)	74	29	39.2

Difference in percentages: 15.3 ± 6.9

Table 17.6
Total severity of rheumatoid arthritis in relation to lateral distribution of joint involvement (see Table 17.1)

Type of involvement	No. of patients	Total severity Mild No.	Total severity Mild Per cent	Total severity Moderate No.	Total severity Moderate Per cent	Total severity Marked No.	Total severity Marked Per cent
Total	252	67	26.6	144	57.0	41	16.3
Bilateral	178	33	18.5	114	64.0	31	17.4
Unilateral	74	34	45.9	30	40.5	10	13.5

Difference in percentages: 27.4 ± 6.1 ; 23.5 ± 6.8
$\chi^2 = 20.24; p < .01$

ments available in regard to the length of time required for the unilateral involvement to become bilateral. Three authors [126, 307, 510] have enumerated the proportion of patients with bilateral joint involvement from the beginning in series numbering respectively 180, 200, and 1,002 patients. In each instance, the proportion was about 50 per cent, a figure somewhat lower than that found in the present series. In two [126, 307], females were present in significantly higher frequency in the group with bilateral onset. In regard to coincidental involvement of corresponding joints, Jones [286] has stated that "in the majority of cases at first the disease is asymmetrical," with symmetry at the onset or rapidly arrived at only in swiftly progressive forms.

17.5   Although over a hundred years have passed since Budd's [62] description of symmetry in rheumatoid arthritis, a plausible explanation of the reasons for or mechanism of this distribution has yet to appear. From an historical point of view, it may be noted that this symmetry has been cited as one point of evidence in favor of the neural origin of rheumatoid arthritis [13, 199, 286, 394, 490]. These authors evidently assumed a bilateral disturbance in the nervous system with peripheral effects on the joints, although many known diseases of the nervous system are unilateral or asymmetrical. Even with the usual bilateral involvement of the posterior roots and cord in tabes, the resultant Charcot joints are more often unilateral [488, 565].

17.6   The nervous system could also participate in a secondary manner in the determination of symmetrical articular localization. With the disease process once established in a single joint, alterations in the physiology of the corresponding joint on the other side might be set up through a contralateral reflex path, with spread across the cord. In this way, the opposite joint might at least be rendered more susceptible to a chemical or infectious agent. An argument against this theory is contained in the fact that successive involvement of the opposite joint is relatively uncommon in the arthritides of known origin. Specific joint infections, with the notable exception of the symmetrical synovitis of of the knees in congenital syphilis, are usually monarticular or, if more than one site is involved, not characteristically symmetrical. Traumatic arthritis, regardless of the severity, is not observed to spread to the corresponding articulation on the other side (although, as pointed out by

Unilateral and Bilateral Joint Involvement

Kelly [295], if rheumatoid arthritis developed in the injured joint, in nearly half of his series of 30 patients the second joint involved was the fellow of the injured one). With the same true of a metabolic disease, like gout, we possess no analogous process in three important joint diseases of recognized cause. However, since the etiologic agent of rheumatoid arthritis is unknown, such a mechanism is possible, being dependent upon a specific attribute of the disease, rather than upon a process common to many joint disorders.

17.7   The fact that the joints make up an organ system which is uniformly distributed to both sides of the body hardly explains the symmetry of lesions in rheumatoid arthritis, although a high frequency of bilateral involvement would be expected. Other bilateral organs, including the lungs, eyes, and kidneys, may suffer from either unilateral or bilateral pathologic changes. Whether one or both of these paired structures is affected would seem to depend more on the individual nature of the etiologic agent or the tissue susceptibility of the host than on the simple fact that they are found on both sides of the body. Arthritis forms no exception to this situation, with primary degenerative joint disease, the symmetrical synovitis of congenital syphilis, the arthritis accompanying disseminated lupus and scleroderma, and pulmonary osteo-arthropathy the only important types, in addition to rheumatoid arthritis, that are usually symmetrical. Unless we assume, without evidence, that the symmetry of rheumatoid arthritis represents a peripheral effect of a bilateral disturbance in the nervous or vascular systems, or both, we must conclude that symmetry constitutes an interesting but unexplained characteristic of the disease, which, to be sure, is of great diagnostic value.

17.8   An interesting discussion of the underlying basis for symmetry in rheumatoid arthritis and other diseases was presented by Sir James Paget [396] in 1842 in the same volume in which Budd's [62] observations on symmetry were published. Symmetrical disease appeared, he believed, under three conditions. The first was degeneration of tissue from age or malnutrition, consistent with what we have since observed in the symmetrical nature of degenerative joint disease. A second was "metastasis" from one joint or organ to the corresponding opposite, a possibility which has been taken up in a preceding paragraph. The third presupposed circulation of a morbid agent, the effects of which are localized in symmetrical tissues. The reason for this localization is that corresponding parts on opposite sides of the body are the only parts with the identical tissue properties which render them susceptible to the harmful agent. If it should be found that such a circulating factor sets in motion the train of pathologic events which result in rheumatoid arthritis, then Paget's third hypothesis should be considered in attempting to explain the symmetrical nature of this disease.

SUMMARY

17.9 In 30 per cent of the patients in the present series the arthritis had been unilateral at the start but in nearly all had become bilateral by the time of admission. Evidence is presented, however, that the arthritis may remain unilateral in a small proportion of cases for as long as five or ten years. The group with unilateral onset showed a predilection for the male sex, an onset under the age of forty, and a milder total severity of arthritis on admission.

17.10 The symmetrical distribution of rheumatoid arthritis, with involvement of corresponding joints on opposite sides of the body, constitutes one of the outstanding clinical features of this disease and a very helpful aid in diagnosis. Theories of the mechanism of symmetry have been reviewed but an adequate explanation of this characteristic must in all probability await the discovery of the etiologic agent.

17.11 Objectives for further study:

1. Investigation of the mechanism of symmetrical joint involvement in rheumatoid arthritis, including observations on corresponding joints in various forms of experimental arthritis as well as in rheumatoid patients with unilateral involvement.

2. Additional data on symmetry in tenosynovitis, nodule formation, atrophy and pigmentation of the skin, and atrophy of muscles.

18

Age of Patients on Hospital Admission and Duration of Disease before Admission

AGE ON ADMISSION

18.1 The patients in the present series were admitted to the hospital at widely varying ages, ranging from 11 years to 72 years. In the accompanying tables and charts, the ages on admission are divided into five-year groups and actual frequencies compared with expected frequencies based on Census figures for the age distribution of the Massachusetts population in 1930. In males (Table 18.1 and Fig. 18.1) admission was most common in the 30–34 age group but there was no significant departure, as shown in the chi-square test, from the Massachusetts population. As presented in Table 6.1, a similar finding was obtained in respect to age at onset in males, with the 25–29 age group most heavily represented. In females, as was the case in regard to age at onset, age on admission differed significantly from the age distribution of the Massachusetts population (Table 18.2 and Fig. 18.2). The marked increase in the 50–54 and 55–59 age groups corresponded to the increase in age at onset in the 50–54 age group (Table 6.2). The decrease from the expected frequency in the 15–19 age group may reflect the generally admitted relative infrequency of rheumatoid arthritis in childhood (par. **6.7**). When the sex ratio for age on admission is computed by decades, a 2:1 ratio, with females predominating, is obtained in the fifth decade and in patients admitted from the age of 60 on. The ratio

Table 18.1

Age on hospital admission—males of present series compared with male population of Massachusetts in 1930

Age group	Census Per cent	Present series No.	Present series Per cent
15–19	12.3	7	6.6
20–24	11.1	14	13.2
25–29	10.4	15	14.2
30–34	10.5	18	17.0
35–39	11.1	9	8.5
40–44	10.0	6	5.7
45–49	8.9	12	11.3
50–54	7.8	8	7.5
55–59	6.6	8	7.5
60–64	5.2	4	3.8
65–69	3.7	3	2.8
70–74	2.4	2	1.9
Total	100.0	106*	100.0

$\chi^2 = 13.31; p > 0.2$

* Patients admitted before the age of 15 were not tabulated because most of those under 12 were assigned to a separate pediatrics service.

Table 18.2

Age on hospital admission—females of present series compared with female population of Massachusetts in 1930

Age group	Census Per cent	Present series No.	Present series Per cent
15–19	11.8	9	5.0
20–24	11.6	18	9.9
25–29	10.9	14	7.7
30–34	10.6	13	7.2
35–39	10.9	21	11.6
40–44	9.4	21	11.6
45–49	8.6	11	6.1
50–54	7.6	27	14.9
55–59	6.5	30	16.6
60–64	5.3	7	3.9
65–69	4.0	7	3.9
70–74	2.8	3	1.7
Total	100.0	181*	100.1

$\chi^2 = 56.13; p < .01$

* See note on Table 18.1.

Age and Disease Duration

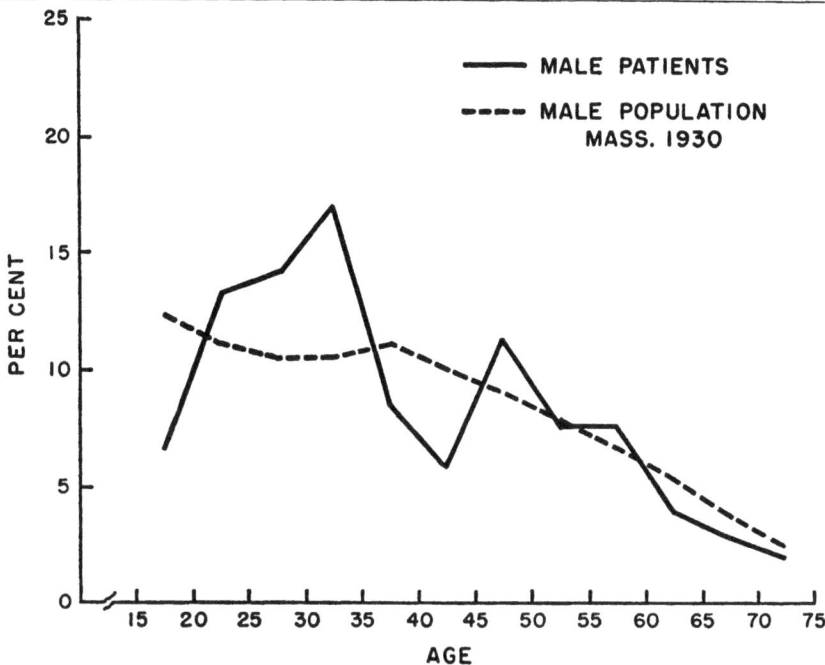

Figure 18.1 Percentage distribution of ages at hospital admission of 106 male patients with rheumatoid arthritis compared with expected frequencies based on the 1930 Massachusetts Census figures. (Although the chart shows an excess of admissions between the ages of 30 and 35 and a decline from the population percentage between the ages of 40 and 45, these variations lack significance, as shown in Table 18.1)

rises to 3:1 in the 50–59 age group, while female predominance decreased markedly in the third and fourth decades. The last finding is related to the 41 spondylitics in the present series, 20 of whom were males aged 20 to 40 at the time of admission. Males in general tended to be admitted at an earlier age than females, with the median age of admission 35 years (37 years with spondylitis excluded) compared with 43 years in women. As noted in Table 5.1, a similar difference was observed in the median age at onset of the two sexes.

18.2   Table 18.3 lists the associations of certain factors with age 40 or over on admission.* That males tended to enter the hospital at a younger age has already been mentioned and may be related to the

* For a complete list of associations, see Table 47 in the Appendix.

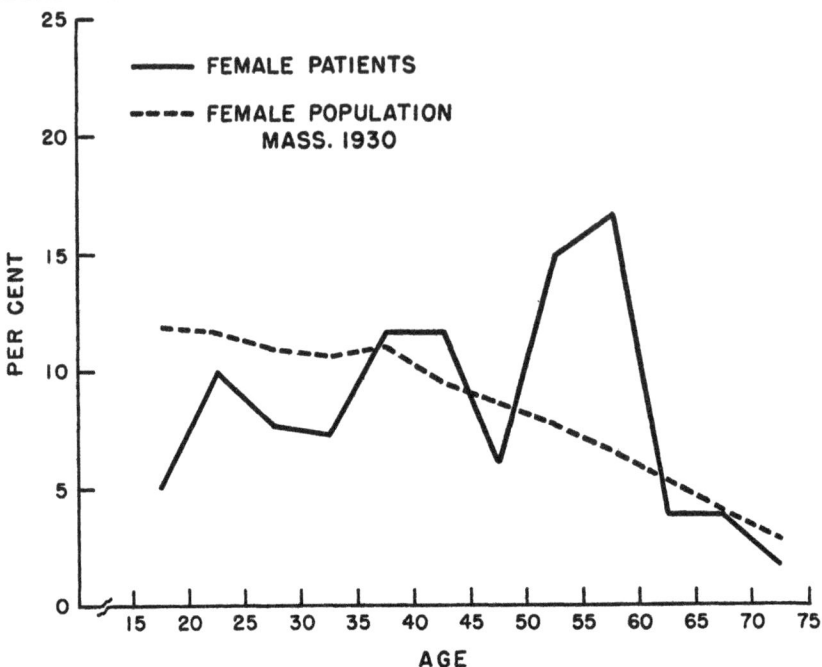

Figure 18.2 Percentage distribution of ages at hospital admission of 181 female patients with rheumatoid arthritis compared with expected frequencies based on the 1930 Massachusetts Census figures

predominance of males among patients with spondylitis. The association of age on admission with age at onset is to be expected and probably accounts for the degree of association recorded in factors preceding or connected with the onset of arthritis. Those listed in the table include prodromata, strain, and infection as precipitating factors, joints first involved, and acute onset. Association of age 40 or over on admission with increased disease duration before admission was one that seemed likely, but, as shown in the table, mutual associations between the two factors were not consistently found. As one example, an intermittent course before admission, which often included prolonged remissions, was related to increased disease duration but not to older age either at onset or on admission. A similar difference was also apparent in the case of spondylitis. That disease activity* showed no tendency to abate

* See definition, par. 4.27.

Age and Disease Duration

Table 18.3
Association of certain factors with duration of rheumatoid arthritis before hospital admission and with age on admission among patients of present series

Factor	Duration (longer)	Admission after age 40
Sex (male)	0	—
Onset after age 40	0	+
Prodromal symptoms	—	+
Strain before onset	0	+
Infection before onset	—	0
Onset acute	—	—
Onset in small or large joints or monarticular	0	0
Admission after age 40	+	
Duration before admission (longer)		+
Intermittent course before admission	+	—
Spondylitis (males)	+	—
Activity of disease	0	0
Total severity (increased)	+	+
Improvement (after discharge)	—	—

Note: + signifies positive association, — negative association, and 0 absence of association.

with increasing age was suggested by the absence of association between this factor and age on admission, but it must be remembered that our patients were primarily admitted to the medical ward for treatment and not for rehabilitation or orthopedic surgery. A more marked total severity* of disease on admission was associated with age 40 or over at hospital entry as well as with longer duration of disease. Follow-up of the patients in the present series also showed that the subsequent course was less favorable in those admitted after reaching 40.

DURATION BEFORE ADMISSION

18.3 The duration of arthritis before admission in the series patients varied from two days to thirty-five years. The length of time that definite joint involvement had been present is shown in Table 18.4, as well as in Figs. 18.3 and 18.4. No significant difference according to sex is shown in this table—the mean duration, 5.1 years, being the same for males and females. If the appearance of prodromal symptoms really marks the onset of the disease, then the short duration recorded in many

* See definition, par. **4.26**.

Table 18.4

Duration of rheumatoid arthritis before hospital admission among males and females of present series

Duration of arthritis	No. of patients	No. of males	No. of females
1 month or less	7	3	4
6 months to 1 month	49	19	30
1 year to 6 months	28	7	21
3 years to 1 year	93	38	55
5 years to 3 years	36	12	24
10 years to 5 years	42	14	28
Over 10 years	38	14	24
Total	293	107	186
Mean duration (years)	5.1	5.1	5.1

patients is only apparent. Actually about two-thirds of those with disease duration of one year or less gave histories of such symptoms. In addition, the patients whose arthritis was of long duration had not infrequently experienced complete or nearly complete remission for considerable periods of time. Such an intermittent course was pursued by nearly half of those whose disease had been present for more than five years. That the diagnosis of rheumatoid arthritis may be difficult in the first few months is freely admitted, so that it should be stated again that in no instance did we include a patient in our series until further observation had made the correct diagnosis reasonably certain. Eventually, 7 patients, all but 1 with less than three months' disease duration on admission, were eliminated from the series of 300 patients originally chosen, because the passage of time made it clear that the diagnosis had been erroneous.

18.4   For the purpose of statistical analysis, the patients were divided into three groups. The first group numbered 84 patients with disease duration of one year or less. The second group was composed of 129 patients with disease duration of five years or less but more than one year, and the third group was composed of 80 patients with disease duration of more than five years. Table 18.3 lists the nature of the association of certain factors with increasing duration as measured by these three groups.* It should again be pointed out that, on account of the

* For a complete list of associations, see Appendix Table 47.

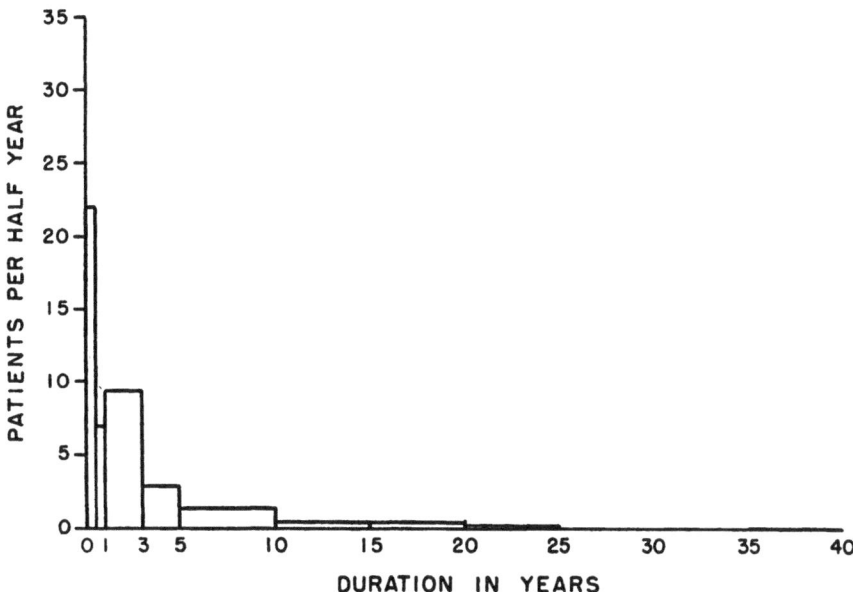

Figure 18.3 Duration of arthritis before hospital admission in group of 107 male patients with rheumatoid arthritis

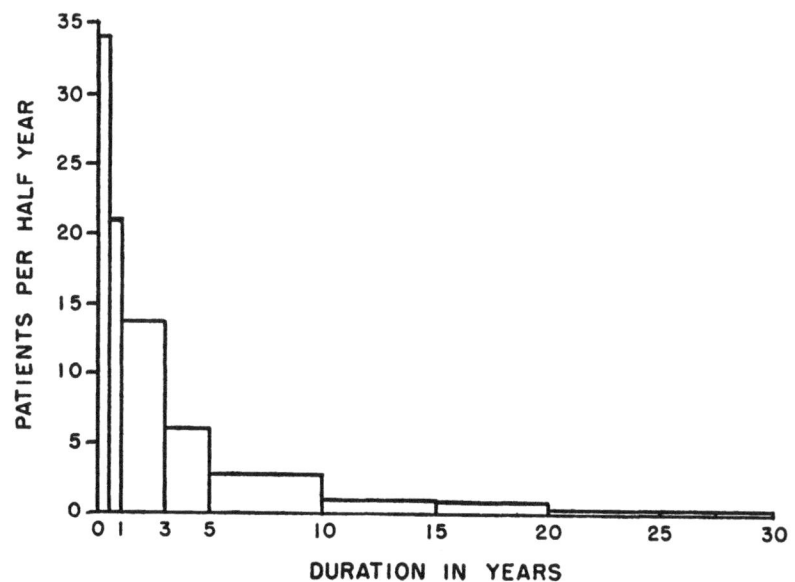

Figure 18.4 Duration of arthritis before hospital admission in group of 186 female patients with rheumatoid arthritis

large number of factors and the relatively small number of patients, no attempt was made to sort out the many inter-relationships among the factors. While the degree of positive or negative association in each instance thus listed is statistically significant according to the chi-square test, the influence of other factors, either tested or as yet undetermined, cannot be excluded with the presently available data. We should thus regard the information presented in this table as merely helping to confirm or refute clinical opinion about the disease and, in certain cases, as being of some value in predicting the future course of a given individual. It is important finally for the reader to realize that this analysis of disease duration cannot arbitrarily be applied to an unselected group of rheumatoid arthritics outside the hospital. In every case the point in the disease course at which the patient was studied was when severity of symptoms, or other unrecorded reasons, led to hospital admission for study and treatment.

18.5   As seemed likely from Table 18.4, no association was noted in respect to sex. The expected finding that age 40 or over on admission was associated with greater duration has already been referred to (par. **18.2**), but age at onset apparently bore no relation to a greater or shorter interval before hospital entry. As mentioned before (par. **13.6**), the higher frequency of prodromal symptoms in those with shorter duration of arthritis may depend merely upon the naturally more exact memory of such patients for more recent events. The relationships among infection as a precipitant, acute onset, and early admission to the hospital have already been discussed (par. **14.10**). The conclusion then reached was that the significance of the association between antecedent infection and early admission might be illusory but that effect of time on the patient's memory was less important than the type of onset. In other words, it seems reasonable to assume that early hospitalization would follow infection associated with an acute, severe type of onset. In the next chapter on "Course of Disease before Admission," the point will be brought out that a progressive disease should naturally lead to earlier admission (par. **19.2**). Conversely, it was found that a course marked by remissions was associated with longer disease duration before hospital entry. While a more marked degree of total severity appeared to be related to the interval between onset and admission, no

Age and Disease Duration

differences were found in regard to disease activity, for reasons already applied to a similar finding in respect to age on admission (par. 18.2). As far as subsequent course is concerned, a direct relationship was evident between disease duration of one year or less and a favorable outcome. Of the 250 patients who received only simple medical and orthopedic therapy, 74.1 per cent of those with duration of one year or less showed improvement in follow-up studies, compared with 43.2 per cent of the remainder (Table 44.6).

SUMMARY

18.6 The age-on-admission distribution of the present series has been compared with the age distribution of the Massachusetts population in 1930. The findings approximate those obtained in regard to age at onset (Chapter 6), with no significant difference in males but a marked increase in females admitted during the sixth decade. Males tended to be admitted at an earlier age, probably due to the age and sex distribution of patients with spondylitis. A more marked total severity of disease on admission and a less favorable subsequent course was related to age 40 or over on admission.

18.7 The duration of arthritis from onset to hospital admission showed a wide variation in our patients. In about one-fourth the duration was one year or less, and in a similar proportion over five years, with the remainder falling between. The relationships between disease duration and certain other factors have been tabulated, but the reader is cautioned that our findings are not necessarily applicable to unselected groups of rheumatoid arthritics outside the hospital. In our series shorter duration appeared to be related to decrease in total severity, and improvement following discharge was observed in about 75 per cent of patients admitted within one year of onset.

18.8 Objective for further study:

Additional long-term follow-up observations on patients seen early in the course of rheumatoid arthritis.

19

Course of Disease before Hospital Admission

19.1 Although rheumatoid arthritis is generally regarded as a chronic, progressive disease, an intermittent form, characterized by relapses and remissions, has been noted by many observers [*251, 252, 286, 333, 427, 434*]. The first part of this chapter will be devoted to a comparison between members of the present series whose course was progressive and those who enjoyed periods of complete or nearly complete freedom from articular symptoms. We have not included in the latter group patients in whom the activity of the disease showed minor fluctuations or variations while the general trend was toward progression but only those experiencing remissions for at least a month. (In each instance, course refers to that pursued before hospital admission, with the data procured from the patients' histories rather than by direct observation.) The rest of the chapter will be concerned with a study of the patients whose disease course was intermittent, including an attempt to classify the patterns of the relapses and remissions experienced by this group.

19.2 Table 19.1 shows in 80 patients, or slightly over one-fourth of the series, that the course was intermittent, while in the remaining 213, the disease process was progressive. The table also demonstrates that each group was made up of almost exactly the same proportion of males and females. When patients with the two types of course were

Disease Course before Admission

Table 19.1
Sex distribution in relation to type of course among patients of present series

Type of course	No. of patients	Percentage of	
		Males	Females
Total	293	36.5	63.5
Intermittent	80	36.2	63.8
Progressive	213	36.6	63.4

compared in respect to age at onset, a higher proportion of patients with onset before the age of forty was found among those who experienced remissions (Table 19.2). A relationship between an acute, severe type of onset and an intermittent course before admission has been shown in a previous table (Table 15.5). Four other differences were found between the progressive and intermittent groups. The first included a relationship between progressive course and initial involvement of small joints and a relationship between intermittent course and monarticular onset (Table 16.11). The second was the relationship between a progressive course and a relatively short duration of arthritis before admission (Table 19.3). This difference was not unexpected, since a patient with progressive disease would be more likely to seek hospital treatment. The mean duration of arthritis before admission also differed in the two groups: 7.3 years for those with an intermittent course compared with 4.4 years for patients whose disease was progressive. An association to be taken up in a subsequent chapter (par. 26.5) was also found between an intermittent course before admission and fever while in the hospital.

19.3   No significant difference was apparent in the two groups

Table 19.2
Onset of rheumatoid arthritis before age 40 in relation to type of course among patients of present series

Type of course	No. of patients	Onset before age 40	
		No.	Per cent
Total	293	177	60.4
Intermittent	80	61	76.2
Progressive	213	116	54.5
		Difference in percentages:	21.7 ±·6.4

Table 19.3

Shorter duration of rheumatoid arthritis before hospital admission (1 year or less) in relation to type of course among patients of present series

Type of course	No. of patients	Shorter duration	
		No.	Per cent
Total	293	84	28.7
Intermittent	80	8	10.0
Progressive	213	76	35.7
	Difference in percentages:	25.7 $\pm$ 5.9	

in respect to a number of other factors. These included the presence or absence of prodromal symptoms, of either strain or infection as precipitants, and of spondylitis. Hence, little prognostic help is to be obtained from our data concerning the factors preceding or associated with the onset of arthritis, although primary small-joint involvement and onset at age forty or over point toward the likelihood of a progressive course. On the other hand, either acute onset, onset before the age of forty, or monarticular onset may foretell the possibility of at least one remission. The total severity* of the arthritis as evaluated after hospital admission was found to be approximately the same irrespective of the course previously pursued. Similarly, the type of course before admission was found to be unrelated to the presence or absence of improvement in a follow-up study of the patients after they left the hospital.†

19.4 The remaining part of this chapter deals with our attempt to classify the differing patterns of the course pursued by the 80 patients who enjoyed one or more remissions before entering the hospital. The first step in this procedure was to construct individual graphs** presenting in a form which could be easily visualized the duration and degree of exacerbations and remissions experienced by each patient (see Fig. 19.1). In these graphs the two phases of the disease were divided by an arbitrarily defined line at which the patient passed from activity toward quiescence or the reverse. Under this line the patient would be considered in remission and, above it, his disease would still show signs of activity.

---

* See definition, par. **4.26**.

† For a complete list of associations, see Table 47 in the Appendix.

** These were constructed from the Hospital and Arthritis Clinic records by Dr. Jean M. Beauregard, whose assistance is gratefully acknowledged.

Disease Course before Admission

19.5 The degree of remission was determined according to data obtained in the history and graded as I (complete), II (major improvement), and III (minor improvement) according to the amount, if any, of residual complaints. In our group of 80 patients, 85 per cent of the remissions charted could be classified as complete. Each patient enjoyed at least one such cessation of arthritic activity, with three exceptions in whom the degree of improvement could be regarded as major but not complete. The evaluation of the degree of activity of the disease when the patient was in exacerbation was made according to a numerical system which seemed suited to the expression of clinical data obtained from history alone without opportunity of direct observation of the patient. The factors utilized are listed in Table 19.4, together with the maximum number of points assigned to each. After examination of the charts constructed from data obtained in this way, the length of exacerbation proved of far greater interest than the degree. For this reason, further explanation in regard to the method employed is deemed unnecessary.

19.6 The charts drawn up for each patient were intended to give an idea of the whole course of the disease before admission. An example portraying the course of one patient's disease before admission is given in Fig. 19.1, in which the duration of the disease is shown on the abscissa, while the state of disease activity at a given time is shown on the ordinate. The line dividing disease activity from remission may also be seen in this figure. Although the data for the graph were arrived at by an arbitrary point score, the reader may see at a glance that

Table 19.4

Factors used in evaluating exacerbation of rheumatoid arthritis and maximum number of points assigned to each factor

Factors	Maximum no. of points
Functional activity	100
Pain and/or tenderness	100
Stiffness	75
Swelling of joints	75
Joint effusion	50
Heat and/or redness of joints	50
Limitation of joint motion	50
Maximum degree of exacerbation	500

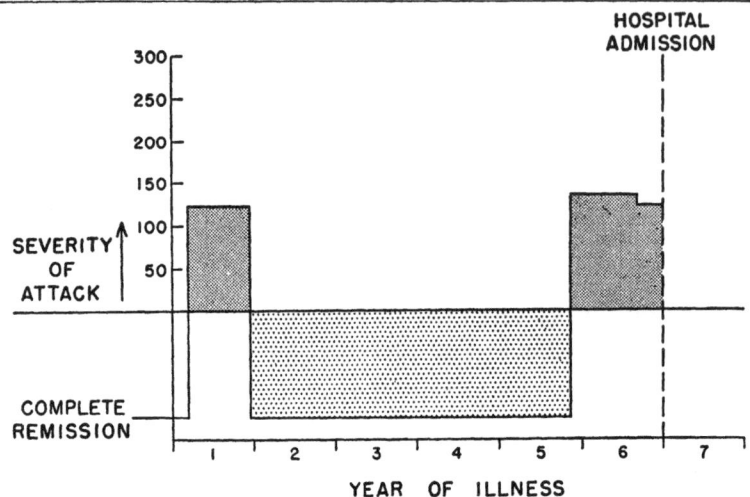

Figure 19.1 Disease course before hospital admission of a typical patient (see par. 19.6). It should be noted that, in this figure and in Figures 19.2–19.5, exacerbations and remissions are expressed in respect to the point of onset in the calendar year

this patient's course consisted of two periods of mild disease activity, one lasting about nine months and the other fourteen months, separated by a complete remission of nearly four years. There is no reason to believe in this instance, or in many others, that there was an instantaneous change from disease activity to remission and the reverse, as the graph seems to imply. The transitions were undoubtedly more gradual but cannot be thus expressed with any degree of accuracy, due to lack of available data in the patients' histories.

19.7 Before going on to a classification of the types of course pursued by the 80 patients, certain features gleaned from a survey of the clinical histories of this group will be briefly stated. In Table 19.5 it may be seen that in the case of both males and females about two-thirds of the course before admission was spent in remission and about one-third in exacerbation. The average length of time spent in each by males was greater than that spent by females. This finding was associated with the longer duration of arthritis in the males. The impression that long remissions may intervene among early attacks of rheumatoid arthritis was thus confirmed.

Disease Course before Admission

Table 19.5

Average duration of rheumatoid arthritis before hospital admission and average number of years and percentage of course spent in remission and exacerbation—comparison of males and females of present series having intermittent course before hospital admission

	Total	Males	Females
No. of patients	80	29	51
Duration			
Average no. of years	7.3	9.0	6.4
Remission			
Average no. of years	5.0	6.0	4.4
Percentage of course	65.4	63.5	66.3
Exacerbation			
Average no. of years	2.4	3.2	2.2
Percentage of course	34.6	36.5	33.7

19.8 For the actual classification or subdivision of the 80 patients in respect to the pattern of their course before admission, what seemed to us the simplest and most useful method was finally adopted. This involved dividing remissions and attacks or exacerbations according to their length. Attacks or remissions lasting one year or less were designated *brief* and those lasting more than one year *long*. As mentioned above, the degree of remission was considered complete in practically all instances. Although the degree of exacerbation, computed according to the method referred to above (par. **19.6**), ranged from less than 50 to 370 points, no relationship to the duration of either the attack or the adjacent remissions was evident. For these reasons, we did not attempt to measure the degree of remission or exacerbation but, in formulating a scheme of classification, merely considered whether the period was brief or long.

19.9 In spite of the apparent simplicity of this method, the well-recognized variability of the course of rheumatoid arthritis necessitated the use of subheadings to indicate minor exceptions to the four main patterns expressed in Table 19.6. The four main headings represent the four possible combinations of attacks and remissions divided according to their length, with graphic examples of each provided in Figs. 19.2, 19.3, 19.4, and 19.5. As may be noted in the table, in half of the 80 patients, both attacks and remissions were mainly brief (Group 1), while

Table 19.6

Patients with intermittent course before hospital admission, divided according to brief (1 year or less) and long (more than 1 year) attacks and remissions of rheumatoid arthritis

Group		No. of patients
I	Brief attacks and brief remissions	40
	No exceptions	22
	Long attack before admission	4
	1 or more long remissions	9
	1 long attack and 1 long remission	5
II	Brief attacks and long remissions	31
	No exceptions	21
	Long attack before admission	6
	1 or more brief remissions	4
III	Long attacks with brief remissions	4
	No exceptions	1
	1 brief attack	3
IV	Long attacks with long remissions	5
	No exceptions	2
	1 or more brief attacks	3
Total		80

in the majority of the remainder, attacks were brief and remissions longer than a year. Long attacks, with either brief or long remissions, occurred in less than one-eighth. It is thus suggested that when an attack of rheumatoid arthritis persists longer than a year, the prospect of a spontaneous remission becomes less likely.

19.10 The average number of attacks experienced by the patients in Group I was slightly over four, a figure almost twice as high as in the remaining groups (Table 19.7). In a few patients, multiple attacks

Table 19.7

Average duration of rheumatoid arthritis before hospital admission and average number of attacks among patients of Groups I–IV (see Table 19.6) and percentage of males in each group

		Group			
	Total	I	II	III	IV
No. of patients	80	40	31	4	5
Average no. of years before admission	7.3	4.9	9.3	6.0	16.0
Average no. of attacks	3.4	4.3	2.5	2.25	2.6
Percentage of males	36.2	27.5	45.0	50.0	40.0

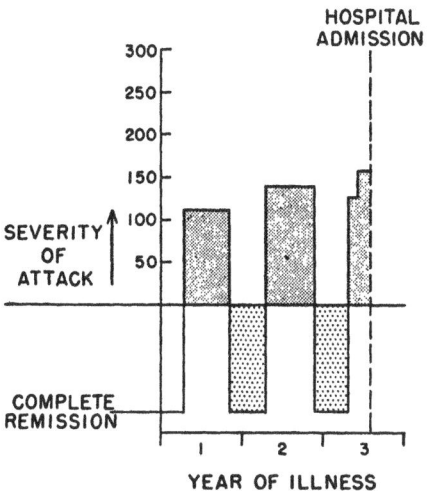

Figure 19.2 Disease course before hospital admission of a patient in Group I (brief attacks and brief remissions)

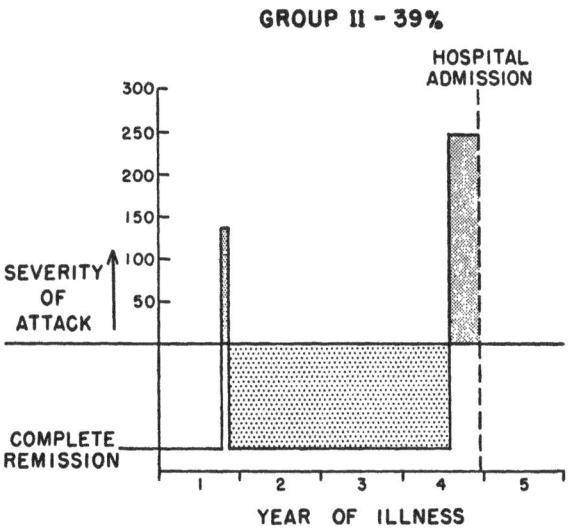

Figure 19.3 Disease course before hospital admission of a patient in Group II (brief attacks and long remissions)

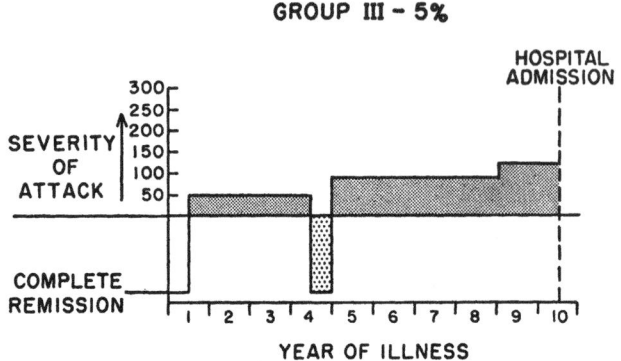

Figure 19.4 Disease course before hospital admission of a patient in Group III (long attacks and brief remissions)

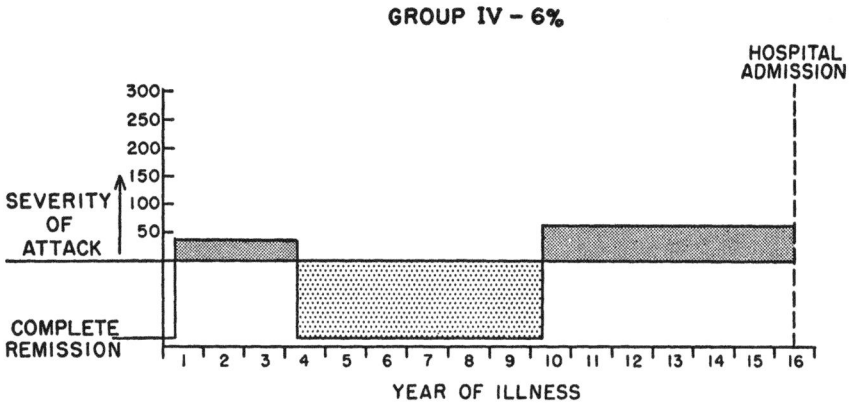

Figure 19.5 Disease course before hospital admission of a patient in Group IV (long attacks and long remissions)

occurred, numbering as high as fourteen, eighteen, and twenty-three in 3 patients. The average duration of the brief attacks in Group I was just over two months, with the average length of brief remissions much longer, slightly over seven months. As shown in Table 19.7, the average duration of arthritis before admission was shortest in Group I, as might be expected in view of the shorter remissions. Although the percentage of males was lowest in Group I, the differences among the four groups in sex distribution were not significant. Group II, comprising those pa-

Disease Course before Admission

tients who had chiefly brief attacks and long remissions, was the second largest, numbering 31 patients (Table 19.6). The differences between this group and Group I in regard to the average number of attacks and the duration before admission are shown in Table 19.7. The average duration of the brief attacks in this group was four months, slightly longer than in Group I. Remissions in general were prolonged, averaging over four years and with the longest nearly twelve years. The most common pattern of attacks and remissions in this group is shown in Fig. 19.3—a brief attack, followed one or more years later by an attack of greater severity which persisted until hospitalization became necessary. Groups III and IV were made up of relatively small numbers of patients (Table 19.6). Remissions in Group IV were as prolonged as in Group II, again averaging over four years. The average length of the attacks in Group IV was over four years, with complete remissions taking place in several cases after attacks lasting from two to five years. Not unexpectedly, the average duration before admission was easily the longest in this group, sixteen years.

19.11 Before concluding this description of course patterns, a few points should be mentioned in regard to the four groups taken together. Although we have referred to the variability in degree of individual attacks, in most patients successive attacks seemed to increase in severity, with the one leading to admission usually receiving a higher point score than earlier exacerbations. There were a few exceptions with apparently decreasing severity of attacks and others in whom all attacks were about equally severe. The average duration of all attacks, 227 in number, preceding the ones leading to hospital admission was over six months. The average duration of all remissions, numbering 226, was over twenty-one months, a finding which provides further evidence that a patient with an intermittent type of course is likely to spend appreciably more time in remission than with active disease.

19.12 Chapter 14 was devoted to so-called "precipitating factors" operative before the onset of the disease and Chapter 20 will deal with factors believed by the patients to have influenced the course once an actual arthritis had developed. Factors associated with exacerbations in the disease and with remissions have also been studied in this selected group of 80 patients whose course was marked by one or more remissions before entry. In about half these patients, factors of possible significance preceded the onset of exacerbation. These factors were gathered from the patients' clinical records and not by systematic questioning. They included, in order of frequency: infection, exposure to cold or dampness, childbirth, surgical operation, and strain. The infections noted were almost entirely of the upper respiratory tract. In a few patients, multiple exacerbations were preceded by upper respiratory infections, with seventeen instances recorded in 1 man and ten in each of 2 women. The unexpected finding of an exacerbation during pregnancy was recorded in 2 women and exacerbation after delivery in 8. About two-thirds of this group, or 55 patients, gave a history of factors associated with remissions in their arthritis. These were, again in order of frequency: heat (chiefly from change of season), increased rest or freedom from strain, surgery (usually for focal infections), and orthopedic measures. Also, 2 patients gained relief from an intercurrent jaundice, and 4 out of 6 females who became pregnant experienced remissions. As will be pointed out in the next chapter, no difference was found in the frequency of patients with an intermittent course whether or not the groups were adversely affected by either strain or intercurrent infection. Similar findings were obtained in regard to the effect of cold, moisture, heat, season of the year, and menstruation. It should be noted that the results just listed were obtained by direct questioning of the patients and not gleaned incidentally from their histories.

19.13 Mention will also be made in the next chapter of the patients' opinions as to the effect of season of the year upon their symptomatology (par. 20.13). Slightly over half noted no difference according to the time of year, while the large majority of the remainder stated that they were better in summer or worse in winter. Another approach to the association of season with exacerbations and remissions was afforded by tabulating such changes, according to month of occurrence, among the 80 patients with an intermittent course. The number of exacerbations starting in each month has been expressed in Table 19.8 and in Fig. 19.6 and the number of remissions in Table 19.9 and in Fig. 19.7. (In each case, rapid fluctuations have been omitted by the elimination of exacerbations not preceded by four months of remission and similarly of remissions not preceded by four months of disease activity.)

Table 19.8

Frequency of exacerbations starting in each month, according to reports by 80 patients with intermittent course before hospital admission

Month	Exacerbations	
	No.	Per cent
January	35	17.1
February	14	6.8
March	28	13.7
April	7	3.4
May	11	5.4
June	9	4.4
July	8	3.9
August	6	2.9
September	18	8.8
October	19	9.3
November	29	14.2
December	21	10.3
Total	205*	100.2

* In order to eliminate rapid fluctuations, exacerbations not preceded by 4 months of remission have been omitted.

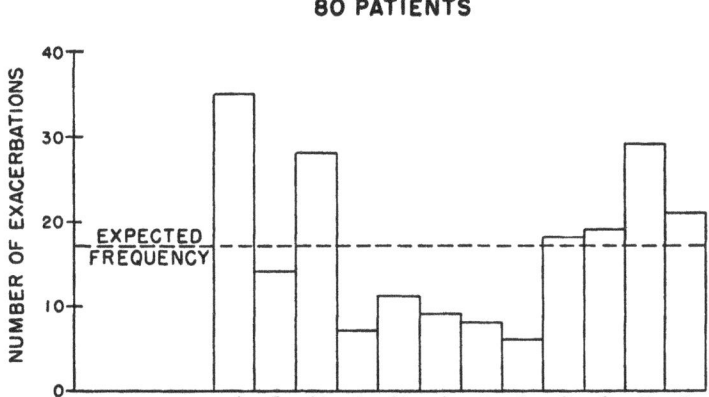

Figure 19.6 Number of exacerbations starting in each month in a group of 80 patients with intermittent course before hospital admission. The expected frequency represents the number of exacerbations that would have occurred each month, if they had been distributed equally throughout 12 months

Table 19.9

Frequency of remissions starting in each month, according to reports by 80 patients with intermittent course before hospital admission

	Remissions	
Month	No.	Per cent
January	7	9.5
February	2	2.7
March	11	14.9
April	4	5.4
May	21	28.4
June	2	2.7
July	6	8.1
August	5	6.8
September	8	10.8
October	2	2.7
November	2	2.7
December	4	5.4
Total	74*	100.1

* In order to eliminate rapid fluctuations, remissions not preceded by 4 months of disease activity have been omitted.

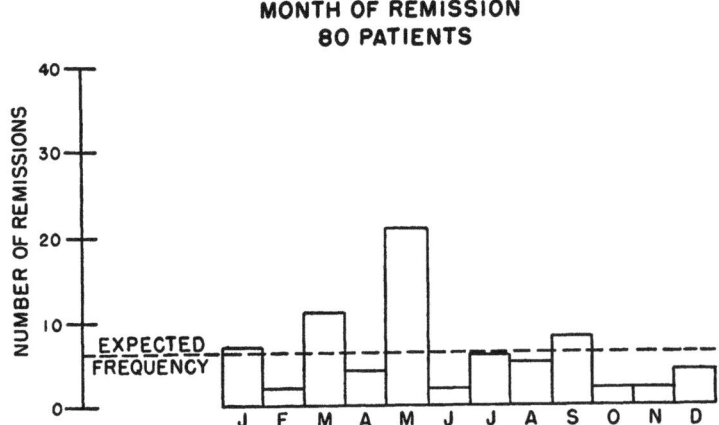

Figure 19.7 Number of remissions starting in each month in a group of 80 patients with intermittent course before hospital admission. The expected frequency represents the number of remissions that would have occurred each month, if they had been distributed equally throughout 12 months

Disease Course before Admission

The patients reported that a consistently higher number of exacerbations began in the fall, winter, and early spring—from September through March. The onset of remissions, however, was fairly evenly distributed throughout the months, with the exception of a peak in May. In Table 19.10 the year has been divided into the warmer and colder months, and in order to set off a seasonal difference in disease activity, figures have been derived from the present series and from other sources [133, 166] in respect to the onset of arthritis as well as to exacerbations and remissions. In one sense, the onset of the arthritis may be regarded as the first severe exacerbation, since in many cases there is evidence of the existence of the disease in the form of prodromal symptoms. In addition to the months of onset reported by the 80 patients with intermittent course, we have studied those of 82 patients with disease duration of one year or less and hence with more accurate memory of the time of onset. The only series in the literature we have been able to find for which the months of onset were tabulated were those studied by Dawson [133] in New York City and Edström [166] in Sweden. Their data are given in Table 19.10, together with our data for the exacerbations and remissions reported by the 80 patients with intermittent course, which serve

Table 19.10

Frequency of onset, exacerbations, and remissions in warm and cold months among rheumatoid arthritics—two groups from present series compared with similar groups reported in the literature

		Onset	
		Percentage of patients	
Source	*No. of patients*	*Nov.–April*	*May–Oct.*
Edström [166]	467	59.0	41.0
Dawson [133]	73	68.4	31.6
Present series—patients with intermittent course	80	80.3	19.7
Present series—patients with duration of 1 year or less	82*	58.5	41.5
		Exacerbations	
Present series	80	65.7	34.3
		Remissions	
Present series	80	38.6	61.4

* The total differs from that given in Table 19.3 because data for onset were lacking in 2 cases.

to confirm the impression given by the histograms in Figs. 19.5 and 19.7. Table 19.11 and Fig. 19.8 show that March was by far the most common month of onset for the 80 patients with intermittent course. Table 19.12 compares the actual frequency of onset in March with the expected frequency, if distribution had been equal throughout the twelve months. The actual frequency was also higher in 56 patients whose onset was abrupt and severe and therefore sharply defined. As a matter of fact, in all five groups, more patients dated their onset in March than in any other month. When exacerbations were considered apart from disease onsets in our 80 patients, the number of attacks was slightly higher in November and January than in March. Some corroboration of the above findings is afforded by data assembled by the U. S. Public Health Service on "Sickness Experience in Selected Areas of the United States" and based on periodic canvasses of households in these areas [*111*]. In the case of "arthritis and chronic rheumatism" the highest monthly rates were found between November and April, with a peak in January and a low point in July.

19.14 From the figures presented, it seems reasonable to make the statement that rheumatoid arthritics in the regions studied are more likely to experience the onset of their arthritis, and, if remittent, a serious worsening during the colder months of the year. The last expression, "colder months of the year," should not lead to the assumption that climatic changes are directly responsible for this difference. Other possibilities, which as yet rest purely on speculation, also deserve consideration. The first is the increased frequency of respiratory infections during the winter months. In the United States attacks of rheumatic fever occur predominantly in the late winter and early spring and are believed to correspond to the seasonal prevalence of hemolytic streptococcus infections. The next, by analogy, is the marked seasonal variation in the incidence of certain infectious diseases, chiefly of virus origin. For example, measles and poliomyelitis occur in epidemic form in distinct seasonal patterns. A third possibility rests upon differing nutritional requirements according to season. Recent studies in pellagra [*449*] indicate that an increased metabolic requirement for water-soluble vitamins in late spring and early summer is responsible for outbreaks of pellagra at this season. Finally, mention should be made of the inactivity and

Table 19.11

Frequency of onset starting in each month, according to reports by 80 patients with intermittent course before hospital admission

Month	Onset	
	No.	Per cent
January	4	5.0
February	10	12.5
March	37	46.2
April	9	11.3
May	6	7.5
June	1	1.2
July	1	1.2
August	3	3.8
September	1	1.2
October	3	3.8
November	5	6.2
December	0	0.0
Total	80	99.9

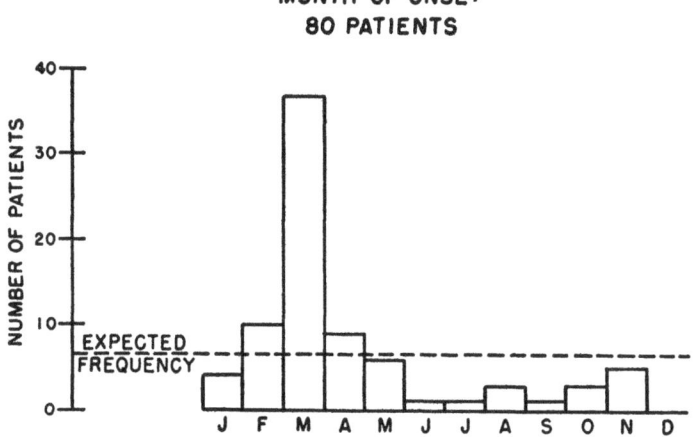

Figure 19.8 Distribution of onset of arthritis according to months in a group of 80 patients with intermittent course before hospital admission. The expected frequency represents the number of onsets that would have occurred each month, if they had been distributed equally throughout 12 months

Table 19.12

Onset of rheumatoid arthritis in March—observed frequency compared with expected frequency of onsets equally distributed over 12 months

Reported in literature	No. of patients	Onset in March	
		Observed no.	Expected no.
Dawson [133]	73	19	6
Edström [166]	467	52	39
Present series			
With acute onset	56	16	5
With duration of 1 year or less	82	14	7
With intermittent course	80	37	7

* The total differs from that given in Table 19.3 because data for onset were lacking in 2 cases.

even atrophy of endocrine organs, including the anterior pituitary and adrenal cortex [456], which occur in certain animals during the winter months.

19.15 A final point of interest was the tendency exhibited by the majority of individual patients to experience exacerbations (as well as onset) in the same quarter of the year. While there were also some whose exacerbations were scattered throughout the year, in certain patients the attacks invariably occurred in the same month. For example, one patient's disease started in March and was followed by six exacerbations over the next fifteen years, all starting in this month. A similar tendency was shown in the case of remissions.

SUMMARY

19.16 Slightly over one-fourth of the series, or 80 patients, experienced at least one complete, or nearly complete, remission before admission. Onset before the age of forty and primary involvement of a single joint favored an intermittent rather than a progressive course, while primary involvement of multiple small joints favored a progressive course. No differences were found in respect to other factors, including the presence or absence of prodromal symptoms, the total severity of the arthritis on admission, and the subsequent course.

19.17 A graphic portrayal according to an arbitrary scheme was constructed from the course pursued before admission by each of the

Disease Course before Admission

80 patients. From these graphs we derived a simple classification of the differing course patterns, based on the length of attacks and remissions. A large majority of the patients reported "brief" attacks (one year's duration or less), with either "brief" or "long" remissions (over one year). A much smaller number of patients reported "long" attacks with either "brief" or "long" remissions. While attacks of over one year were thus much less likely to be followed by remissions, instances were recorded of complete remissions after periods of two to five years of active disease. As a whole, the group with intermittent course spent about twice as much time in remission as in exacerbation.

19.18 Remissions occurred throughout the year, with a peak in May, but exacerbations were more frequent during the colder months, a distribution corresponding to the available figures for the season of onset of rheumatoid arthritis. In our series, as well as in two others reported in the literature, onset occurred most frequently in the month of March. The majority of the 80 patients exhibited a tendency to experience exacerbations or remissions in the same quarter of the year.

19.19 Objectives for further study:

1. Additional observations on the month of onset in patients seen early in the course of their disease. The onset of prodromal symptoms should be noted as well as that of the actual arthritis. Geographical variation in the seasonal distribution of onset would be of particular interest.

2. A search for causes in patients with exacerbations occurring in the same quarter of the year, to include investigation of anniversaries of potentially upsetting events, such as the death of a near relative.

3. The relationship of the possible causes listed in par. **19.14** to the onset or worsening of rheumatoid arthritis in the colder months of the year.

20

Factors Which Patients Believed to Have Influenced the Course of Their Disease

20.1 As part of the study of the course of the disease before admission, each patient was questioned in regard to the apparent effect of certain factors upon the progress of his arthritis. Sufficient data for analysis were obtained in the case of strain, intercurrent acute infections, season of the year, and the climatic or environmental factors of heat, cold, and moisture or dampness. The influence of menstruation and pregnancy in women was also recorded. In regard to three other possibly influential factors—latitude, altitude above sea level, and proximity to bodies of water—the information acquired was too meager to warrant consideration. The same was true of the effect of the allergic states, but later on in the present chapter reference will be made to the observations of others on this subject.

20.2 It is evident that the patients' answers in regard to the factors considered might fall into four categories, depending upon whether the apparent effect was adverse, beneficial, or neutral or, in certain instances, whether the patient was exposed to the factor under consideration during the course of his illness. The results obtained from the questionnaire will be outlined below, with each factor taken up separately. The reader should finally be reminded that we have recorded patients' impressions which were in no wise backed up by objective observations and that, especially in the case of heat, cold, moisture, and

Factors Believed to be Influential

season, the individuals questioned may have been influenced by the traditional ideas about the effect of these factors upon joint disease.

STRAIN

20.3 Of the entire series, 209 patients, or about 70 per cent, gave a history of being under strain at some point in the course of their arthritis. Of the latter group, 125 or 60 per cent, felt that the disease was affected adversely in this way, while the remainder noted no effect. In no instance was a favorable response recorded. The type of strain was not defined in our data, so that figures are not available to differentiate the physical from the mental variety. As already mentioned when strain was taken up as a precipitating factor (par. **14.4**), it seems probable that a combination of the two was frequently present. It should also be brought out that a patient under strain may become more aware of pain and hence believe his disease course to be adversely affected [278].

20.4 No sex differences were observed in the patients with and without strain during the course of their disease, but, as shown in Table 20.1, a smaller proportion of males was encountered in the group adversely affected by this factor. Otherwise the two groups showed no significant differences when comparisons were made in respect to age on hospital admission (under or over forty), duration of disease on admission, presence or absence of spinal involvement, type of onset, and course before admission, but patients with marked total severity on admission more often considered themselves unaffected by strain (Table 20.2). The occurrence of strain as a precipitating factor appar-

Table 20.1

Apparent effect of strain on course of rheumatoid arthritis among patients of present series divided according to sex

Apparent effect of strain	Strain in course		
	No. of patients	Percentage of males	Percentage of females
Total	209	39.2	60.8
Adverse	125	33.6	66.4
None	84	47.6	52.4
		Difference in percentages:	14.0 ± 6.9

Table 20.2
Total severity of rheumatoid arthritis among patients of present series divided according to apparent effect of strain on course

Apparent effect of strain	No. of patients	Total severity of arthritis*					
		Mild		Moderate		Marked	
		No.	Per cent	No.	Per cent	No.	Per cent
Total	209	48	23.0	127	60.8	34	16.3
Adverse	125	32	25.6	79	63.2	14	11.2
None	84	16	19.0	48	57.1	20	23.8
					Difference in percentages:		12.6 ± 5.3

$$\chi^2 = 6.1; p < .05$$

* See definition, par. **4.26**.

Table 20.3
Frequency of worsened symptoms of rheumatoid arthritis following infection among patients of present series divided according to apparent effect of strain on course

Apparent effect of strain	No. of patients with both strain and infection in course	Worsened after infection	
		No.	Per cent
Total	156	34	21.8
Adverse	85	27	31.8
None	71	7	9.9
	Difference in percentages:		21.9 ± 6.6

ently had no influence on subsequent fluctuations in the course of the arthritis following exposure to strain. Table 20.3, however, demonstrates an association between an increase in symptoms following strain and a similar change following an intercurrent infection.

INTERCURRENT INFECTIONS

20.5 Our data indicate that intercurrent infections were believed to play a less important role than strain in association with alterations in the course of the disease before hospital admission. Although 182 patients, or 62 per cent of the series, admitted to intercurrent infections during their arthritis, only 48 of these, or about one-fourth, believed that such illnesses had exercised an adverse effect. No changes were re-

Factors Believed to be Influential

ported by the remaining 134 patients. However, as mentioned in a previous section (par. 10.4), attacks of intercurrent jaundice, presumably infectious in nature but separately recorded, apparently instituted temporary remissions of rheumatoid arthritis in 2 out of 4 patients of the present series. Data from direct observation of 37 patients who contracted infections while hospitalized for rheumatoid arthritis were collected by Järvinen [*278*]. No apparent effect on the arthritis was observed in one-third of this group, but it became worse in two-thirds—a larger proportion than that obtained by interrogation of our patients.

20.6 As in the case of strain, little difference in most respects was observed between the group of patients apparently made worse by infection and those whose course was unchanged. No sex or age differences were found, and no associations between a worsening of symptoms following intercurrent infections and disease duration, spinal involvement, or type of course before hospital admission. When the two groups were divided according to total severity of the arthritis on admission, a greater percentage of those with mild severity was encountered in the group on whom infection seemed to exert an adverse influence, although the difference was not significant by the chi-square test (Table 20.4). The findings in this table point in the same direction as those in Table 20.2, where the relationship between total severity on admission and strain in course is considered. While it is possible that those with a milder disease were more likely to experience fluctuations in course and assign strain or infection as causes, no association was noted between intermittent course and a mild degree of severity (par. 19.3) or between severity and adverse effects of cold and moisture (par. 20.12).

Table 20.4

Total severity of rheumatoid arthritis on hospital admission among patients of present series divided according to apparent effect of infection on course

Apparent effect of infection	No. of patients	Total severity of arthritis					
		Mild		Moderate		Marked	
		No.	Per cent	No.	Per cent	No.	Per cent
Total	182	45	24.7	105	57.7	32	17.6
Adverse	48	18	37.5	23	47.9	7	14.6
None	134	27	20.1	82	61.2	25	18.7

$$\chi^2 = 5.6; 0.1 > p > .05$$

20.7 The converse of Table 20.3 is expressed in Table 20.5 which indicates that a greater proportion of patients seemingly made worse by strain appeared among those similarly affected by infection. A group of 27 patients is thus set forth who believed that their course was adversely affected by stress, whether in the form of infection or strain. In comparison with the remainder of the series, this small group showed a higher frequency of prodromal symptoms, of infection as a precipitating factor, and of onset of arthritis before age forty. Otherwise, no essential differences emerged. Two rather close associations with an apparently adverse influence of intercurrent infections were also encountered—acute onset of a severe form of arthritis (Table 20.6) and the presence of infection as a precipitating factor (Table 20.7). As mentioned previously (pars. **14.10** and **15.3**), an association between history of antecedent infection and acute onset was found among our patients. The subtables accompanying Tables 20.6 and 20.7 demonstrate that neither an acute

Table 20.5

Frequency of apparent worsening of symptoms of rheumatoid arthritis following strain among patients of present series divided according to apparent effect of infection on course

Apparent effect of infection	No. of patients with strain and infection	Worsened after strain	
		No.	Per cent
Total	156	84	53.8
Adverse	35	27	77.1
None	121	57	47.1
	Difference in percentages:	30.0 ± 9.5	

Table 20.6

Frequency of acute onset of rheumatoid arthritis among patients of present series divided according to apparent effect of infection on course

Apparent effect of infection	No. of patients	Acute onset	
		No.	Per cent
Total	182	31	17.0
Adverse	48	17	35.4
None	134	14	10.4
	Difference in percentages:	25.0 ± 6.3	

Factors Believed to be Influential

Table 20.6A

Frequency of acute onset of rheumatoid arthritis among patients of present series with infection as a precipitant divided according to apparent effect of infection on course

Apparent effect of infection	No. of patients with infection as a precipitant	Acute onset No.	Per cent
Total	32	12	37.5
Adverse	18	9	50.0
None	14	3	21.4
	Difference in percentages:	28.6 $\pm$ 17.6	

Table 20.7

Frequency of infection as a precipitant in rheumatoid arthritis among patients of present series divided according to apparent effect of infection on course

Apparent effect of infection	No. of patients	Infection as a precipitant No.	Per cent
Total	182	32	17.6
Adverse	48	18	37.5
None	134	14	10.4
	Difference in percentages:	27.1 $\pm$ 6.4	

Table 20.7A

Frequency of infection as a precipitant among patients with acute onset of rheumatoid arthritis divided according to apparent effect of infection on course

Apparent effect of infection	No. of patients with acute onset	Infection as a precipitant No.	Per cent
Total	31	12	38.7
Adverse	17	9	53.0
None	14	3	21.4
	Difference in percentages:	31.6 $\pm$ 17.6	

onset nor an antecedent infection is related in a significant degree to intercurrent infection with adverse effect, if the influence of the other factor is eliminated. We are thus justified in stating merely that a relationship exists among the three factors, with speculation as to its nature inadvisable in the absence of further information.

MENSTRUATION AND PREGNANCY

20.8 Information is available in regard to the apparent effect of menstrual periods on arthritic symptoms in 107 females of the present series, with the results shown in Table 20.8. Less than one-third stated that they felt worse at the time of their periods, while the remainder, with the exception of 2 women who claimed to feel better, noted no effect. Of 15 women who became pregnant after the disease had started, all but one experienced a distinct betterment in symptoms during the period of gestation.

Table 20.8

Apparent effect of menstrual periods on symptoms of rheumatoid arthritis among females of present series

Apparent effect of menstrual periods	Patients	
	No.	Per cent
Adverse	33	30.8
None	72	67.3
Favorable	2	1.9
Total	107	100.0

ALLERGY

20.9 Remissions in rheumatoid arthritis have been described following reactions, considered to be allergic in nature, to gold therapy [276]. One member of the present series was observed to enjoy a striking amelioration of symptoms following bouts of urticaria brought on by various chemical and physical agents [464]. Alternation in activity of bronchial asthma and rheumatoid arthritis in patients with both disorders has been mentioned in the literature [239]. An especially careful study of 12 such individuals has been recently published by Järvinen [276], who found uniformly that an improvement in the arthritis coincided with the onset of asthma and that an increase in activity of the joint disease occurred when the attack of asthma ceased. Records are available in regard to the relationship between rheumatoid activity and attacks of bronchial asthma for a total of 6 patients seen in this clinic, 3 of whom were members of the present series. In 2 of these a definite alternation of disease manifestations was observed, in 2 others the al-

Factors Believed to be Influential

ternation was inconstant, and in the remaining 2 the activity of both disorders ran parallel. It is thus not possible to confirm Järvinen's observations from this small experience.

COLD, MOISTURE, AND HEAT

20.10   As shown in Table 20.9, only half the patients of the present series gave the answers traditionally expected in regard to the effect of cold, moisture or dampness, and heat on the course of their arthritis. A surprisingly large proportion, in fact, claimed no increase in symptomatology from cold or moisture and no benefit from heat. (In the questioning, no distinction was drawn between heat as a climatic phenomenon and heat supplied to the patient by artificial means.) The table also includes a few patients who were apparently made worse by heat and felt better in the presence of cold or dampness—members of a small group well known to physicians who treat rheumatoid arthritis. A sex difference was observed in the case of each environmental factor, since a significantly smaller proportion of males than females was adversely affected by cold or moisture and improved by heat. This difference was confined to patients under forty in the case of cold and heat but applied to both younger and older patients where moisture was concerned. In general, no age difference was found, with the one exception that a larger proportion of females past the age of forty stated that dampness increased their symptoms.

20.11   The mechanism of the influence of environmental changes upon the symptomatology of rheumatoid arthritis is not entirely known, but there are reasons to believe that alterations in vasomotor tone may be largely responsible [168, 377, 430]. Our data furnish some

Table 20.9

Apparent effect of cold, moisture, and heat on course of rheumatoid arthritis before hospital admission among patients of present series (see par. 20.2)

Operative factor	No. of patients	Apparent effect					
		Adverse		None		Favorable	
		No.	Per cent	No.	Per cent	No.	Per cent
Cold	286	142	49.7	131	45.8	13	4.5
Moisture	286	164	57.3	112	39.2	10	3.5
Heat	285	21	7.4	115	40.4	149	52.3

corroboration of this belief as shown in Table 20.10. In each case, a much higher proportion of patients with vasomotor symptoms was found among those responding favorably to heat and unfavorably to cold and moisture than in the remainder. These findings remained consistent when the patients were divided according to sex except for the absence of association between vasomotor symptoms and adverse response to moisture among males. As will be described in Chapter 22, the patients were questioned in regard to four vasomotor symptoms: cold extremities, paresthesias, cyanosis of extremities, and attacks of vascular spasm. When considered individually, the first two were found to contribute chiefly to the strength of the associations in Table 20.10. In the group of 12 patients who were seemingly improved on exposure to cold and worsened by heat, the proportion giving a history of vasomotor symptoms was significantly smaller than in the remainder.

20.12 To conclude the analysis of the influence of environmental factors on the course of rheumatoid arthritis, two groups of patients were formed. The first was made up of those who noted unfavorable effects from cold and moisture, and the second of those who were apparently unaffected or improved by these factors. In neither group was the effect of heat considered. As shown in Table 20.11, a greater proportion of females was encountered in Group I, but the difference was significant only in patients who were under forty when admitted to the hospital. Further comparison of Groups I and II gave approximately equal findings in regard to age (under and over forty), duration of disease before admission (less or more than one year), total severity of arthritis on admission, and the presence or absence of spondylitis. As might be expected from previous data (Table 20.10), a much larger percentage of Group I gave a history of vasomotor symptoms, with qualifications similar to those noted in the preceding paragraph. The remaining patients in the series constituted a third group, those apparently made worse by either cold or moisture but not by both. In general this group resembled Group I (those adversely affected by both environmental factors) as far as the associations mentioned above are concerned, including 1 with a history of vasomotor symptoms. In regard to the last, the association was stronger in patients who noted an

Table 20.10

Frequency of vasomotor symptoms among patients of present series divided according to apparent effect of cold, moisture, and heat on course of rheumatoid arthritis (see par. 20.2)

Apparent effect of cold*	No. of patients	Patients with 1 or more vasomotor symptoms	
		No.	Per cent
Total	286	190	66.4
Adverse	142	113	79.6
None or favorable	144	77	53.5
Apparent effect of moisture†			
Total	286	190	66.4
Adverse	164	122	74.4
None or favorable	122	68	55.7
*Apparent effect of heat***			
Total	285	189	66.6
Favorable	149	113	75.8
None or adverse	136	76	56.0
* Difference in percentages:			26.1 ± 5.6
† Difference in percentages:			18.7 ± 5.7
** Difference in percentages:			19.8 ± 5.6

Table 20.11

Sex distribution of patients apparently made worse by both cold and moisture (Group I) and of patients apparently unaffected or improved by these factors (Group II) irrespective of the effect of heat (see par. 20.12)

Group	No. of patients	Males		Females	
		No.	Per cent	No.	Per cent
Total	198*	67	33.8	131	66.2
I	110	28	25.5	82	74.5
II	88	39	44.3	49	55.7
				Difference in percentages:	18.8 ± 6.8

* The remaining 88 patients constitute a third group, those apparently made worse by either cold or moisture but not by both (see par. **20.12**).

adverse effect of cold than in those who seemed unfavorably influenced by moisture.

SEASON

20.13 Information was obtained from 236 patients in regard to the effect of season upon their joint symptoms (Table 20.12). In the remainder, the duration of disease was not sufficiently long for the formation of an opinion in regard to seasonal variations. Slightly over half noted no difference according to the time of year, while the majority of the remainder gave the expected answers that they were better in summer or worse in winter. Only 3 patients felt worse in spring or fall when the season changed. A small number gave an unexpected reply that warm weather affected their arthritis adversely or cold weather favorably.*

Table 20.12

Apparent effect of season of the year on course of rheumatoid arthritis among patients of present series

Apparent effect of season	Patients	
	No.	Per cent
None	125	53.0
Better in summer	37	15.7
Worse in summer	7	3.0
Better in winter	7	3.0
Worse in winter	43	18.2
Better in spring	1	0.4
Worse in spring	1	0.4
Better in fall	0	0.0
Worse in fall	2	0.9
Affected by more than 1 season	13	5.5
	236	100.1

COMMENT

20.14 In 1930 Ghrist and Hench [205] published a study of relapses in rheumatoid arthritis, based upon careful questioning of 35 patients. As was the case in our series, more than one factor was blamed

* See pars. 19.13 and 19.14 for additional data on the relationship of season to the course of the arthritis.

Factors Believed to be Influential

by many of the patients. The results are, in general, comparable to ours in that strain, either mental or physical, and cold or dampness were more frequently cited by the patients as causes for exacerbations than intercurrent infections. As in our series, the majority felt better in a warm environment or in summer and worse in a cold environment or in winter, with the reverse experienced by a few. In a more recent British investigation [320] of the clinical features of rheumatoid arthritis, about 60 per cent of the patients found that the severity of their disease varied with climatic conditions, chiefly in the expected direction. Our finding was also confirmed that about half of those studied would not admit that season or weather had any effect upon their symptoms. A careful study [430] of the relation of weather changes to the symptomatology of a large group of patients with rheumatoid arthritis indicated that climatic conditions exert a more striking influence upon arthritic pain and stiffness. Among 300 patients with rheumatoid arthritis observed for varying periods over the course of a year, Rentschler and his colleagues [430] encountered only 7 per cent consistently unaffected by storms or other weather phenomena. The effect of barometric pressure was considered to be more important than changes in temperature or humidity, with the majority feeling better when the barometer was rising and worse when it fell. An interesting corollary to our own and other studies dealing with the influence of cold, moisture, and heat on rheumatoid arthritis exists in the use of "micro-climate" as a therapeutic instrument. Edström and others [168] kept 18 patients with this disease in a ward with a constant temperature of 89.6°F. (32°C.) and 35 per cent humidity for periods averaging 100 days. In all, clinical improvement was noted along with disappearance of vasomotor symptoms and signs and an elevation of the skin temperature of the extremities.

20.15 As long as the pathogenesis of rheumatoid arthritis remains obscure, attempts to explain the influence of the diverse factors considered in this section upon the course of the disease rest largely upon speculation. Both strain and infection rank high as factors associated with the actual onset of the arthritis (but not necessarily of the disease) and with exacerbations or increases in symptomatology. While there is some indication that the patient whose arthritis is apparently precipitated by infection may later be vulnerable to relapses following intercurrent infections, no such relationship is apparent in the case of strain. In fact, as shown above, patients whose disease seems adversely affected by one of these factors are likely to note a similar influence from the other.

20.16   The ameliorating effect of pregnancy upon the course of rheumatoid arthritis has been convincingly described by Hench [255], although the mechanism is still unestablished. The reasons for the increase in symptomatology at the time of menstruation in certain women remain undisclosed. Theoretically they might involve a hormonal mechanism, an enhancement of pain sensitivity at this time, or merely an increase in articular swelling associated with fluid retention.

20.17   As mentioned before (par. 20.11), a possible explanation of the effect of climatic conditions upon the symptomatology of rheumatoid arthritis may lie in alterations in the vasomotor phenomena so important in the clinical picture of this disease. The patients in Edström's [168] series who improved in a warm, dry environment also evidenced disappearance of vasomotor symptoms and signs. Rentschler and others [430] describe a patient who, after a lumbar sympathectomy, ceased to feel increased pain in his legs during the climatic changes brought on by a storm but continued to feel pain in his arms. It is interesting to note in the present series that females, for whom a higher frequency of vasomotor symptoms was recorded (par. 22.4), more consistently reported that their symptoms were adversely affected by cold and dampness and relieved by heat.

SUMMARY

20.18   The patients' impressions of the effect of various factors upon the course of their arthritis were studied. Strain and climatic conditions, including cold, moisture, and heat, appear to exert an influence upon the symptomatology more frequently than intercurrent infections. In the last instance, our data suggest that patients whose arthritis was precipitated by infection are more prone to subsequent exacerbation in association with intercurrent infectious illnesses. No essential difference was found between the 27 patients who believed their course adversely affected by both strain and infection and the remainder. From records available on 6 patients in this clinic, it has not been possible to confirm

Factors Believed to be Influential

Järvinen's observations on the alternation in activity of rheumatoid arthritis and bronchial asthma in patients with both disorders. In female patients the ameliorating effect of pregnancy has been confirmed as well as, in about one-third, the adverse influence of menstruation.

20.19   About half the patients in our series experienced a worsening of symptoms with cold and moisture and improvement with heat. In addition to the large proportion whose disease was apparently uninfluenced by climatic conditions, a paradoxical effect was reported by a few. Explanation of how the factors studied are operative in producing their effects awaits a more complete knowledge of the pathogenesis of rheumatoid arthritis. Our data, however, do supply some additional evidence in favor of the concept that cold, heat, and dampness exert their effects through alterations in vasomotor tone.

20.20   Objectives for further study:

1. Observations on the effect of intercurrent infection in patients whose onset was preceded by infection, including the use of prophylactic chemotherapy.

2. Forward observations on the relationship between activity in rheumatoid arthritis and asthma in patients with both conditions.

3. Direct measurements of alterations in vasomotor tone as related to climatic changes, including temperature, humidity, barometric pressure, and atmospheric electricity.

21

Constitutional Symptoms

21.1 In a disease like rheumatoid arthritis, which is clearly systemic rather than confined to the joints, general or constitutional symptoms would be expected and indeed have been frequently mentioned in clinical accounts of this disorder [52, 208, 251, 271, 514, 571]. As pointed out before (par. 13.2), such symptoms may be prominent in the prodromal phase and long precede the development of an actual arthritis, following which time they may become more pronounced. In this chapter, certain symptoms of a general nature and not directly related to the vascular or nervous system will be taken up. The list includes headache, weakness or fatigue, anorexia, and weight loss—each patient having been questioned in regard to the presence of such symptoms at any time in the course of the arthritis prior to hospital admission. Data will also be presented in regard to the patients' weights on admission in comparison with the average, or "normal," weights for individuals of corresponding age, sex, and height.

21.2 From Table 21.1 it seems reasonable to consider that weakness or fatigue, anorexia, and weight loss are characteristic of rheumatoid arthritis since the frequency of these symptoms was overwhelmingly higher in patients than controls. Headache, on the other hand, occurred equally in both groups and thus need not be regarded as a symptom of the disease, unless clearly linked to arthritis of the cervical spine or

Constitutional Symptoms

Table 21.1

Frequency of constitutional symptoms among 293 rheumatoid arthritics and 293 controls

Symptom	Patients		Controls	
	No.	Per cent	No.	Per cent
Headache	72	24.6	67	27.7*
Weakness or fatigue	234	79.9	62	21.2
Anorexia	153	52.2	22	7.5
Weight loss	228	77.8	43	14.7

* Figured on 242 controls, since 51 with eye disease were excluded.

temporo-mandibular joints. The most common of the three symptoms was generalized weakness or fatigue, which was reported by 80 per cent of the patients. In the one other series [157] which includes a tabulation of this symptom, only about half the patients complained of general weakness. Slightly more than 50 per cent of our patients admitted to loss of appetite. By comparison, 32.6 per cent of Lewis-Faning's [320] patients and 10.9 per cent of his matched controls complained of anorexia. The lower percentage obtained in Lewis-Faning's patients may be due to the fact that no patients with disease duration of more than five years were included, while over one-fourth of our patients were admitted with duration of more than five years. The large proportion of our patients who claimed weight loss was not surpassed in four reports [157, 320, 325, 478], where the percentages given were 25.5, 53.5, 57, and 72.4, respectively. In a series of 132 American soldiers with rheumatoid arthritis studied in 1943 [463], 87 per cent gave a history of one or more of the three constitutional symptoms, fatigue, anorexia, and weight loss. The corresponding figure for the present series was 95.2 per cent.

21.3   In Table 21.2 the period of weight loss in patients with this symptom has been set down in respect to the actual onset of arthritis: 33 patients, or 11.9 per cent of the series, had lost weight before definite joint symptoms appeared, a figure much lower than that secured by Eaton [157], who listed 36 per cent of his 173 patients as underweight when the disease began. As shown in the table, weight loss appeared or continued in most of our patients after the onset of arthritis. Table 13.1 shows the frequency of certain prodromal symptoms, including

Table 21.2

Weight loss in relation to onset of rheumatoid arthritis among patients of present series

Time	Patients	
	No.	Per cent
Before onset only	4	1.8
Before and after onset	29	12.7
After onset only	179	78.5
Not recorded	16	7.0
	228	100.0

weakness or fatigue and appetite loss, for the entire series. The following list shows the proportion of patients with each constitutional symptom who had also experienced it in the prodromal period: fatigue—53.8 per cent, anorexia—28.1 per cent, and weight loss—12.7 per cent. Loss of weight and appetite thus seem more prone to appear with the arthritis than to precede it in the prodromal phase of the disease, a conclusion also suggested by the data in one other series [320].

21.4 The associations between certain factors and the three constitutional symptoms are listed in Table 21.3.* While their significance must remain inconclusive due to interrelationships among the factors tested as well as among the three symptoms, brief comments are warranted. Both weakness and anorexia were more common among females, while weight loss showed no sex difference. Each symptom was found with approximately the same frequency in patients above and below the age of forty, a result confirmed by Lewis-Faning [320] in the case of anorexia. As would be expected from data presented in the preceding paragraph, weakness alone was associated with prodromata. Strain as a precipitating factor, but not infection, was associated with weakness, an example of the lack of mutual relationships with other factors shared by the two precipitants. The relationships between an acute, severe onset, and weakness and anorexia have been previously commented upon (par. 15.4), as have those between constitutional symptoms and either a monarticular or unilateral distribution of joint involvement at onset (par. 16.14). Among the three symptoms themselves, positive associations were present except between weakness and

* For a complete list of associations, see Appendix Table 47.

Constitutional Symptoms

Table 21.3

Association of various factors with weakness, anorexia, and weight loss among patients of present series

Factor	Weakness	Anorexia	Weight loss
Sex (male)	—	—	0
Prodromal symptoms	+	0	0
Strain before onset	+	0	0
Infection before onset	0	0	0
Onset acute	+	+	0
Onset monarticular	0	—	0
Onset unilateral	0	—	0
Age on admission	0	0	0
Duration before admission (longer)	0	0	0
Intermittent course before admission	0	0	0
Weakness		+	0
Anorexia	+		+
Weight loss	0	+	
Vasomotor symptoms			
(cold extremities and paresthesias)	+	+	0
Vasomotor signs	0	0	0
Nervousness and/or emotional upsets	+	+	0
Muscular atrophy	+	+	+
Fever	0	0	0
Spondylitis (in males)	0	+	0
Total severity (increased)	0	+	+
Improvement (after discharge)	0	0	0

Note: + signifies positive association, — negative association, and 0 absence of association.

weight loss, where the degree of association was not significant. As in the case of prodromal symptoms (par. 13.9), it has been suggested that constitutional symptoms may actually be due to emotional disturbances [527]. The associations between weakness and strain as a precipitant and between nervousness and both weakness and anorexia lend a little support to this concept, which remains unsubstantiated by the presently available psychiatric studies on rheumatoid patients. Weakness and anorexia were related to two out of the four vasomotor symptoms studied, but not to objective signs of vasomotor instability, both of which will be discussed in detail in the next chapter. Muscular atrophy was associated with all three constitutional symptoms and marked total severity* of disease on hospital admission with two of them. These

* See definition, par. 4.26.

relationships might be expected, since both constitutional manifestations and muscle wasting were taken into account in classifying each patient in regard to total disease severity on admission. No differences were observed between those with spondylitis and patients with peripheral joint involvement alone, except in the case of anorexia. The absence of association between a febrile hospital course and weight loss suggests that increased metabolism from fever is not operative in the loss of weight which so commonly accompanies rheumatoid arthritis. Finally, the presence or absence of constitutional symptoms was apparently not of prognostic assistance, either in regard to the patient's course before admission or after he had left the hospital.

21.5   Data are available in regard to weight on admission to the hospital from 237 patients whose heights were also measured, thus permitting comparison with tables for average, or "normal," weight for age and sex [55]. The results, expressed in percentage of standard weight, are shown in Table 21.4. Nearly half the patients varied from the standard weights by not more than 10 per cent, while the remainder were divided between those under (35.9 per cent) and over (21.5 per cent) the normal weight for individuals of corresponding age, sex, and height. In discussing these figures, it must first be remembered that the percentages are not derived from the whole series and that information about the 56 patients not included is unobtainable. However, a notably large proportion of the patients were of normal or more than normal weight. Thus, while nearly 80 per cent of our series gave a history of weight loss, many patients must either have had very small losses or have been so overweight before onset that their weights remained within the normal range even after considerable losses. Eaton's [157] figures for patients' weights at onset of their arthritis are in keeping with this assumption, since, while 36 per cent were underweight at this time, 30 per cent were of normal weight and 34 per cent above normal. In Lewis-Faning's series [320], over half of the patients were estimated by the examiner to be underweight compared with only one-sixth of the controls. By actual measurement, while the mean height was essentially the same in both groups, the average weight of the patients was 125 lbs. compared with 139 lbs. in the controls. That a substantial portion of the patients were of greater than normal weight at the onset of their arthri-

Constitutional Symptoms

Table 21.4

Weights of patients of present series recorded on hospital admission (see par. 21.5) and compared with standard tables for sex, height, and age [55]

Percentage of standard weight	Patients No.	Per cent
Less than 70	10	4.2
70–79	27	11.4
80–89	48	20.3
90–99	64	27.0
100–109	37	15.6
110–119	25	10.5
120–129	13	5.5
130–139	6	2.5
140 and over	7	3.0
	237	100.0
70–89	85	35.9
90–109	101	42.6
110–140 or more	51	21.5

tis is borne out by the finding that half of those who were considered normal or overweight when examined gave a history of losing weight during the course of their disease. It may thus be concluded that being underweight does not especially predispose an individual to the development of rheumatoid arthritis but that those of average or above-average weight seem equally liable.

21.6 Although fatigue and anorexia are characteristic and sometimes disabling symptoms of rheumatoid arthritis, no reasonable explanation of the mechanism of their production is at hand. At most, their presence emphasizes the constitutional or systemic nature of the disease and is often helpful in differential diagnosis. The cause or causes of weight loss are similarly obscure. That nearly half of those claiming weight loss did not admit to anorexia suggests that diminished food intake due to poor appetite is not the important factor. Muscular atrophy, although found in two-thirds of those who lost weight, may contribute to but hardly accounts for the marked and rapid loss in certain cases. Evidence is lacking to implicate either fever (par. 26.3) or an increase in basal metabolism as a cause of weight loss. However, a metabolic defect must be present in many instances, as indicated by studies showing a negative nitrogen balance in rheumatoid arthritis [*441*] and by examples seen in our clinic of patients who fail to gain weight, in the absence of fever, when actually ingesting a total number of calories far in excess of their theoretical needs. The nature of this metabolic defect awaits further investigation—a type of research, which, if successful, might go far toward unraveling the pathologic physiology of rheumatoid arthritis.

SUMMARY

21.7   By means of controls, we have shown that fatigue, anorexia, and weight loss are characteristic constitutional symptoms of rheumatoid arthritis. Of the three, fatigue was more often present before as well as after the actual onset of arthritis among the patients of our series. While the large majority gave a history of weight loss, at least half were of normal or more than normal weight on admission and the conclusion can be drawn that those of average and above-average weight are as liable to the development of rheumatoid arthritis as the undernourished. No explanation is as yet available for the production of the symptoms fatigue and anorexia in rheumatoid arthritis, nor for the characteristic weight loss accompanying the disease.

21.8   Objectives for further study:

1. More detailed observations in regard to fatigue and anorexia as constitutional symptoms, to include their relationship to variations in disease activity.

2. The pathogenesis of weight loss in patients in whom neither fever nor decreased caloric intake is apparently responsible.

3. Psychogenic factors in relation to the mechanism of the production of fatigue and anorexia.

22

Vasomotor Symptoms and Signs

22.1 From the earliest available clinical descriptions of rheumatoid arthritis to the most recent, symptoms and signs consistent with increased vasomotor tone have received prominent mention. By some, vasomotor manifestations have been looked upon as predisposing to the development of a severe type of disease or even as important factors in the pathogenesis of the arthritis [570]. The present chapter will summarize the pertinent literature on this subject and will analyze the data gained from questioning and examination of 293 patients and corresponding controls. The first part of the section will be concerned with vasomotor symptoms and the second with signs.

VASOMOTOR SYMPTOMS

22.2 Each patient and control was asked whether or not one or more of the following symptoms had been present (in the case of the patients at any time in the course of the arthritis and in the controls without specification as to time of occurrence): cold extremities from a subjective standpoint; cyanosis in the form of "blue" hands or feet; paresthesias of the extremities, variously described as numbness and tingling, stinging, burning, or sensation of pins and needles; and vascular spasm. The last has been recorded by several authors [286, 338, 476], most vividly perhaps by Jones [286], who described attacks not only in the hands and feet but also in the nose, ears, and genitals, in addition to constricted visual fields due to retinal vasospasm. Paresthesias have been included under the heading of vasomotor symptoms, although it might seem equally reasonable to classify them among the neurologic symptoms, to be taken up in the next chapter. Symptoms of this nature are surely mediated through sensory nerve endings and may occur in diseases of the peripheral and central nervous system as well as in vasomotor disorders, such as Raynaud's syndrome. In the latter instance, as well as in rheumatoid arthritis, it is possible that they result from alterations in blood supply to the peripheral nerves or their endings, although the inflammatory infiltration of the peripheral nerve sheaths in rheumatoid arthritis may furnish a more reasonable explanation. Still another possibility is that of interaction between sympathetic and sensory fibers in peripheral nerves, as has been demonstrated in animals between the motor and sensory fibers of a nerve that has been cut or injured [221]. Such mechanisms probably explain the pain and sensory symptoms of causalgia, as well as their relief by sympathetic block [149]. At least three other authors [333, 338, 476] have assumed that paresthesias in rheumatoid arthritis are largely of vasomotor origin, and patients have frequently associated these sensations with other manifestations obviously due to vasomotor instability. Some degree of numerical confirmation is also available in that among both patients and controls, each of the other three vasomotor symptoms occurred with significantly greater frequency when paresthesias were present. In fact, 78 per cent of the patients with a history of paresthesias also noted cold extremities.

22.3   As shown in Table 22.1, the distribution of vasomotor symptoms among our patients covered a wide range—over half reported cold extremities but about one-tenth reported vascular spasm. It is evident from the table that each symptom was elicited from a significantly higher number of patients than controls and that a much greater proportion of patients than controls admitted to at least one. When the two groups were divided according to sex and to age on hospital admission (under forty or forty and over), vasomotor symptoms, both individually and collectively, were found with significantly greater frequency among patients than controls in each of the four subgroups so formed. Table 22.2 thus demonstrates that rheumatoid arthritics are

Table 22.1

Frequency of vasomotor symptoms among 293 rheumatoid arthritics and 293 controls

Symptom	Patients		Controls		Difference in percentages
	No.	Per cent	No.	Per cent	
1 or more present (total)	196	66.9	70	23.9	43.0 ± 4.1
Distribution of symptoms					
Cold extremities	161	54.9	44	15.0	39.9 ± 3.9
Paresthesias	102	34.8	27	9.2	25.6 ± 3.4
Cyanosis	61	20.8	11	3.8	17.0 ± 2.6
Vascular spasm	33	11.3	8	2.7	8.6 ± 2.1

Table 22.2

Vasomotor symptoms in rheumatoid arthritis—patients of present series divided according to sex and to age at hospital admission and compared with corresponding controls

	Patients				
	Males (107)		Females (186)		Difference in percentages
Symptom	No.	Per cent	No.	Per cent	
1 or more present (total)	62	57.9	134	72.0	14.1 ± 4.4
A Under 40*	35	54.7	60	75.0	20.3 ± 8.0
B 40 or more†	27	62.8	74	69.8	7.0 ± 8.6
Cold extremities	47	43.9	114	61.3	17.4 ± 6.1
Paresthesias	23	21.5	79	42.5	21.0 ± 5.8
Cyanosis	19	17.8	42	22.6	4.8 ± 4.9
Vascular spasm	8	7.5	25	13.4	5.9 ± 3.8
	Controls				
1 or more present (total)	13	12.1	57	30.6	18.5 ± 5.2
A Under 40*	11	17.2	24	30.0	12.8 ± 7.0
B 40 or more†	2	4.7	33	31.1	26.4 ± 7.4
Cold extremities	9	8.4	35	18.8	10.4 ± 4.4
Paresthesias	6	5.6	21	11.3	5.7 ± 3.5
Cyanosis	1	0.9	10	5.4	4.5 ± 1.2
Vascular spasm	2	1.9	6	3.2	1.3 ± 1.9

* Comprising 64 males and 80 females.
† Comprising 43 males and 106 females.

generally liable to the development of vasomotor symptoms irrespective of sex or age. As shown in the table, a history of one or more vasomotor symptoms was elicited more often among females than males (with the difference significant only in patients under forty on admission). With regard to individual symptoms, this difference was significant only in respect to cold extremities and paresthesias. These results were nearly duplicated in the controls, the exceptions being that a significant sex difference was found only in the frequency of cold extremities and cyanosis and that a significant difference between males and females with one or more vasomotor symptoms existed only in controls forty and over. The suggestion thus arises that the female sex is more susceptible to symptoms usually considered of vasomotor origin. As pointed out in a previous section (par. 5.4), the prevalence of migraine and Raynaud's syndrome, both of which might be termed vasomotor neuroses, is much higher among females. One author has even gone so far as to associate the preponderance in women of rheumatoid arthritis to the increased vasomotor tone inherent in this sex [377].

22.4 In neither patients nor controls was the influence of age apparent on the frequency of vasomotor symptoms. In both males and females the proportion with such symptoms was approximately the same regardless of age—a finding that was confirmed when the four vasomotor symptoms were tested individually. Cyanosis and vascular spasm, however, were more common in patients with disease onset under the age of forty. The constitutional symptoms, weakness and anorexia, were associated with two of the four vasomotor symptoms, cold extremities and paresthesias, while a history of prodromata was associated with cold extremities and vascular spasm. These two constitutional symptoms and a history of prodromata, both occurred, like the vasomotor symptoms, more often among females, but further analysis made it seem less likely that the higher frequency of these symptoms among females was responsible for the associations. The same was true of the association between a history of nervousness and the presence of individual vasomotor symptoms (except cyanosis). This last association suggests the possibility that "nervous" patients may have been more aware of vasomotor manifestations or that the symptoms were aggravated by emotional causes. In addition it adds some support to the thesis that vasomotor symptoms are largely due to emotional disturbances

Vasomotor Symptoms and Signs

[527]. When males having spondylitis were compared with those having peripheral joint involvement alone, only cyanosis among the four vasomotor symptoms was reported less frequently by those with spinal localization of their disease.

22.5 The following aspects of the disease were noted with approximately equal frequency among patients with and without vasomotor symptoms: infection or strain as precipitating factors; an acute, severe onset; and fever or an increase in pulse rate while in the hospital. The distribution of primary joint involvement was similar in the two groups and duration of disease was apparently unrelated to the presence or absence of vasomotor symptoms. The only relationship found between a vasomotor symptom and total disease severity* on hospital admission was the association of increasing severity with a history of cold extremities, and no associations were found between vasomotor symptoms and the course of the disease before admission or after discharge. Hence our data failed to demonstrate that inquiry in regard to these symptoms may be helpful in formulating a prognosis.†

VASOMOTOR SIGNS

22.6 The finding by the examiner of both cold and moist hands or feet was regarded as objective evidence of increased vasomotor tone. While the proportion with cold, moist extremities was significantly higher among patients than controls (Table 22.3), the frequency of this finding was less than the percentage in each group giving a history of one or more vasomotor symptoms. It should be noted that our data were derived from a single examination of each individual and not by the use of the more exact methods of determining vasomotor activity employed by others [343, 377, 570]. When both patients and controls were divided into subgroups according to sex and age, essentially the same difference obtained. When male and female patients were compared according to age on hospital admission, objective evidence of increased vasomotor activity was found more frequently among females of the younger age group and among males of the older age group (Table 22.4). The finding with respect to the younger age group was consistent with that shown in Table 22.2 for vasomotor symptoms.

* See definition, par. 4.26.
† For a complete list of associations, see Appendix Table 47.

Table 22.3

Vasomotor signs in rheumatoid arthritis—patients of present series compared with controls

	No.	Vasomotor signs	
		No.	Per cent
Patients	293	97	33.1
Controls	293	27	9.2
Difference in percentages:			23.9 ± 3.4

Table 22.4

Frequency of vasomotor signs among patients of present series divided according to sex and to age on hospital admission

		Vasomotor signs	
All ages*	No.	No.	Per cent
Total	293	97	33.1
Males	107	39	36.4
Females	186	58	31.2
Under age 40 on admission†			
Total	144	54	37.5
Males	64	18	28.1
Females	80	36	45.0
Age 40 or more on admission**			
Total	149	43	28.9
Males	43	21	48.8
Females	106	22	20.7
* Difference in percentages:			5.2 ± 5.6
† Difference in percentages:			16.9 ± 8.1
** Difference in percentages:			28.1 ± 8.2

Among controls of both age groups similar tendencies were observed, but the differences were not wide enough to be significant (Table 22.5). As might be expected, older male patients evidenced vasomotor signs more often than younger, while the reverse was true of females. This distribution was duplicated in the female controls, but not in the male controls. The latter finding is the only indication we have encountered in our data that, in males at least, age differences in respect to vasomotor signs may be related to the disease rather than to the sex.

22.7   No constant association was found either among patients or among controls between individual vasomotor symptoms and the presence of cold, moist extremities. Vasomotor signs were associated

Vasomotor Symptoms and Signs

Table 22.5
Frequency of vasomotor signs among controls divided according to sex and to age at admission to study

	No.	Vasomotor signs	
		No.	Per cent
*All ages**			
Total	293	27	9.2
Males	107	9	8.4
Females	186	18	9.7
Under age 40 on admission†			
Total	144	20	13.9
Males	64	6	9.4
Females	80	14	17.5
*Age 40 or more on admission***			
Total	149	7	4.7
Males	43	3	7.0
Females	106	4	3.8

* Difference in percentages: 1.3 ± 3.5
† Difference in percentages: 8.1 ± 5.8
** Difference in percentages: 3.2 ± 3.7

with cold extremities and vascular spasm among patients but only with cold extremities among controls. It should again be noted that our data in regard to the vasomotor tone of the extremities was gathered from a single examination. In neither group was a history of paresthesias related to the finding of vasomotor signs—possibly a point against considering this symptom necessarily of vasomotor origin. As with vasomotor symptoms, the frequency of various disease factors was figured for those with and without objective evidence of vasomotor activity. No important differences were found and in particular no information of prognostic assistance was encountered.*

COMMENT

22.8 In general, figures in the literature are in keeping with those obtained from our data on both patients and controls and bear out the assumption that vasomotor phenomena form an integral part of the clinical picture of rheumatoid arthritis. The mechanism of their production is presumably that of sympathetic overactivity, perhaps dependent upon the anatomic changes that have been demonstrated in sympathetic

---
* For a complete list of associations, see the Appendix Table 47.

ganglia in this disease [367]. Nearly half of Douthwaite's [150] patients gave a history of cold hands and feet since puberty, while Stewart [502] found a frequency of paresthesias among his patients comparable to that obtained from ours. In a recent British study [320], with an approximately equal number of matched controls, a significantly greater proportion of patients gave a history of cold hands and feet, chilblains, and vascular spasm. This study also brought out the important point that in most cases vasomotor symptoms were present both before and after the onset of arthritis. The frequency of vascular spasm was reported in another study [478] as 15 per cent, a figure close to the one obtained in the present series. In regard to objective changes, cold extremities were recorded for about 75 per cent of Smith's [478] patients, a higher proportion than was recorded for our patients, in whom a moist as well as a cold skin was required for inclusion in the group with vasomotor signs. In one other series [320] matched controls as well as patients were examined. No evidence of increased vasomotor activity was noted in 88 per cent of the controls and in 45 per cent of the patients. Cold fingers were recorded for 15 per cent of the patients and only 5 per cent of the controls.

22.9 In two studies [377, 570] the vascular response to exposure to heat and cold in rheumatoid arthritics and controls was observed by means of skin temperature recordings. The conclusions are in essential agreement: that the blood flow is frequently attenuated in the limbs of patients with rheumatoid arthritis, presumably through increased vascular tone. A similar response was found in some normal individuals, more often in females than males. Conversely, it was pointed out in one study [570] that this vascular "defect," since it may be absent in well-marked cases, is not essential to the development of rheumatoid arthritis of severe degree. In our own series, vasomotor manifestations, either subjective or objective, were not recorded in more than one-fourth of the patients. Both clinical and skin temperature studies are thus in accord regarding the association between vasomotor instability and rheumatoid arthritis. The data from neither source, however, allow the assumption that increased vasomotor tone, either inherent or acquired, plays an important role in the pathogenesis of rheumatoid arthritis or even determines the greater liability of females to the acquisition of this condition. Differences in the frequency of vasomotor symptoms and signs

Vasomotor Symptoms and Signs

in respect to sex and age, as observed among our patients, probably merely reflect similar differences in the liability of the population at large to the development of peripheral vascular disease. To cite two well-known examples, Raynaud's syndrome is found almost exclusively in younger women, while obliterating arteriosclerosis of the legs occurs predominantly in older men.

SUMMARY

22.10 Evidence of vasomotor instability, both subjective and objective, was encountered with significantly greater frequency among rheumatoid arthritics than among controls. Although the inclusion of paresthesias among symptoms of vasomotor origin may be questioned, some data are available to warrant such a tentative classification. Females admitted before the age of forty and males entering the hospital after reaching this age were in general more likely to display vasomotor instability. Such differences in respect to age and sex are probably not confined to rheumatoid arthritics but merely reflect a similar distribution of susceptibility to vasomotor disorders in the population at large. No important differences were found in the characteristics or severity of the arthritis whether or not vasomotor instability was present. For about one-fourth of the patients, no evidence of a vasomotor defect was recorded by means of either history or physical examination. This negative finding, corroborated elsewhere by quantitative studies, constitutes one important argument against regarding vasomotor changes as essential to the development of rheumatoid arthritis.

22.11 Objectives for further study:

1. Observations on vasomotor symptoms and signs as related to exacerbations and remissions, as well as further observations on the effect of suppressive therapy with cortisone and other agents [29, 72, 569a].

2. Elucidation of the mechanism of alterations in the peripheral circulation in rheumatoid arthritis, including the use of interruption of sympathetic innervation of the limbs and of newer drugs acting on the autonomic nervous system.

3. The pathogenesis of paresthesias in rheumatoid arthritis, whether they are dependent upon primary alterations in the peripheral nerves or secondary to sympathetic overactivity.

23

Neurologic Symptoms and Signs

23.1 That neurologic manifestations form an integral part of the clinical picture in rheumatoid arthritis has long been recognized. At times, such symptoms and signs may precede any obvious arthritis or so dominate the picture as to suggest strongly the diagnosis of a primary neurologic disorder. Both patients and controls were therefore systematically questioned and examined in regard to clinical features in which the nervous system might have been involved. Muscular atrophy was included, although the pathogenesis of this often disabling condition is by no means settled. The results of an inquiry into the frequency of patients giving a history of nervousness and/or emotional upsets have also been outlined in this section.

NEUROLOGIC SYMPTOMS

23.2 Patients and controls were questioned about four symptoms of probable neurologic origin: muscular twitching [*92, 286, 333, 403*]; vertigo [*403*], or more properly giddiness; tremor [*286, 333*]; and tinnitus [*403*]. (Paresthesias were included among vasomotor symptoms from considerations set forth in par. 22.2.) All have been mentioned in the literature in association with rheumatoid arthritis. No specification was made as to the time of occurrence of these symptoms when a control was questioned, but the patients were confined to the interval

Neurologic Symptoms and Signs

between the onset of arthritis and the time of interrogation. As shown in Table 23.1, the frequency of each symptom was higher among patients than among controls, but the difference lacked significance in the case of tinnitus. For this reason, it was decided to exclude tinnitus from detailed statistical consideration, although the possibility remains that the difference would have been significant had the controls been questioned in regard to periods comparable with the duration of arthritis in patients. In the single series [403] encountered in the literature in which tinnitus was regarded as a common symptom, patients with both rheumatoid arthritis and degenerative joint disease were included without differentiation. It should also be mentioned that in some of the patients with this symptom, the tinnitus may be due to salicylism or related to involvement of the cervical spine or temporo-mandibular joints.

23.3 The remaining three symptoms, twitching, vertigo and tremor, were found with equal frequency in males and females among both patients and controls, while tinnitus was more common in female patients. Some differences were observed between older and younger patients, with vertigo and tremor admitted to more often by patients aged forty or more on hospital admission and tinnitus more often by patients of the younger group (Table 23.2). Among controls, only vertigo occurred with higher frequency in the older group. In addition to age and sex, associations between other disease factors and the three neurologic symptoms was determined. The significance of such associations must remain inconclusive due to interrelationships among the factors tested

Table 23.1

Frequency of neurologic symptoms among 292 patients* of present series and corresponding controls*

Symptom	Patients		Controls		Difference in percentages
	No.	Per cent	No.	Per cent	
1 or more present (total)	134	45.9	63	21.6	24.3 ± 3.9
Twitching	83	28.4	24	8.2	20.2 ± 3.2
Vertigo	61	20.9	36	12.3	8.6 ± 3.1
Tremor	64	21.9	22	7.5	14.4 ± 2.9
Tinnitus	48	16.4	37	12.7	3.7 ± 2.9

* Information was not obtained from 1 patient, and a corresponding control was therefore omitted.

Table 23.2

Frequency of neurologic symptoms among 292 patients* of present series divided according to age on hospital admission

	Age on admission				Difference in percentages
	Under 40 (144)		40 or more (148)		
Symptom	No.	Per cent	No.	Per cent	
1 or more present (total)	54	37.5	82	55.4	17.9 ± 5.8
Twitching	36	25.0	47	31.8	6.8 ± 5.5
Vertigo	17	11.8	44	29.7	17.9 ± 4.8
Tremor	20	13.9	44	29.7	15.8 ± 4.8
Tinnitus	33	22.4	15	10.1	12.3 ± 4.4

* See note, Table 23.1.

as well as among the three symptoms. Only a few findings of clinical interest will be mentioned here, but all the results of the tabulation are available in Appendix Table 47. In the first place, each of these three symptoms showed a significant degree of association with both of the others. (Tinnitus was found associated with only one of the three, vertigo.) There was thus a tendency for more than one neurologic symptom to be reported by a single patient. As shown in Table 23.3, a history of nervousness and/or emotional upsets was associated with each of the three neurologic symptoms, but not with tinnitus. As with vasomotor symptoms (par. 22.4), the possibilities may be mentioned that the nervous individual might be more aware of minor symptoms or even that emotional factors might play a part in their production. Vasomotor symptoms and signs were related most consistently among the three to vertigo. The suggestion is thus raised that this symptom may result from vasomotor instability of the cerebral circulation. In male patients the three neurologic symptoms occurred with equal frequency among those with spinal and those with peripheral involvement. No significant associations were found between any of the three neurologic symptoms and a history of prodromal symptoms, strain or infection as precipitating factors, type of onset, duration of arthritis before hospital admission, and distribution of primary joint involvement. Only tremor was associated with two of the constitutional symptoms, weakness and anorexia. Finally, may the presence or absence of one or more of these symptoms aid in prognosis? Vertigo is apparently not helpful; a history of twitching was associated with increased total

Table 23.3
Frequency of neurologic symptoms among 292 patients* of present series with and without nervousness and/or emotional upsets

	Nervousness and/or emotional upsets				
	With (177)		Without (115*)		Difference
Symptom	No.	Per cent	No.	Per cent	in percentages
1 or more present (total)	106	59.9	30	26.1	33.8 ± 6.0
Twitching	66	37.3	17	14.8	22.5 ± 5.4
Vertigo	47	26.6	14	12.2	14.4 ± 4.9
Tremor	53	29.9	11	9.6	20.3 ± 4.9
Tinnitus	27	15.3	21	18.3	3.0 ± 4.4

* See note, Table 23.1.

severity* of disease on admission; but tremor was associated with a progressive course before admission, an increased total severity after hospital entry, and a less favorable subsequent course.†

NERVOUSNESS AND/OR EMOTIONAL UPSETS

23.4 Both patients and controls were directly questioned in regard to a history of nervousness and/or emotional upsets. As shown in Table 23.4, one or both of these symptoms was admitted to by a larger proportion of patients than controls. The differences were not great and, when both groups were divided according to sex, significant only in females. It should be admitted that, among patients with rheumatoid arthritis severe enough to require hospitalization, factors provocative of increased emotional tension are often operative and that a patient would be more likely to admit his nervousness than a control. On the other hand, no time of occurrence of such symptomatology was specified in the case of the controls, while the patients were limited to the periods covered by their disease duration. As might be expected, these symptoms were reported more frequently by females than males, a distribution also found among the controls (Table 23.4). There was also a higher frequency of nervousness among males with spondylitis than among those with peripheral involvement alone. Reference has already been made to the associations between nervousness and strain as a precipitating factor (par. 14.6); the constitutional symptoms, weak-

* See definition, par. 4.26.
† For a complete list of associations, see Appendix Table 47.

Table 23.4

Nervousness and/or emotional upsets in rheumatoid arthritis—patients of present series divided according to sex and compared with corresponding controls

	No. in each group	Nervousness and/or emotional upsets present				Difference in percentages
		Patients		Controls		
		No.	Per cent	No.	Per cent	
Total	292*	177	60.6	142	48.6	12.0 ± 4.1
Males	107	50	46.7	37	34.6	12.1 ± 6.7
Females	185	127	68.6	105	56.8	11.8 ± 5.0
Differences in percentages:			21.9 ± 5.9		22.2 ± 6.1	

* See note, Table 23.1.

ness and anorexia (par. 21.4); vasomotor symptoms (par. 22.4); and neurologic symptoms (par. 23.3). Certain implications of these associations have also been mentioned, including the likelihood of a nervous individual's being aware of minor symptomatology and the possibility of the aggravation or even the production of such symptoms on an emotional basis. No differences were found in regard to the following factors: age on admission; prodromal symptoms (par. 13.9); infection as a precipitant (par. 14.11); type of onset; duration of arthritis before hospital admission; and elevation in pulse rate. Nervous patients apparently did as well in regard to their disease as the remainder, as shown by the absence of association of nervousness with either a progressive or a remittent course before admission, degree of total severity after admission, and either a favorable or unfavorable subsequent course.*

23.5 One author, Eaton [157], studied the frequency of nervous symptoms among patients with rheumatoid arthritis. The proportion considered "nervous, excitable, restless, or timid" was comparable to the proportion of patients in the present series who gave a history of nervousness—or about half the patients studied. What might be regarded as a control group, patients with hypertrophic arthritis, did not differ significantly from the rheumatoids in this respect. It should be emphasized that in Eaton's series, as in ours, results were drawn from superficial questioning or observation and do not warrant comparison with reports on patients with rheumatoid arthritis whose personality structures have been subjected to detailed psychiatric study [236, 283, 328,

* For a complete list of associations, see Appendix Table 47.

Neurologic Symptoms and Signs

527]. The results of such studies have thus far revealed a consistent personality pattern, but one which is admittedly nonspecific and also encountered in ulcerative colitis, bronchial asthma, Raynaud's syndrome, and chronic dermatitis [328]. In spite of obvious objections—that a relatively small number of patients were examined, that some may have been chosen on account of emotional problems accompanying their arthritis, and that adequate control data are lacking—this approach to the study of the disease warrants further attention.

NEUROLOGIC SIGNS

23.6 Patients and controls were examined for objective tremor and activity of tendon reflexes (knee and ankle jerks), but the presence or absence of muscular atrophy was recorded only for the patients. The last admittedly represents such a common feature of rheumatoid arthritis as to render control observations superfluous. In our series muscular atrophy was obvious in nearly two-thirds, and the proportion might easily have been higher had careful measurements been carried out.

23.7 The results shown in Table 23.5 demonstrate a higher frequency of exaggerated tendon reflexes among the arthritics but no difference in regard to tremor. However, since tremor has been shown by electromyographic studies [373] to constitute a genuine manifestation of rheumatoid arthritis, statistical analysis of this neurologic sign was carried out along with the others. No sex differences were observed in either patients or controls, except that tremor was more frequent in male patients. Muscular atrophy alone among the three neurologic signs studied was found more often in patients admitted after the age of forty.

23.8 Few differences were noted between the patients with exaggerated reflexes and the remainder of the group. Patients giving a his-

Table 23.5
Frequency of neurologic signs among 293 rheumatoid arthritics and 293 controls

Sign	Patients		Controls		Difference in percentages
	No.	Per cent	No.	Per cent	
Tremor	22	7.5	19	6.5	
Exaggerated reflexes	96	32.8	50	17.1	15.7 ± 3.3
Muscular atrophy	186	63.5	—	—	

tory of nervousness and/or emotional upsets were found to have an increased frequency of such reflexes, while no difference was evident in respect to tremor or muscular atrophy. Increased nervous tension, then, may be a factor in determining hyperactivity of tendon reflexes in rheumatoid arthritis, but no relationship was discovered between increased reflex activity and strain as a precipitating factor. A history of tremor was found in association with all three neurologic signs, but neurologic symptoms and signs were otherwise unrelated. (One might expect an association between exaggerated reflexes and a history of muscular twitching, both of which have been deemed examples of the increased muscular irritability [*199, 286, 549*] seen in rheumatoid arthritis.) We were also unable to confirm the finding by two authors [*86, 199*] of an association between increased tendon reflex activity and muscular atrophy. Duration of arthritis, distribution of primary joint involvement, and spondylitis compared with purely peripheral arthritis were apparently unrelated to the state of the tendon reflexes. The course before admission and the total severity of arthritis as estimated on admission were likewise not associated with the activity of the reflexes, but the course after leaving the hospital was found to be less favorable among patients with exaggerated reflexes. Except for an excess of males, the small group with objective tremor largely conformed to the remainder of the series. No information of prognostic value was apparent from either the presence or absence of this physical sign.

23.9 Table 23.6 lists the nature of the association of certain factors with muscular atrophy. In general those related to increased disease severity on hospital admission and to an unfavorable subsequent course were found in association with loss of muscle substance. They include age over forty (both at onset and on admission), longer duration of disease, constitutional symptoms (weakness, anorexia, and weight loss), and subcutaneous nodules. We might expect, then, as was actually the case, an association between muscular atrophy and an unfavorable course after leaving the hospital. Since the degree of muscular atrophy was undoubtedly taken into account in the estimate of disease severity on admission, the association found between the two is really dependent upon definition. Another group of constitutional symptoms, those of vasomotor origin, were noted more frequently among patients with

Neurologic Symptoms and Signs

Table 23.6
Association of various factors with muscular atrophy among patients of present series

Factor	Muscular atrophy
Sex (male)	0
Age at onset over 40	+
Prodromal symptoms	0
Onset acute	0
Joints first involved	0
Onset unilateral	0
Age on admission over 40	+
Duration before admission (longer)	+
Course before admission	0
Weakness	+
Anorexia	+
Weight loss	+
Vasomotor symptoms	+
Lymphadenopathy	+
Splenomegaly	+
Nodules	+
Spondylitis (in males)	0
Total severity (increased)	+
Improvement (after discharge)	—

Note: + signifies positive association, — negative association, and 0 absence of association.

muscular atrophy, although not associated with increased disease severity or poor prognosis. The two remaining positive associations listed in the table were with lymphadenopathy and splenomegaly, manifestations of rheumatoid arthritis to be taken up in a subsequent chapter. As shown in the table, the frequency of muscular atrophy on admission was not related to the distribution of primary joint involvement, to type of onset (whether acute or gradual), to course before admission (whether intermittent or progressive), or to the presence or absence of spondylitis.*

COMMENT

23.10 The neural theory [13, 199, 286, 394, 490] represents a now nearly forgotten item in the ever-changing pattern of speculative thought in regard to the etiology and pathogenesis of rheumatoid ar-

* For a complete list of associations with muscular atrophy and other neurologic signs, see Appendix Table 47.

thritis, although in recent years attention has again been directed toward histologic changes in the nervous system as indicative of the systemic nature of the disease [368]. Abnormalities in the spinal fluid have also been noted [330], as well as derangements found in electroencephalograms and psychometric tests [318]. A sizable part of the argument for the neural theory has rested upon the commonly observed neurologic manifestations which have been treated in this chapter. While a number of authors have listed twitching, vertigo, tremor, and tinnitus among the common symptoms of rheumatoid arthritis, numerical data have been furnished only by Smith [478] in regard to twitching. Nearly two-thirds of his patients admitted to this symptom, a much higher figure than ours. In the same series, muscular atrophy and objective tremor were observed with approximately the same frequency as in the present series. Five references [86, 122, 157, 199, 478] have been encountered in which the frequency of exaggerated tendon reflexes was given, with percentages varying from 37 to 79 per cent. Any comparison between these figures and ours (32.7 per cent) is of course unprofitable, since the difference between a normal and an exaggerated tendon reflex has in each case been dependent upon the judgment of the observer. We have noted increased reflex activity on the diseased side, along with others [86, 157, 199, 286, 333, 549], but we neglected to obtain numerical data on this point. Clonus [86, 122, 199, 286, 333, 518] has also been observed in our patients, once in association with an acutely involved ankle joint. Garrod [199] noted abnormal plantar reflexes in a few patients. We were unable to duplicate this finding during the course of the present study, but have since observed several patients with true spasticity suggesting pyramidal tract involvement—possibly a manifestation of the arthritis. Electromyographic studies undertaken by this clinic [368] have otherwise failed to show the characteristics of upper motor neurone lesions, including spread of tendon reflexes, of the type observed in 1 case by Garrod [199]. The absence of tendon reflexes in rheumatoid arthritis has been mentioned in the literature [157, 286, 518] and was noted in 6 of our own patients. But the significance of this observation may be questioned, since tendon reflexes were also absent in 5 of the controls. In general, the tremor observed in our patients has been coarse and associated with muscle wasting, weakness, and arthritis in the arm

Neurologic Symptoms and Signs 279

and hand concerned. The origin of the tremor has not been defined, but it resembles that found in fatigue states [373]. It occasionally furnishes some difficulty in diagnosis, especially in respect to Parkinson's disease, since the latter may be accompanied by skeletal symptoms. One patient in our series was found to have both rheumatoid arthritis and Parkinsonism.

23.11 A number of theories have been advanced as to the mechanism of muscular atrophy in rheumatoid arthritis. They have been discussed in full elsewhere [368] but may be briefly mentioned at this point. Disuse has generally been discarded as a sole factor, since the atrophy may appear before the development of arthritis [151, 286] or in relation to joints still maintaining full function. A postulated reflex mechanism from the involved joints has been supported by animal experimentation [428]. Another theory supposes a central inhibitory state in the spinal cord occasioned in part by pain [373]. Direct involvement of muscle and nervous tissue by the disease process has also been demonstrated [368].

SUMMARY

23.12 Of four neurologic symptoms cited in the literature in association with rheumatoid arthritis, twitching, vertigo, and tremor were found with greater frequency among patients than among controls, while no significant difference was noted in respect to tinnitus. An association between vertigo and vasomotor instability suggests that this symptom may be of vascular origin. Subjective tremor was found to be related to an increased total disease severity on admission and to a less favorable course both before and after hospitalization. A history of nervousness, emotional upsets, or both was obtained slightly more often in the arthritic than in the control group. Female sex distribution, constitutional and vasomotor symptoms, neurologic symptoms, strain as a precipitating factor, and exaggerated tendon reflexes were more common among the "nervous" patients. Hyperactive tendon reflexes were observed in about one-third of the patients, and muscular wasting was observed in about two-thirds, but no association was found between these two neurologic signs. Muscular atrophy was found more frequently among older patients and those with disease of longer duration.

It was also related to increased total severity* of disease on hospital admission and an unfavorable subsequent course.

23.13   Objectives for further study:

1. Additional observations on nervous system involvement in rheumatoid arthritis, to include clinical, electroencephalographic, and psychometric examinations as well as histologic.

2. The mechanism of muscular atrophy in rheumatoid arthritis and other forms of joint disease.

* See definition, par. **4.26**.

24

Cardio-respiratory Symptoms and Signs

24.1 The patients of the present series were questioned in regard to certain cardio-respiratory symptoms occurring either before or after the onset of arthritis, but since the controls were not similarly questioned the significance of the data in Table 24.1 is not apparent. Both patients and controls were given physical examinations, with the results shown in Table 24.2. Here, however, the significant difference with respect to rales cannot be explained because in the control group physical examination was not supplemented by roentgenographic examination. X-ray examination of the chest was routine on admission to the hospital, and the abnormal findings obtained in this way for the patients of the present series are given in Table 24.3. Tuberculosis, bronchiectasis, and pleurisy will be discussed below, but the interpretation of less specific findings remains in doubt due to the lack of comparable roentgenograms for the control group. Insufficient evidence was brought to light during the course of the present study to corroborate the recent reports [38, 41, 170, 322, 353] of pulmonary infiltration constituting a systemic manifestation of rheumatoid arthritis, although several patients have since been seen in whom this possibility has been suspected.

24.2 Pleurisy was diagnosed in 5 patients and in 3 of the controls (without the aid of x-ray films), while 9 additional patients and 5 controls gave a history of one or more attacks (par. **10.4**). In 2 of the pa-

Table 24.1
Frequency of cardio-respiratory symptoms among 293 rheumatoid arthritics

	Patients	
Symptom	No.	Per cent
None	178	60.8
Cough	43	14.7
Sputum	32	10.9
Dyspnea	53	18.1
Palpitation	55	18.8

Table 24.2
Frequency of abnormal pulmonary signs among 293 rheumatoid arthritics and 293 controls

	Patients		Controls		Difference
Sign	No.	Per cent	No.	Per cent	in percentages
Consolidation	11	3.8	4	1.4	2.4 ± 1.3
Emphysema	10	3.4	13	4.5	
Rales (without consolidation)	34	11.6	17	5.8	5.8 ± 2.3
Pleurisy	5	1.7	3	1.0	

Table 24.3
Abnormal findings in chest x-rays of 293 rheumatoid arthritics

	Patients	
Finding	No.	Per cent
Old pleurisy	18	6.1
Old or "inactive" tuberculosis	16	5.5
Increased lung markings	9	3.1
Diminished radiance or atelectasis	8	2.7
"Active" tuberculosis	5	1.7
Bronchiectasis	2	0.7
Enlarged hilar glands	1	0.3
Silicosis	1	0.3
Pleural effusion	1	0.3

Cardio-respiratory Symptoms and Signs

tients pleurisy was associated with tuberculosis or bronchiectasis, but in the remaining 3 it presumably constituted a systemic manifestation of rheumatoid arthritis. In 2 of the rheumatoid patients pleuritic pain associated with a friction rub established the diagnosis; in 1 a small pleural effusion was demonstrated by x-ray and by aspiration. In the last patient, who was running a high, spiking fever, articular signs were meager and the pleurisy formed the most prominent feature of this phase of her illness. As early as 1860 Fuller [*195*] referred to pleurisy as one of the accessory manifestations of rheumatoid arthritis, and McCrae [*333*] diagnosed the condition clinically in 2 per cent of 319 patients. Inflammation of the pericardium [*227, 249, 333, 505*] and peritoneum [*227*] have also been noted in rheumatoid arthritis, but neither was encountered among our patients during their first hospitalization.

24.3 Active pulmonary tuberculosis was diagnosed in 5 patients at the time of hospital admission. In all of these the pulmonary disease probably antedated the arthritis. It may be mentioned here that 4 other patients, whose pulmonary changes were regarded as "inactive" at admission on clinical and roentgenologic grounds, subsequently developed active tuberculosis—all but 1 of them more than ten years later. The combination of rheumatoid arthritis and pulmonary tuberculosis was formerly believed to be extremely rare [*403*], but a few years ago Fletcher and Lewis-Faning [*187*] found the frequency of phthisis to be 4.3 per cent among 254 rheumatoid patients, while autopsy studies of 61 patients by Fingerman and Andrus [*179*] revealed active tuberculosis in the lungs of over 10 per cent.

24.4 Bronchiectasis was found in 4 patients. In 1 of them symptoms of this condition followed the development of arthritis, and in the remainder preceded it. Reference should also be made to the finding that a history of pneumonia was reported more often by patients than by controls (par. **10.6**).

24.5 In Table 24.4 the frequency of heart disease in patients and controls is set forth, with the figures for both valvular disease and other types essentially the same in the two groups. Of the 6 patients with valve lesions, 5 gave a history of probable rheumatic fever in childhood. Of more interest in regard to the concept of "rheumatoid" heart disease is the later finding that 5 additional patients developed valvular disease

Table 24.4
Frequency of heart disease among 293 rheumatoid arthritics and 293 controls

Valvular disease, presumably rheumatic	No.	Per cent	Remarks
Patients	6	2.0	5 with history of rheumatic fever; 2 had spondylitis. 3 with mitral valve affected; 1 with aortic, 2 with both.
Controls	4	1.4	3 with history of rheumatic fever; 4 with mitral valve affected.
Hypertensive or arteriosclerotic disease			
Patients	19	6.5	
Controls	19	6.5	

while under observation following their hospital discharge. The diagnoses made in these patients were as follows: aortic regurgitation (in 2 patients, 1 of whom also developed spondylitis); mitral regurgitation (in 1 patient); mitral stenosis (in 1 patient); and aortic regurgitation and aortic stenosis, presumably calcareous in type (in 1 patient). A sixth patient was readmitted within a few months and died of a fulminating pancarditis and aortitis, with autopsy findings characteristic of "rheumatoid" rather than rheumatic etiology. Although he had symptoms referred to the spine, the diagnosis of spondylitis was not established. The experience gained from the study of the present series has not been of material assistance in settling the status of the valvular lesions in rheumatoid arthritis—whether they represent an association between rheumatic heart disease and rheumatoid arthritis or whether they actually constitute, along with myocarditis and pericarditis, systemic manifestations of the disease. For further discussion of this subject, the reader is referred to the introductory section, pars. 2.6–2.12.

SUMMARY

24.6 Pleurisy, which may be regarded as one of the systemic manifestations of rheumatoid arthritis, was diagnosed in 5 patients and in 1 was accompanied by an effusion. Pulmonary tuberculosis was found on admission or through follow-up in 9 patients (a frequency of 3.1 per cent), while bronchiectasis was present in 4 patients. The frequency on admission of valvular and other types of heart disease was essentially the same among patients and controls; 5 additional patients developed signs of valvular heart disease during the follow-up period.

24.7   Objectives for further study:

1. Clinical and pathologic observations on pulmonary lesions in rheumatoid arthritis, including those developing in patients exposed to dust [353].

2. The nature of the cardiac involvement found in patients with rheumatoid arthritis.

25

Gastro-intestinal Symptoms

25.1 The gastro-intestinal tract has been included in the total clinical picture of rheumatoid arthritis in a number of ways. The high frequency of dyspeptic symptoms and disorders of bowel function has been commented upon in early accounts of the disease [*271, 286, 510, 518*] and, at one period, absorption of noxious material from the colon was regarded as a link in the pathogenesis of the arthritis [*214, 310*]. The gallbladder has also been indicted as an occasional focus of infection [*258, 288, 560, 566*], while more recent studies have shown a disturbance of liver function in a high proportion of patients [*327, 358, 426, 438, 560*]. There remains in addition the association, present in 3 of our patients, between idiopathic ulcerative colitis and rheumatoid arthritis, which has been discussed in the introductory section (par. **2.105**) and will not be reviewed here. The frequency of hepatomegaly or liver disease among patients of the present series, as well as the results of x-ray examination of the gallbladder and colon, will be taken up subsequently (Chapters 30, 35, and 36).

25.2 As shown in Table 25.1, a higher frequency of vomiting, constipation, diarrhea (with ulcerative colitis excluded), and anorexia was obtained from the patients' histories than from the controls', with no significant difference in respect to nausea (unaccompanied by vomiting), flatulence, and abdominal pain. As is usually the case in medi-

Gastro-intestinal Symptoms

Table 25.1
Frequency of gastro-intestinal symptoms among 293 rheumatoid arthritics and 293 controls

	Patients		Controls		Difference
	No.	Per cent	No.	Per cent	in percentages
Nausea (total)	44	15.0	29	9.9	5.1 ± 2.7
Nausea with vomiting	33	11.3	19	6.5	4.8 ± 2.4
Abdominal pain	28	9.6	28	9.6	0.0
Flatulence	62	21.2	66	22.5	1.3 ± 3.3
Constipation	113	38.6	43	14.7	23.9 ± 3.7
Diarrhea (ulcerative colitis excluded)	8	2.7	1	0.3	2.4 ± 1.0
Anorexia	153	52.2	22	7.5	44.7 ± 3.8

cal practice, a history of constipation was more often elicited from females than from males and from patients who were forty or over on admission compared with the younger group. Similar findings were obtained from the much smaller number of controls with this symptom. Nausea, with or without vomiting, was also more frequent among females (not duplicated in the controls), with no apparent difference in regard to age on admission. Since both nausea and constipation were more often recorded for females, the apparent association of the two symptoms in our series remains of doubtful significance and cannot be defined by further analysis of the data. One other comparison was made between those with constipation and those without it in regard to the total severity* of the arthritis on admission, but no significant differences were found. Of the last two symptoms listed in Table 25.1, 6 of the 8 patients with diarrhea were females, while anorexia has already been taken up in Chapter 21 as a constitutional symptom.

25.3 Llewellyn Jones [286] noted the frequency of digestive tract disturbances preceding or accompanying rheumatoid arthritis, with abdominal pain after meals, persistent vomiting, and weight loss in some patients, perhaps similar to the "gastric crises" cited by Spender and Garrod [491]. Actual figures in regard to gastro-intestinal symptoms are few, but in one paper [510], a history of dyspepsia was given by 37 of 200 patients, a somewhat higher percentage than that found in the present series; and in another [150], 30 per cent of the patients told

* See definition, par. **4.26.**

of bilious attacks in childhood. Two authors set down the frequency of constipation among their patients, the one [478], 30.4 per cent, quite close to ours, and the other [150], 82 per cent, thus making constipation a nearly consistent finding in this group of patients with rheumatoid arthritis. The 8 patients with diarrhea in the present series, though few in number, lend support to previously expressed clinical opinions that diarrhea is an occasional symptom of rheumatoid arthritis [90, 286]. Millard Smith [477] encountered 6 patients in his series of 102 with an idiopathic diarrhea preceding exacerbations in the disease, while Clark [90] noted in some of her patients a persistent and troublesome diarrhea alternating with constipation.

25.4 A history of peptic ulcer was given by none of our patients at the time of admission and by only 1 of the controls. This disease appeared subsequently in 5 male and 4 female patients, or 4.7 and 2.2 per cent of the series. Data from 357 additional patients with rheumatoid arthritis observed in this clinic show even higher percentages: 7.5 per cent for 173 males, 3.8 per cent for 184 females, and 5.6 per cent for the whole group. Figures are not yet available for the frequency of peptic ulcer among a population comparable to the 650 patients with rheumatoid arthritis just mentioned. In a study of 13,885 employees, chiefly clerical workers and over two-thirds females, observed over a ten-year period, Jennison [282] found that the frequency of peptic ulcer was 3.4 per cent among males, 0.7 per cent among females, and 1.48 per cent among the total group. These percentages are undoubtedly lower than the actual incidence because of the probability that some of the employees with ulcer failed to come to the company clinic for treatment or diagnosis. According to Ivy, Grossman, and Bachrach [273], a reasonably accurate figure for the autopsy prevalence of peptic ulcer is not yet available, although figures from carefully studied large series range from 5 to 10 per cent. The preceding data suggest that peptic ulcer occurs among patients with rheumatoid arthritis at least as often as among the general population.

25.5 The nature of the relationship between rheumatoid arthritis and the gastro-intestinal manifestations described in this chapter remains obscure. Pathologic study has failed to disclose lesions which might justify the inclusion of the digestive tract in the widespread sys-

Gastro-intestinal Symptoms

temic involvement of this form of arthritis [284, 289]. The autonomic imbalance probably responsible for the vasomotor symptoms in rheumatoid arthritis may be concerned with the increased frequency of constipation and diarrhea. Aspirin and other salicylates may sometimes play a part in the production of dyspeptic symptoms or even of peptic ulcer. Finally, emotional factors, either concerned in the development of the arthritis or consequent to the impact of the disease upon the personality of the patient, may be related to the occurrence in rheumatoid arthritis of peptic ulcer and ulcerative colitis, as well as less specific disturbances of the digestive tract.

SUMMARY

25.6 Among gastro-intestinal symptoms, anorexia, vomiting, constipation, and diarrhea were encountered with higher frequency among patients than among controls. The available evidence suggests that peptic ulcer occurs among rheumatoid arthritics at least as often as among the general population.

25.7 Objectives for further study:

1. Additional search for pathologic changes in the gastro-intestinal tract and related autonomic nerves of rheumatoid patients coming to autopsy.

2. The association of peptic ulcer and rheumatoid arthritis in a population study.

3. Clinical and histologic observations on Whipple's disease as a possible member of the connective-tissue disease group.

26

Fever

26.1 Prior to the establishment of rheumatoid arthritis as a disease entity, some difference of opinion existed in regard to whether fever should be considered a commonly associated symptom. During the period when the "infectious" was separated from the "pure, atrophic" type of chronic arthritis, fever was considered to be characteristic of the former, but rarely if ever present in the latter [213, 397]. Since the discarding of this artificial division, it is safe to say that fever is now well recognized as a frequent accompaniment of rheumatoid arthritis [13, 97, 183, 199, 251, 286, 325, 333], with great variation in degree not only among different patients but also within the course of a single individual's disease. Since the observations recorded in this section represent only those made while the patients were hospitalized, it is clear that in most instances they present the state of body temperature during only a small fraction of the patients' total illness.

26.2 For purposes of analysis the patients of the present series were divided into three groups (Table 26.1). The first includes those without fever during their entire hospital stay. The second is made up of those with "rare" fever (oral temperature 99° to 100°F.) not occurring on more than one day a week, and the third of those with "frequent" fever, occurring on more than one day a week. Over one-third of our patients were found to have no rise in temperature during their hospital

Fever

Table 26.1
Body temperatures recorded during hospitalization for patients of present series

Group	Fever	Patients No.	Per cent
I	Afebrile	112	38.2
II	"Rare"* and not over 100°F. (oral temperature)	110	37.5
III	"Frequent"†	71	24.2
	Total	293	99.9
Type and degree of fever in Group III			
	Not over 100°F.	31	10.6
	On "rare" days over 100°F.	18	6.1
	Higher temperature at first, later same as Group II	6	2.0
	Daily rise to 99°–100°F.	8	2.7
	Same, with "rare" rise to 100°–101°F.	2	0.7
	Same, with "frequent" rise to 100°–101°F. and "rare" rise above 101°F.	3	1.0
	Daily rise to 100°–101°F.	1	0.3
	Intermittent from afebrile to above 101°F.	2	0.7

* "Rare" refers to rise in temperature not more than once a week.
† "Frequent" refers to rise in temperature more than once a week.

stay. As mentioned above, the lack of fever, even in severe cases, has been referred to by others [213, 286, 333, 397, 518]. However, in only 8 of the 112 afebrile cases was the total severity* of the arthritis considered marked, and it must be again mentioned that our observations cover only a brief period of the disease course, in most instances a month or less. Symes [518] also pointed out that fever is usually limited to the early stages of the attack and that the temperature often remains "subnormal" even though symptoms are severe. As far as our patients are concerned, it has not been possible to corroborate this clinical impression, since the proportion of those with and without fever while in the hospital remained essentially the same irrespective of the duration of the arthritis. The second group, containing also slightly over one-third of the patients, consisted in those with a slight rise (not over 100°F.) occurring not more than once a week. Such rises in temperature have doubtless often been disregarded and might even be overlooked without careful scrutiny of the charts. It is possible that a group of controls,

* See definition, par. **4.26**.

either in good health or with nonfebrile illnesses, might demonstrate a similar infrequent, slight rise in temperature. Until the findings for such a group are available, it seemed preferable to separate these patients from the afebrile group, with the realization that the frequency and degree of their fever may be insignificant. The third, and smallest group, comprising about one-fourth of the series, was further subdivided according to the type and degree of fever recorded. In the majority of the 71 patients of this group, as set forth in the table, rises in temperature were intermittent and of relatively slight degree; 14 had continuous fever, with a daily rise, in most cases usually not over 100°F. Only 3, with fever at times over 101°F., resembled patients mentioned in the literature [13, 133, 183, 286] with fever as high as 105°F. Since the conclusion of the study we have encountered some patients with high fever as a presenting symptom. At times, articular findings have been minimal, and so have led to exhaustive diagnostic studies and even a trial of antibiotic therapy.

26.3 In our study of fever in rheumatoid arthritis we also made a statistical comparison between those with no fever or a slight degree (Groups I and II, Table 26.1) and the remainder with a more definite febrile course. No differences were found in regard to sex or to age at onset or age on admission. In particular, no association was found between onset of disease or hospital admission at an early age (under twenty) and the presence of fever, as postulated by one author [366]. Reference has been made above to the apparent lack of effect of disease duration on the presence or degree of fever. Similarly no differences were discovered in respect to the presence or absence of prodromal symptoms, vasomotor symptoms or signs, infection or strain as a precipitating factor, or a history of weight loss. The last finding does not eliminate fever as one factor in loss of weight, since some of the patients may of course have been febrile during the periods when weight was lost prior to hospital admission. The concept of an atypical form of rheumatoid arthritis, involving one or a few joints often in an asymmetrical fashion and often with fever (par. 16.13), is not furthered by the present data. No relationship was evident between "frequent" fever and any of the following factors: monarticular or unilateral onset; initial involvement of large rather than small joints; unilateral joint involvement on hospital

Fever

Table 26.2

Total severity of rheumatoid arthritis on admission in relation to fever during hospital stay among patients of present series (see Table 26.1)

Group	No. of patients	Total severity of arthritis					
		Mild		Moderate		Marked	
		No.	Per cent	No.	Per cent	No.	Per cent
Total	293	72	24.6	172	58.6	49	16.8
I and II	222	60	27.0	137	61.7	25	11.3
III	71	12	16.9	35	49.3	24	33.8
Difference in percentages:			10.1 ± 5.9		12.4 ± 6.2		22.5 ± 5.1
$\chi^2 = 19.88; p < .001$							

admission; or spinal involvement as opposed to involvement confined to the peripheral joints.

26.4   Table 26.2 shows an association between increasing severity of arthritis on admission and the presence of frequent fever during hospital stay. This association may depend partly on definition, since fever was included among the constitutional manifestations taken into account in the estimation of total disease severity.* But it is also evident in this table that the presence of fever was not consistently associated with increased severity. The group with "frequent" fever included some with mild total severity, and the groups with little or no fever included some with marked severity. As far as the subsequent course of the arthritis was concerned, a febrile state in the hospital apparently made no difference. Nor was there any association between a febrile hospital course and the presence of lymphadenopathy (par. 30.4), splenomegaly (par. 30.6), subcutaneous nodules (par. 33.3), or anemia (par. 38.3).

26.5   Two not unexpected associations were discovered in the course of our comparison. Patients with an acute, severe type of onset (often febrile at the start) were more prone to have "frequent" fever while in the hospital. Similar findings were encountered in the case of patients with an intermittent rather than a progressive course before admission. Such patients may correspond to those described by earlier writers [97, 183, 286] with intermittent febrile and afebrile periods running parallel to exacerbations and remissions and, as in the case of

---

* See definition, par. 4.26.

our patients, a final febrile exacerbation leading to hospital entrance. However, the nature of the relationships of fever in the hospital to type of onset and course before admission is obscured by the presence of an association between an acute onset and an intermittent course (par. 15.5). Further treatment of the data does not permit clarification of the mutual relationship existent among the three factors.*

26.6 While fever is mentioned frequently in clinical descriptions of rheumatoid arthritis, only three authors give actual figures as to the frequency of this symptom. Due to varying criteria for fever, comparison with the present figures is not relevant, but the percentages with fever according to the authors' standards may be mentioned. In one series [325], fever was listed as a symptom in 43 per cent of 28 children, while in two adult series numbering about 100 patients each, fever was recorded in 68 per cent of one group [97] and in 42 per cent of another [366].

26.7 Any explanation of the mechanism of fever in rheumatoid arthritis probably awaits the discovery of the etiology of this disease, although certain possibilities may be briefly reviewed at this time. In the first place, there is no evidence of an increased heat production, as measured by studies of basal metabolism. Interference with heat loss, as by decreased peripheral circulation, remains a possible factor, although our findings show no association between vasomotor symptoms or signs and frequent fever. If we presume that the usual mechanism in febrile disease is operative—i.e., a disturbance of the thermoregulatory mechanism in the hypothalamus—the question arises as to how this heat-regulating center is affected. No pathologic alterations have as yet been demonstrated in the hypothalamus similar to those found in peripheral nerves, spinal cord, and autonomic nervous system [367]. Tissue injury is believed to be the common denominator in most fevers, whether or not of infectious origin, with the heat regulating center affected either through afferent nerves or by a substance discharged into the blood stream from the site of injury. Tissue injury clearly takes place in rheumatoid arthritis and may well be the underlying cause of the frequently associated fever. In rheumatoid patients with high fever but little or no evidence of an active arthritis, extra-articular tissues may

* For a complete list of associations, see Appendix Table 47.

Fever

form the site of injury, in line with the well-recognized systemic nature of the disease. Although an infectious process is undoubtedly the most common cause of a febrile state, non-infectious conditions may also be responsible for an increased body temperature. These include (to cite a few examples) diseases due to immune mechanisms (serum sickness), sudden interference with blood supply (coronary thrombosis), a metabolic disease like gout, certain neoplasms and even endocrinopathies such as Addisonian crisis and thyroid storm. One can only conclude that no one of the present hypotheses as to the etiology of rheumatoid arthritis is materially strengthened or weakened by the fact that fever is a common manifestation.

SUMMARY

26.8 During a period of hospital observation which, in most cases, was brief compared with the total disease course, one-third of our patients were afebrile, one-third had fever not over 100°F. not more than once a week, and the remainder more frequent rises in body temperature of inconsistent pattern. Neither younger patients nor those with a relatively recent onset of arthritis were more likely to run a febrile course. A significant, but by no means constant association, was found between fever and arthritis of marked total severity,* but the patients' subsequent course was apparently unrelated to the presence or absence of fever while in the hospital. The mechanism of fever in rheumatoid arthritis remains obscure. Possibly it can be explained by tissue injury, as in other febrile diseases of both infectious and noninfectious origin.

26.9 Objectives for further study:

1. Observations on the relationship between body temperature and fluctuations in symptomatology and disease activity, based on long-term daily temperature recordings.

2. The effect of antipyretic agents on fever in rheumatoid arthritis.

* See definition, par. 4.26.

27

Pulse Rate

27.1 In two early clinical descriptions, written about a hundred years ago, tachycardia was mentioned by both Charcot [*80*] and Graves [*222*] as a characteristic finding in rheumatoid arthritis. Succeeding authors [*133, 150, 199, 249*] have rarely failed to mention the occurrence of an increased pulse rate in this disease, and some [*97, 157, 333, 366, 490*] have set down figures in regard to its frequency among observed patients. In general, there has been a recent tendency to dismiss tachycardia as a fairly common manifestation with relatively unimportant diagnostic value.

27.2 Nevertheless, the frequency of increased pulse rate was included in the present study. Whenever possible, the rates chosen for analysis were taken under basal conditions—that is, at the time of the routine basal metabolism test, which was carried out on all but 17 per cent of the patients. Otherwise, the average pulse rate was estimated from the clinical charts kept during their hospital stay. A pulse rate over 90 was considered a tachycardia and was recorded for 45 patients, or 15.4 per cent of the series. (In all but 8 of these, the tachycardia was present under basal conditions.) Pulse rates were not taken when the controls were examined, but the results of one study [*320*] in which controls were used is available in the literature. Pulse rates of 80 or over were found in 47 per cent of 279 patients compared with 27 per cent

Pulse Rate

of a corresponding number of controls. Rates of 90 or over were recorded with about equal frequency among the two groups. In other reports, the proportion of patients with pulse rate of over 90 varies from 13.6 per cent [366] to 67 [97, 333] and even 80 per cent [490].

27.3 No differences in the occurrence of tachycardia were found in regard to disease duration, sex, or age. The last point has been confirmed by Morris [366]. Similarly, the following aspects of the disease were found with approximately equal frequency among those with pulse over 90 and the remainder: an intermittent course before admission, bilateral joint involvement, a history of prodromal symptoms, spondylitis, anemia, and nervousness and/or emotional upsets. The association between tachycardia and an acute type of onset was found to be dependent upon mutual association between both factors and a febrile hospital course. But the presence or absence of tachycardia showed no relationship to the total severity* of the arthritis on hospital admission nor to an unfavorable subsequent course—findings which are at variance with those of several other authors [97, 183, 222, 286], who have cited rapid pulse rate as a sign of severity or even of poor prognosis. Of special interest was our failure to note an association between tachycardia and vasomotor symptoms or signs, since autonomic imbalance would constitute a plausible explanation of the rapid heart action occurring in rheumatoid arthritis.†

27.4 Table 27.1 shows the proportion of patients with "frequent" fever among those with and without tachycardia. Over half of those with a rapid pulse rate were also included in the group of 71 patients who had fever of significant degree. This finding strongly suggests that fever may often be responsible for an increased pulse rate in rheumatoid arthritis, with the corollary that fever may occur in this disease without an accompanying rise in pulse. In this connection, it should be remembered that most of the determinations of heart rate in our series were made in the early morning, when the body temperature would be less likely to be increased. Bannatyne [13], without supporting data, stated that he believed fever to be the common cause of tachycardia in rheumatoid arthritis. The only detailed study we have encountered of

* See definition, par. 4.26.
† For a complete list of associations, see Appendix Table 47.

Table 27.1

Frequency of "frequent" fever among patients of present series with and without tachycardia

Patients	No.	"Frequent" fever	
		No.	Per cent
Total	293	71	24.2
With tachycardia*	45	26	57.8
Without tachycardia	248	45	18.1
	Difference in percentages:		39.7 ± 7.0

* Pulse rate over 90.

the relationship between these two aspects of the disease was made by Morris [366] in 1910. Among 95 patients whose charts were observed over an extended period, 32.6 per cent had pulse rates of over 90 during their week of highest fever, while only 13.6 per cent showed tachycardia during the week when their temperature was lowest. The difference is significant and suggests that the pulse rate in rheumatoid arthritis tends to vary with the body temperature. Morris' additional finding— that increased pulse rate sometimes occurs among patients with minimal fever or even with normal temperature—is supported by our figures and the statements of various other writers [133, 183, 286, 333, 397, 490]. Comments have been made [150, 157] in regard to instability of pulse rate in individual patients with rises on slight exertion or excitement. No data are available for our patients in this regard. Reference has been made, in addition, to occasional patients with persistent high pulse rates, ranging from 120 to 140, without obvious cause such as fever, thyrotoxicosis, or carditis [199, 286, 333, 490]. We have also observed such patients, but it is our impression that they make up a very small proportion of the total group.

27.5 As mentioned above, fever is most probably the important factor in the causation of tachycardia in a significant proportion of rheumatoid arthritics. Associated cardiac involvement may account for an increased pulse rate in others, as may the severe anemia which is occasionally encountered. In the remainder the mechanism of accelerated heart action is still to be explained. In certain patients overactivity of the sympathetic nervous system, which is often demonstrably present in rheumatoid arthritis, may be partially responsible. It is not yet known

Pulse Rate

whether this overactivity originates in higher centers of the central nervous system, by reflex pathways from painful joints, or in the anatomical changes demonstrated in the ganglia themselves [367]. An equal possibility that must be thought of lies in underactivity of the vagal mechanism which restrains the heart rate, a speculation which suggests neuropathologic investigation in this direction. Hormonal mechanisms or endocrine imbalance resulting in increased production of adrenalin should also be mentioned, although there is no available evidence of their influence in the production of tachycardia in rheumatoid arthritis. A last but not least likely possibility in some patients is that the increased pulse rate may be of functional origin and dependent upon a constant state of emotional tension.

SUMMARY

27.6 A pulse rate of over 90 was found in 15 per cent of the patients of the present series, having been determined under basal conditions in most instances. Tachycardia is often associated with fever in rheumatoid arthritis but may also accompany a normal temperature; in the latter instance, the mechanism of an increased pulse rate has not been explained. Possible factors include carditis, autonomic imbalance, and emotional tension.

27.7 Objective for further study:

The mechanism of tachycardia in rheumatoid arthritis. For possible factors see par. 27.5.

28

Blood Pressure

28.1 While the statement has been frequently made that the blood pressure is abnormally low in rheumatoid arthritis [*187, 213, 251, 306, 514*], only one other study offers data comparable to ours. In this study, which utilized a series of about 500 British patients and an equal number of matched controls, no differences could be demonstrated between patients and controls in regard to either systolic or diastolic blood pressure. The data were presented as a percentage distribution of varying levels of blood pressure in each of the two groups, without subdivision according to sex or age. The results of blood pressure determinations for our patients and controls are shown in Table 28.1, which differs from the British tabulation in that systolic pressures only were considered and that three instead of nine groupings of blood pressure levels were employed. In distinction to the British report, significant differences are evident between patients and controls. As may be noted in the table, a higher percentage of patients than controls was found in the group with systolic pressure less than 110, with the reverse true in that with pressure over 140. Subdivision of our groups according to sex and age, brought out only one significant difference—as might be expected, systolic pressure of 140 or over occurred more often among

Blood Pressure

Table 28.1
Systolic blood pressure in rheumatoid arthritis—patients of present series compared with controls

Systolic pressure	Patients No.	Patients Per cent	Controls No.	Controls Per cent	Difference in percentages
Less than 110	40	13.7	15	5.1	8.6 ± 2.4
From 110 to 140	209	71.3	193	65.9	5.4 ± 3.5
Greater than 140	44	15.0	85	29.0	14.0 ± 3.3
Total	293	100.0	293	99.9	

Table 28.2
Systolic blood pressure determinations for 293 rheumatoid arthritics and 293 controls divided according to sex and to age groups and compared with findings of Master et al. [346] for 15,706 subjects

Age groups	No. of patients and controls	Mean Pressures Patients	Mean Pressures Controls	Mean Pressures Master et al.	Median pressures Patients	Median pressures Controls
Males						
10–19	8	121.4	123.3	120.2	114	120
20–29	29	118.6	123.4	124.0	120	120
30–39	27	121.8	132.2	126.6	120	130
40–49	18	128.9	138.1	129.5	132	140
50–59	16	120.8	139.1	136.1	120	140
60–	9	146.1	158.5	141.8	140	154
Total	107					
Females						
10–19	14	118.5	115.8	116.0	120	110
20–29	32	113.5	125.2	116.2	110	125
30–39	34	120.1	125.6	122.0	120	130
40–49	32	123.7	137.6	128.8	120	130
50–59	57	138.8	160.9	138.0	140	152
60–	17	148.1	159.0	144.0	145	160
Total	186					

female patients and controls aged forty or over. Patients with mild, moderate, and marked total disease severity* were distributed equally among the three blood pressure groups listed in the table.

28.2 Outlining our data in another way, Table 28.2 shows a consistently higher pressure among controls when means and medians are

---
* See definition, par. **4.26**.

figured for each decade by sex. It should also be noted that the differences between controls and patients tend to become greater with increasing age. As a further comparison, the table includes the results compiled by Master, Dublin, and Marks [346] from examinations made of over 15,000 American industrial workers and applicants for employment during World War II. These last figures are only slightly higher than the systolic pressure reading for the patients of the present series but are lower than the readings for controls, especially those over forty years of age. Essentially the same findings were obtained in regard to diastolic pressures, as recorded in Table 28.3. It thus seems reasonable to believe that our control group contained an undue proportion of hypertensives, most of them beyond the age of forty, and that the differences between patients and controls, shown in Tables 28.2 and 28.3, rest upon a hypertensive tendency of the controls, who were mainly hospital employees, rather than upon hypotension among the patients.

Table 28.3

Diastolic blood pressure determinations for 293 rheumatoid arthritics and 293 controls divided according to sex and age groups and compared with findings of Master et al. [346] for 15,706 subjects

Age groups	No. of patients and controls	Males				
		Mean pressures			Median pressures	
		Patients	Controls	Master et al.	Patients	Controls
10–19	8	68.7	73.0	74.1	68	72
20–29	29	71.8	77.3	76.9	70	80
30–39	27	77.0	83.7	79.4	76	80
40–49	18	76.2	78.1	81.6	75	80
50–59	16	76.4	85.0	83.7	76	84
60 and more	9	79.4	87.7	84.5	75	90
Total	107					
		Females				
10–19	14	74.7	70.7	71.8	70	74
20–29	32	72.8	78.3	72.7	70	80
30–39	34	75.8	82.7	76.4	80	80
40–49	32	79.7	84.8	80.5	79	84
50–59	57	79.9	92.8	83.5	80	88
60 and more	17	80.1	90.1	85.0	79	89
Total	186					

Blood Pressure

An additional factor, which may actually be of more importance, is that since the controls were ambulatory they came to the office for examination, while the patients were examined after varying periods of bed rest in the hospital. This difference may not have existed in the British study, since about two-thirds of the controls were hospital patients.

28.3   In 1954 a study of the blood pressures of 320 patients with rheumatoid arthritis was reported by Turner and Lansbury [538]. As the series comprised ambulatory as well as hospitalized patients, the possible hypotensive effect of bed rest on the latter was eliminated by selecting the blood pressure readings taken at the time of hospital admission. As shown in Table 28.4, the mean systolic pressure for each age group from 30 on was found consistently lower than in the present series. The same was true of the mean diastolic pressures. In fact, as the authors point out, the average diastolic pressures remained unchanged for all decades at a level of about 75 mm. of mercury. Patients with

Table 28.4

Mean blood pressure determinations in rheumatoid arthritis—patients of present series compared by age groups* with two series from the literature

Age groups	Present series		Turner and Lansbury [538]		Master et al. [346]
	No. of patients	Blood pressure	No. of patients	Blood pressure	Blood pressure
Systolic pressures					
20–29	61	115.9	29	115	120.1
30–39	61	120.9	68	113	124.3
40–49	50	125.6	82	118	129.2
50–59	73	138.8	86	127	137.1
60 or more	26	147.4	55	129.8	142.9
Total	271		320		
Diastolic pressures					
20–29	61	72.3	29	74	74.8
30–39	61	76.3	68	73	77.9
40–49	50	78.3	82	74	81.1
50–59	73	79.1	86	77	83.6
60 or more	26	79.8	55	73.6	84.8
Total	271		320		

* In each series males and females have been lumped together.

spondylitis were not included in the 1954 study, but if males with spondylitis are omitted from the present series, the levels of systolic and diastolic pressure in the remaining males are essentially unchanged. No explanation is at hand for the differing results in the two series, since it is not possible to make a comparison in regard to sex distribution, disease severity, duration, and other factors which might influence the findings.* Since the readings utilized in the present series were obtained after varying periods of hospitalization and bed rest was presumably operative in a number of cases, it is all the more difficult to account for the lower values obtained by Turner and Lansbury [538].

28.4 The frequency in our patients of systolic blood pressure at a hypotensive level, as defined by Master and others [346], may be partly attributed to the effect of bed rest. In comparison with only 3 controls, 19 patients were found to have abnormally low readings—a significant and interesting difference. In 10 of these the blood pressure was under 100 systolic and in one only 85. The findings for this rather limited group of patients thus conform with the striking data of the literature [150], which have contributed to the acceptance of a clinical belief that hypotension is a characteristic of rheumatoid arthritis. As far as could be determined, the 19 patients with hypotension did not differ from the remainder of the series in any important respects, including sex, age, duration, and severity of disease and the frequency of constitutional and vasomotor symptoms. In that the majority were more than 10 per cent below average weight, malnutrition, which is recognized as a cause for hypotension [144], may have been a contributing factor.

28.5 Although a clinical impression exists that rheumatoid arthritis is rarely associated with serious hypertension occurring at a relatively early age [398, 467], figures are not yet at hand to confirm this belief. Only 5 of our series patients were found to have an abnormally high systolic pressure for their age [346], compared with 24 of the controls. (The determining factor here may again rest on the fact that the controls were ambulatory and the series hospitalized.) In the absence of

---

*In a Finnish study of 541 hospitalized patients with rheumatoid arthritis [279], recently published by Järvinen, the mean arterial pressure was slightly *higher* than in a control series from the literature [237]. The highest systolic pressures were noted in patients with very active disease.

Blood Pressure

glomerular nephritis or renal amyloidosis, untimely death from severe hypertension occurred in only 2 of the rheumatoid arthritics thus far encountered in our clinic, and both these patients were males with spondylitis. That equal numbers of patients and controls with diastolic pressures over 100 (9.0 and 10.0 per cent, respectively) were recorded in the British study [320] may be brought up in rebuttal, but our finding would seem to warrant further investigation of an antagonism between rheumatoid arthritis and severe essential hypertension. The possibility is at least suggested by the fact that agents such as corticotropin and cortisone, which suppress rheumatoid activity, number hypertension among their side effects, as well as by recent observations [153, 408] that the hypotensive drug hydralazine (Apresoline) may cause a rheumatic and febrile syndrome resembling a connective tissue disease.

28.6   In spite of the disagreement as to whether or not hypotension constitutes a clinical feature of rheumatoid arthritis, speculations as to possible causes should be mentioned. What may be termed primary hypotension, with systolic pressures as low as 90, is well recognized as occurring among the healthy population and may indeed account for some of the patients with rheumatoid arthritis and a low blood pressure. Malnutrition among rheumatoid patients may be another factor in the production of lowered arterial tension. The hypotension commonly found in a chronic, wasting, febrile disease such as pulmonary tuberculosis may be brought in by way of analogy. Disordered functions of the adrenal cortex or anterior pituitary should also be mentioned as possible mechanisms of hypotension, but they have yet to be established in rheumatoid arthritis. Finally, the reader is referred to the paper by Turner and Lansbury [538] for an interesting hypothesis involving the possible significance of diastolic hypotension in the pathogenesis of rheumatoid arthritis.

SUMMARY

28.7   Evidence that hypotension constitutes a characteristic clinical attribute of rheumatoid arthritis [538] was not obtained in the present study nor in a recent British report, where controls matched as to sex and age were also employed. Whether or not the blood pressures of most rheumatoid arthritics merely follow the age and sex variations noted in the general population, an abnormally low arterial tension may be present in certain patients. Clinical experience also suggests that severe degrees of essential hypertension are unusually rare in patients with rheumatoid arthritis.

28.8 Objectives for further study:

1. Further observations directed toward establishing whether or not low diastolic pressure constitutes a clinical feature of rheumatoid arthritis.

2. The validity of the clinical impression of an antagonism between this disease and severe essential hypertension.

3. Clinical and laboratory investigation of the rheumatic syndromes produced by hypotensive agents.

29

Eyes

29.1   While this chapter is chiefly concerned with the ocular lesions generally regarded as systemic manifestations of rheumatoid arthritis, certain other eye abnormalities were recorded for both patients and controls. As shown in Table 29.1, arcus senilis, pupillary abnormalities, and retinal arteriosclerosis were found with approximately equal frequency in the two groups. The frequency of arcus senilis was investigated with the idea of possibly discovering a sign of premature aging among the patients, while irregularity, inequality, or faulty reaction of the pupils were looked for as neurologic manifestations of the disease [286]. The slightly higher frequency of arteriosclerosis of the fundi among the controls is in keeping with the belief set forth in the preceding chapter on blood pressure that this group contained an undue proportion of hypertensives.

29.2   The association of inflammatory eye disease with rheumatoid arthritis was commented upon at least as far back as 1860, when Fuller [195] noted such conditions in 7.7 per cent of 323 patients. Confirmatory evidence has since appeared to make it reasonably certain that the eye shares in the systemic involvement of this disease. In the first place, three types of ocular disease are rarely found in patients without rheumatoid arthritis: "band" keratopathy [569] (found less often in adults than in children, in whom it constitutes the most common eye lesion,

Table 29.1

Frequency of ocular abnormalities among 293 rheumatoid arthritics and 293 controls

Abnormality	Patients No.	Per cent	Controls No.	Per cent	Difference in percentages
Arcus senilis	22	7.5	17	5.8	1.7 ± 2.1
Pupillary	19	6.5	16	5.5	1.0 ± 1.9
Arteriosclerosis of fundi	49	16.7	64	21.8	5.1 ± 3.2

and occasionally due to toxicity from vitamin D therapy); keratoconjunctivitis sicca (usually a part of Sjögren's syndrome) [499]; and scleromalacia perforans [542]. Study of the scleral nodules in the last condition reveals a microscopic picture identical with that of the subcutaneous rheumatoid nodule [544]. In regard to iritis (or more properly uveitis, for the entire uveal tract is usually affected), the most extensive study thus far undertaken was carried out in 1946 by Sorsby and Gormaz [487], who looked for past or present signs of this condition in the eyes of 332 patients with rheumatoid arthritis, 53 with ankylosing spondylitis, 147 with rheumatic fever, and 695 controls without arthritis. In each group of patients with arthritis, iritis was diagnosed with a significantly higher frequency than among the controls but signs of this condition were entirely absent among patients with rheumatic fever. These figures strongly support a more than coincidental relationship between iritis and rheumatoid arthritis. Signs of iritis or a definite history of one or more attacks were noted in only 5 of our patients during their hospital stay, but 7 others (or a total of 4.1 per cent) later developed iritis. This figure more nearly corresponds to the frequency of iritis among rheumatoid arthritics of other series, as shown in Table 29.2. In addition, 2 patients developed scleritis and 4 keratitis, all following their initial period of hospitalization. No patients with keratoconjunctivitis sicca were encountered in the present series, but this condition was not specifically looked for. Stenstam [499], who carefully examined the eyes of 434 rheumatoid patients, found a frequency of 10.6 per cent.

29.3   That iritis may precede the actual development of arthritis has been noted [443], but it is more likely to occur after the joint disease has been present for some time. In 1 of our patients iritis developed after

Table 29.2

Eye lesions in rheumatoid arthritis—present series compared with representative series from the literature

Source	Type of lesion	No. of patients	Frequency of lesion No.	Per cent
Fuller [195]	"Inflammatory," including conjunctivitis	323	25	7.7
Sorsby and Gormaz [487]	Iritis	332	15	4.5
Short [463]	"	132	4	3.0
Berens et al., [36]	"	83*	2	2.4
Buckley [59]	"	150*	8	5.3
Sorsby and Gormaz [487]	"	53*	3	5.7
Scott [455]	"	300*	20	6.7
Lockie and Norcross [325]	"	28†	1	3.6
Present series	"	293	12	4.1
Fingerman and Andrus [179]	Scleromalacia (autopsies)	61	2	3.3
Present series	Scleritis	293	2	0.7
Stenstam [499]	Keratoconjunctivitis sicca	434	46	10.6

* With rheumatoid spondylitis.
† With juvenile rheumatoid arthritis.

the disease had been present for twelve years, while the median duration of joint involvement before the eyes were affected was four years. Others [133, 345] have commented upon the varying severity of rheumatoid iritis—mild and self-limited and leaving no detectable residual in one patient but relentlessly progressing to total blindness in another. In our series 3 patients lost the sight of one eye in this way and 3 lost the sight of both; the last-mentioned were the only ones with a bilateral process. In another series [487] the iritis was unilateral and relatively mild in 12 patients, and bilateral in 3 patients; 2 of the latter became blind. From these two studies of relatively small groups of patients with rheumatoid iritis, the suggestion is drawn that, in distinction to the cornea and sclera, the uveal tract is affected symmetrically in a minority of cases but then with marked severity. More recent observations in this clinic on a larger number of patients with iritis have shown that, while initial involvement is rarely bilateral, the chance that both eyes will eventually become affected is about two to one.

Table 29.3

Frequency of iritis among patients of present series with and without spondylitis

		Iritis present	
Patients	No.	No.	Per cent
Total	293	12	4.1
With spondylitis	41	8	19.5
Without spondylitis	252	4	1.6
	Difference in percentages:	17.9 ± 3.4	

29.4 A clinical impression has prevailed for some time that iritis (but not other ocular lesions of rheumatoid arthritis) may often be associated with the spinal type of this disease. Such an impression is fostered by the finding in the present series that 7 of the 12 with iritis were males and 8 had spondylitis (Table 29.3). A study of the percentages in Table 29.2 demonstrates a slightly higher frequency of this condition in the three series made up entirely of spondylitics. No definite difference is evident, however, in the carefully studied groups of Sorsby and Gormaz [487]. Before this clinical impression, which has been strengthened in our recent experience, can be either established or disproved, more extensive studies including spinal x-rays are indicated in a larger number of rheumatoid patients with and without iritis.

SUMMARY

29.5 Arcus senilis, pupillary abnormalities, and retinal arteriosclerosis were found with equal frequency among patients and controls. Inflammatory eye lesions, involving the uveal tract, the cornea, and the sclera may be regarded as systemic manifestations of the rheumatoid process. The uveal tract was the most common site of ocular involvement in our series, which was composed largely of adults; about 4 per cent were affected at some time during the course of their disease. An association between iritis and spondylitis was suggested but not established.

29.6 Objectives for further study:

1. The frequency of iritis in patients with and without spinal involvement.

2. Further observations on keratoconjunctivitis sicca as an early manifestation of rheumatoid arthritis.

30

Lymph Nodes, Spleen, and Liver

30.1 From time to time series of patients with rheumatoid arthritis and lymph node enlargement, splenomegaly, and leukopenia—singly or in combination—have been collected with a view to the establishment of separate syndromes. Those which have gained a place in the literature include Still's disease, Still-Chauffard syndrome (adult Still's disease), and Felty's syndrome. Arguments against such a partition of rheumatoid arthritis have already been set forth (par. 2.28) and need not be repeated in the present chapter, which is concerned with enlargement of the lymph nodes, spleen, and liver in rheumatoid arthritis.

30.2 Differing criteria for determining the degree of lymph node enlargement which may be deemed abnormal are undoubtedly reflected in the varying figures given in the literature (from 17.8 to 96 per cent) for the frequency of enlarged nodes in rheumatoid arthritis. In the present study it was left to the judgment of the observer to determine whether or not the nodes of a given individual were enlarged in comparison with others of similar age and habitus. Since the patients and controls were examined by the same observers, it is believed that the difference is significant in regard to lymph node enlargement in the two groups, as shown in Table 30.1. The frequency of lymph node enlargement among our patients (29.4 per cent) is very close to that obtained from a combined series drawn from the literature (36 per cent

Table 30.1

Frequency of enlargement of lymph nodes, spleen, and liver among 293 rheumatoid arthritics and 293 controls

Enlargement	Patients		Controls		Difference in percentages
	No.	Per cent	No.	Per cent	
Lymph nodes	86	29.4	26	8.9	20.5 ± 3.4
Spleen	19	6.5	6	2.0	4.5 ± 1.7
Liver	22	7.5	26	8.9	1.4 ± 2.3

of 530 adult patients) and somewhat lower than that obtained from a series of 84 children (46 per cent). One may conclude, then, that lymph node enlargement constitutes a common manifestation of rheumatoid arthritis, occurring in about one-third of adult patients.

30.3 The next table, 30.2, demonstrates that lymph node enlargement was found more often among males of the present series. A similar distribution in the control group suggests that this sex difference is not peculiar to rheumatoid arthritis. On the one hand, it might be accounted for by the greater susceptibility of males to minor infection of the extremities from occupational injuries, and on the other, by the greater ease with which nodes can usually be palpated in males because of their smaller amount of adipose tissue. The second reason may also explain the finding of a higher frequency of enlarged nodes among females under forty compared with older females. A striking association was found between lymph node enlargement and impaired nutrition, as shown in Table 30.3. In addition, a history of weight loss was given by a higher percentage of patients with enlarged nodes than by those without. Weight loss was also more common among patients with disease of

Table 30.2

Lymph node enlargement in rheumatoid arthritis—patients of present series divided according to sex and compared with controls

Sex	No. in each group	Lymph nodes enlarged			
		Patients		Controls	
		No.	Per cent	No.	Per cent
Total	293	86	29.4	26	8.9
Male	107	39	36.4	15	14.0
Female	186	47	25.3	11	5.9
Difference in percentages:			11.1 ± 5.5		8.1 ± 3.4

Lymph Nodes, Spleen, and Liver

Table 30.3

Weights of 237 rheumatoid arthritics* on hospital admission in relation to presence or absence of lymph node enlargement

Percentage of standard weight	Patients			
	With enlarged nodes		Without enlarged nodes	
	No.	Per cent	No.	Per cent
70–89	42	62.7	43	25.3
90–109	19	28.4	82	48.2
110–140 or more	6	9.0	45	26.5
	67	100.1	170	100.0

* Data are not available in regard to the weights of 56 patients, in whom the proportion with enlarged nodes was approximately the same as in the remainder.

marked total severity,* but lymph node enlargement was found in about the same proportion of patients irrespective of the severity of the disease. Nodes would of course be more easily felt in thin patients, a fact which may be chiefly responsible for the higher frequency of enlargement reported for such individuals.

30.4   Statements have appeared in the literature [83, 97, 192] to the effect that lymph node enlargement is related to disease activity. We have been unable to confirm this relationship, since patients with mild, moderate, or marked disease activity† on hospital admission were distributed equally among those with and without enlarged nodes. Furthermore, in our series, no associations were found between lymph node enlargement and acute onset, "frequent" fever, or "early" cases, with disease duration of one year or less. Another statement [561] which we failed to verify from the patients' course before admission was that in patients with enlarged nodes the course was usually marked by exacerbations and remissions. Other attempts to discover differentiating points between the group with enlarged nodes and the remainder were unsuccessful, including a failure to find associations with a history of prodromal symptoms; infection preceding the onset of arthritis; primary involvement either in large joints, small joints, or a single joint; spinal or peripheral distribution of arthritis; and unilateral rather than bilateral involvement at onset. There was also no difference in total disease

---

* See definition, par. 4.26.

† See definition, par. 4.27.

severity* on hospital admission or in subsequent course between those with and without enlarged nodes.†

30.5 Splenomegaly was considered to be present if the organ could be palpated. On this basis only a small proportion of our patients had splenic enlargement (6.5 per cent), but the frequency was higher than that found in the control group (Table 30.1). Results from the literature are shown in Table 30.4, where the frequency of splenic enlargement is generally recorded as somewhat greater than in our series. The table also confirms the usually accepted belief that splenomegaly is more likely to be found in children with rheumatoid arthritis than in adults with this disease. The results in two rather small autopsied series are also shown in the table; in each instance a splenic weight of 200 gm. or more was regarded as enlargement. The difference in the two percentages may be accounted for by the fact that, in the second series, 6 cases of splenomegaly were due to chronic passive congestion. A previous communication from this clinic [521] pointed out the likelihood of finding an extraneous cause for splenic enlargement in rheumatoid patients if the search were made. Such a cause was present in 2 of our patients—in the one pernicious anemia and in the other toxic cirrhosis of the liver.

30.6 No important differentiating points could be made out between the patients with palpable spleens and the remainder. Sex or age on admission apparently had no influence, nor, as in the case of lymph node enlargement, were we able to confirm reports in the literature [150, 333, 356] of associations between splenomegaly and acute onset, onset within one year of admission, or disease activity. A palpable spleen was recorded for 2 patients with spondylitis, both with peripheral joints also affected. As shown in Table 30.5, an association was found between enlargement of the lymph nodes and the spleen, which bears out the clinical impression of previous observers [333, 354]. No relationship was observed between splenomegaly and either infection as a precipitating factor or fever while in the hospital. Although anemia was not associated with splenic enlargement, in 3 out of the 5 patients with leukopenia the spleen was palpable (see par. 38.7). Finally the presence

---

* See definition, par. **4.26**.

† For a complete list of associations, see Appendix Table 47.

Table 30.4

Splenomegaly in rheumatoid arthritis—present series compared with representative series from the literature

Source	Adults		
	No. of patients in series	Splenomegaly present	
		No.	Per cent
Total	889	95	10.7
Waterhouse [554]	50	3	6.0
McCrae [333]	166*	30	18.1
Coates and Delicati [97]	100	21	21.0
Dawson [133]	Not given		10–15
Freund [192]	280	22	7.9
Present series	293	19	6.5
	Children		
Total	120	34	28.3
Still [504]	19	9	47.3
Waterhouse [554]	17	4	23.5
Lockie and Norcross [325]	28	4	14.3
Coss and Boots [121]	56	17	30.4
	Autopsies (adults)		
Fingerman and Andrus [179]	61	16	26.2
Baggenstoss and Rosenberg [8]	24	14	58.3

* A few children included.

Table 30.5

Frequency of splenomegaly among patients of present series with and without enlarged lymph nodes

Patients	No.	Splenomegaly present	
		No.	Per cent
Total	293	19	6.5
With enlarged nodes	86	11	12.8
Without enlarged nodes	207	8	3.9
	Difference in percentages:		8.9 ± 3.2

or absence of splenomegaly apparently had no effect on either the total disease severity* on hospital admission or the course of the arthritis after discharge.†

30.7   Table 30.1 demonstrates almost the same frequency of liver enlargement among patients and controls and suggests that, while hepatomegaly may be an occasional manifestation of rheumatoid arthritis, the hepatic enlargement can usually be traced to an extraneous cause. (In our series the criterion for liver enlargement was a palpable edge, which, of course, sometimes merely indicates that the organ is in a low position.) No characteristic lesions of the liver have been discovered in post mortem examinations of rheumatoid patients [8, 179, 327], although fatty changes, chronic passive congestion (in some cases resulting in hypertrophy, in others atrophy), "serous hepatitis," and central necrosis have been found. At times amyloidosis secondary to rheumatoid arthritis may also account for hepatomegaly as well as presumably unrelated diseases, including cirrhosis, which was present in 2 of our patients. In two recent publications [327, 372], liver biopsies have been reported for a total of 50 patients with rheumatoid arthritis. Amyloidosis was found in 4 and cirrhosis or hepatitis in 3. In the remainder, the changes were slight and nonspecific and limited to varying degrees of focal necrosis, fatty infiltration, and periportal inflammation. As was pointed out in a previous chapter (par. 10.4), the proportion of patients giving a history of hepatitis did not exceed the proportion of controls. The statement seems justified, then, that, in spite of reports of altered liver function for a sizable proportion of patients with rheumatoid arthritis [327, 358, 426, 438, 560], the role of the liver in this disease is still to be defined.

30.8   In contrast to the liver, the lymph nodes and spleen may be regarded as commonly sharing in the systemic involvement of rheumatoid arthritis. This statement is based upon the frequency with which enlargement of these organs has been encountered among rheumatoid arthritics rather than upon histologic findings consistent with a rheumatoid process. Nonspecific inflammatory changes have been consistently reported in both nodes [333, 359, 561] and spleen [512], except for the few instances in which lymph node biopsies revealed a

---

* See definition, par. 4.26.
† For a complete list of associations, see Appendix Table 47.

Lymph Nodes, Spleen, and Liver

histologic picture resembling that of giant follicle lymphoma [*370*]. At times, nodes may show more than slight or moderate enlargement and suggest an additional diagnosis, which usually remains unverified by biopsy. No study was made in the present series as to the prevalence of enlargement in nodes which drain areas of joint inflammation. Opinions [*333, 504, 554*] differ as to whether or not the nodes are usually satellite; certainly generalized lymph node enlargement is often found without relation to the site of the arthritis. It is still possible, however, in such instances that lymphadenopathy may be secondary to extra-articular rheumatoid lesions. Nothing new about the nature of rheumatoid arthritis has been revealed by the associated findings in regard to the lymph nodes and spleen. An infectious process had been postulated by earlier writers, but one may easily compile a long list of noninfectious conditions which are commonly accompanied by lymphadenopathy or splenomegaly. The data in this chapter also fail to support the recognition of separate syndromes in patients with lymphadenopathy, splenomegaly, or both when their symptoms otherwise correspond to the clinical picture of rheumatoid arthritis.

SUMMARY

30.9   Lymph node enlargement was found in about one-third of our patients. The higher frequency in male patients may not be peculiar to rheumatoid arthritis, since a similar difference was present in the control group. A palpable spleen was recorded in 6.5 per cent of the patients, a percentage significantly greater than that noted in the controls. Splenomegaly was found more frequently in patients with lymphadenopathy than in those without it, but the data presented in this chapter fail to support the creation of separate syndromes on the basis of enlargement of lymph nodes, spleen, or both. Despite the finding of altered liver function in patients with rheumatoid arthritis, neither clinical nor pathologic evidence is as yet sufficient to warrant the inclusion of liver involvement among the systemic manifestations of this disease.

30.10   Objectives for further study:

1. The relationship of regional lymph node enlargement to involved joints.

2. Liver involvement as a systemic manifestation of rheumatoid arthritis, to include tests of liver function as well as liver biopsies.

31

Skin, Nails, and Tongue

31.1 Atrophy of the skin has been noted in rheumatoid arthritis by a number of observers [13, 133, 199, 286, 333, 478]. Descriptions of the appearance of the skin in such instances have generally agreed that it looks and feels thin; may be pink, smooth, and shiny; and may lack hair growth and wrinkles. Such changes in the skin are usually confined to the extremities, below the elbows and knees. Atrophic skin was recorded for 92, or 31.4 per cent, of the patients in our series and for only 18, or 6.1 per cent, of the controls. Atrophy of the nails, consisting chiefly in longitudinal ridging and brittleness, has also been described in rheumatoid arthritis [13, 199, 478]. Such changes were noted in 50, or 17.1 per cent, of the patients, but were not looked for in the controls.

31.2 Table 31.1 lists the nature of the association between atrophy of the skin and nails and certain factors which seemed of clinical interest. It should again be noted that mutual associations among factors may actually account for some apparent associations, but with the data at hand it has not been possible to sort out such interrelationships. The comments which follow should be read with these reservations in mind. The increased frequency of atrophy of the skin among females and among patients aged forty or over was duplicated in the control group, of whom it was found that all but 2 with atrophic skin were females and all were forty or over. That skin atrophy should represent a manifesta-

Skin, Nails, and Tongue

Table 31.1
Association of various factors with atrophy of skin and nails

Factor	Atrophic skin	Atrophic nails
Sex (male)	—	0
Prodromal symptoms	0	0
Onset in small joints	0	0
Onset bilateral	0	0
Age on admission over 40	+	+
Duration before admission (longer)	+	+
Intermittent course before admission	0	0
Vasomotor symptoms	0	0
Vasomotor signs	0	0
Muscular atrophy	+	+
Spondylitis (in males)	—	0
Extent of joint involvement	+	+
Total severity (increased)	+	+
Improvement (after discharge)	—	—
Atrophy of nails	+	
Atrophy of skin		+

Note: + signifies positive association, — negative association, and 0 absence of association.

tion of disease of marked severity,* extensive joint involvement,† and relatively long duration is to be expected. Of more interest, perhaps, is the fact that 12 patients with disease of mild severity and 14 with duration of one year or less were found to have atrophic skin. The association between skin and muscular atrophy mentioned by a previous observer [333] was confirmed in our series. Vasomotor symptoms (with the exception of cyanosis) and cold, moist extremities were not more characteristic of those with skin atrophy than of the remainder. Only 4 patients with spondylitis showed skin atrophy, and all but 1 of these had involvement of the peripheral joints (other than shoulders and hips) as well as the spine. In this patient skin atrophy was confined to the back and chest. No association was noted between skin atrophy and the following: history of prodromal symptoms, initial involvement of small joints, bilateral onset, or course before hospital admission. However, patients with atrophic skin less often showed improvement after discharge.

* See definition, par. 4.26.
† See definition, par. 4.22.

31.3 Nail atrophy was also more common among older patients and among those with arthritis of longer duration before hospital admission. There was also a tendency for nail changes to be associated with muscular atrophy and with marked severity of disease. Like those with atrophic skin, patients with atrophic nails had a less favorable course after discharge from the hospital. Finally, a strong association was evidenced between atrophy of the skin and a corresponding process in the nails.

31.4 No adequate explanation has yet been furnished for atrophic changes in the skin or nails in rheumatoid arthritis. By analogy with similar skin changes in known diseases of the central and peripheral nervous systems, it has been supposed that nervous influences are at work, possibly through reflex pathways from the joints [13, 81, 199, 212]. Our data give no support to a second theory, that circulatory disturbances due to alterations in vasomotor tone are responsible [285, 445]. However, the finding by Curtis and Pollard [125] of inflammatory changes in the corium, along with atrophy of the epithelium, in biopsies from patients with rheumatoid arthritis makes it seem less necessary to postulate an intermediary effect of the nervous or circulatory system. Thus, we may conclude that skin changes, at least, represent another example of the widespread systemic involvement of rheumatoid arthritis.

31.5 In addition to atrophy of the skin, other cutaneous manifestations have been noted in association with rheumatoid arthritis. The abnormal pigmentation described by Spender [490] and others [13, 52, 150, 178, 286, 333] was encountered in only 2 of our patients. In 1 of them the pigmentation was so marked as to suggest the possibility of Addison's disease, a diagnosis not confirmed at autopsy. Erythematous rashes were not noted among the patients of the present series but have since been seen not infrequently in our clinic, especially among children [23]. Writing in 1898, Bannatyne [13] was one of the first to mention purpuric spots in rheumatoid arthritis. Although none of our patients apparently developed such spots during their first hospitalization, a few have subsequently done so. In a recent study of 500 patients with nonthrombopenic purpura [132], rheumatoid arthritis was the underlying disease in 4 per cent. Another as yet unexplained cutaneous finding in

Skin, Nails, and Tongue

rheumatoid arthritis is redness of the thenar and hypothenar eminences and finger tips, so-called liver palms [133]. Such a manifestation has been rare in our experience but was not especially looked for in the present study.

31.6   Table 31.2 lists the frequency of skin disease among patients and controls, with the omission of such intercurrent infections as scabies and epidermophytosis. Except for psoriasis, no differences were noted between the two groups. Vitiligo, described by one author [133] as a manifestation of rheumatoid arthritis, was found in 3 patients but also in 2 controls. We were unable to confirm a previous report [312] of an association between herpes zoster and the onset or localization of the arthritis. The association between rheumatoid arthritis and psoriasis has been discussed at length in the introductory section (par. 2.31), where reasons are given for the inclusion of patients with this combination in the present series. As shown in Table 31.2, the frequency of psoriasis was significantly higher among patients than among controls. The proportion of our patients with psoriasis (3.4 per cent) is approximately that observed in three other series [139, 150, 552]. The data from these series support the clinical impression that psoriasis and rheumatoid arthritis occur together more frequently than would be expected by chance.

31.7   Atrophic changes in the mucous membranes of the tongue were found in 28 patients and in 18 controls, a difference falling short

Table 31.2

Frequency of skin diseases among 293 rheumatoid arthritics and 293 controls

Disease	Patients		Controls		Difference in percentages
	No.	Per cent	No.	Per cent	
Psoriasis	10*	3.4	2	0.7	2.7 ± 1.2
Acne	8	2.7	13	4.4	
Eczema	6	2.0	7	2.4	
Herpes zoster (by history)	4	1.4	8	2.7	
Vitiligo	3	1.0	2	0.7	
Carotinemia	2	0.7	0	0.0	
Pigmentation	2	0.7	0	0.0	
Keratoses	2	0.7	1	0.3	

* Psoriasis was subsequently found in 5 additional patients.

of statistical significance. In this respect our data thus tend to support a statement by Bayles and his coworkers [27], who concluded, on the basis of excretion levels, that arthritic patients do not suffer from thiamin, riboflavin, or nicotinic acid deficiency when maintained on a diet usually considered adequate in respect to these factors. The figures in regard to atrophy of the tongue also suggest that if, as some think, rheumatoid patients are unable to utilize adequately ingested iron in the formation of hemoglobin [381, 444], such lack of utilization is not reflected by changes in the mucous membrane of the tongue.

SUMMARY

31.8 Atrophy of the skin was recorded for nearly one-third of our patients and atrophic changes in the nails for about one-sixth. Both these conditions were apparently more common among older patients and among those with relatively long-standing and severe arthritis. A significantly higher proportion of patients than controls had psoriasis (3.4 per cent), which suggests a more-than-chance association with rheumatoid arthritis. Other skin diseases, including vitiligo, occurred with equal frequency among series and controls. There was no significant difference between patients and controls in regard to atrophy of the tongue.

31.9 Objectives for further study:

1. Additional observations on the histopathology of the skin in rheumatoid arthritis.

2. Chemical and histologic studies on the nails of rheumatoid subjects.

32

Edema, Varicosities, and Clubbing

32.1   Edema for which no extraneous cause could be found has been reported occasionally in patients with rheumatoid arthritis [*13, 199, 286, 333*]. In most instances the edema was described as pitting, although Jones [*286*] referred to solid edema, with dry overlying skin, resembling myxedema. While the role of disuse and dependency in severely crippled patients has been recognized [*333*], no explanations or even speculations have been forthcoming in regard to other mechanisms for edema in rheumatoid patients. In our study, as shown in Table 32.1, the difference between patients and controls with respect to edema was not quite significant until persons with swelling due to extraneous causes were omitted from both groups. Varicosities headed the list of causes, but in some of the patients edema could be traced to severe anemia, heart failure, phlebitis, and nephritis. The group of 14 patients with unexplained edema was equally divided as to sex, but only two were less than forty years of age. We found no evidence that the arthritis was more active or severe in this group than in the remainder of the series. In no case did it seem reasonable to attribute the edema to immobility with consequent loss of muscle activity or to sitting for long periods with feet dependent. Involvement of related joints (in one case the hands and wrists, in the rest the ankles or feet) was noted in 12 of the 14 patients. The last finding suggests an inflammatory process originat-

Table 32.1

Frequency of edema and varicosities among 293 rheumatoid arthritics and 293 controls

	Patients		Controls		Difference
Edema	No.	Per cent	No.	Per cent	in percentages
Total	28	9.6	16	5.5	4.1 ± 2.2
Not due to extraneous cause	14	4.8	2	0.7	4.1 ± 1.3
Varicosities					
Total	24	8.2	43	14.7	6.5 ± 2.6

ing from an active arthritis in the underlying joints. The higher frequency of varicose veins found among controls (Table 32.1) requires some comment. While varicose veins may have been overlooked in bed patients, it is also possible that the nonarthritic individuals were able to pursue occupations requiring much standing on their feet and were thus rendered more liable to the development of noticeable varicosities.

32.2 Although the formation of edema in rheumatoid arthritis has been recognized for nearly one hundred years, the pathogenesis remains unexplained. Lymphatic obstruction has not been demonstrated, but it is possible that a large knee-joint effusion might occasionally interfere with the venous return in the leg or, as suggested in one paper [377], venous as well as arterial constriction might take place in a rheumatoid person. When extraneous causes are eliminated and dependency or disuse is not operative, it does not seem unreasonable to regard edema as an occasional manifestation of rheumatoid arthritis, with a mechanism perhaps analogous to the formation of joint effusions. Histologic evidence of a high degree of edema has been found in biopsy studies of early articular and extra-articular rheumatoid lesions [305]. Study of patients with edema and rheumatoid arthritis seems worthy of pursuit, especially in regard to description of the edema fluid.

32.3 Pulmonary osteo-arthropathy has frequently been mistaken for rheumatoid arthritis, thus delaying investigation of the patient for the primary process, usually a thoracic neoplasm. Clubbing, which nearly always accompanies osteo-arthropathy, is of great help in diagnosis and was looked for in the patients of the present series. Of the 3 patients in whom clubbing was found, 2 had unrelated pulmonary disease

Edema, Varicosities, and Clubbing

—bronchiectasis and tuberculosis, respectively. In the 1 remaining patient, no cause was found, in spite of a fifteen-year follow-up and investigation of the patient's family for a hereditary basis. No similar patients have been encountered in our clinic. Clubbing should thus continue to be regarded as a highly important factor in distinguishing between generalized pulmonary osteo-arthropathy and rheumatoid arthritis.

SUMMARY

32.4 Edema which could be regarded as a manifestation of rheumatoid arthritis was found in about 5 per cent of our patients. In nearly all instances, the patient was over 40 and underlying joints were the seat of an active arthritis. The frequency of varicose veins was higher among the controls, a finding which may be related merely to the inability of many of the patients to stand for long periods. Unexplained clubbing was recorded in only 1 of the patients.

32.5 Objective for further study:

The mechanism of edema formation in rheumatoid arthritis, including a description of the edema fluid.

33

Nodules

33.1 Both clinically and histologically, the subcutaneous nodule must be considered one of the characteristic lesions in rheumatoid arthritis. Although the association was mentioned by a number of the early writers [13, 174, 246], comprehensive descriptions of the histology have appeared only recently and have led to some disagreement in regard to microscopic resemblance to the nodules of rheumatic fever [35, 107, 136]. In the present study subcutaneous nodules were found on hospital admission in 34 patients (11.6 per cent) but in only 2 of the corresponding controls (0.7 per cent). Subsequent development of nodules was noted in an additional 28 patients during a follow-up period amounting in many instances to ten years or more—a cumulative frequency of 21.3 per cent. In other series [30, 97, 320, 333] the frequency of nodules has varied from 6 to 12.2 per cent, with the highest figure (20 per cent) reported by Dawson and Boots [136]. These authors admit that their patients cannot be regarded as unselected, since certain ones were undoubtedly referred to them on account of their interest in this phase of the disease. In one study [320] with 532 matched controls the frequency was less than 1 per cent, as in our controls.

33.2 No differences in the frequency of nodules were discovered when our patients were divided by sex or grouped according to age at disease onset and age on hospital admission (less or more than forty

Nodules

years of age). Typical nodules have been found in children with rheumatoid arthritis [121] and have been verified by biopsy in one eighty-year-old patient [35]. As was pointed out before [35, 136], the elbow represents the most common site for nodule formation. In about 80 per cent of our patients with nodules at least one was found at the elbow. In all but 3 of these patients with nodules about the elbow, the corresponding wrist joints were involved in the arthritic process. According to Collins [107], a painful wrist causes the patient to bear weight more often on the elbow and thus to subject it to an unusual amount of trauma. In any case, it is generally believed that irritation and minor trauma, particularly over bony prominences, may often constitute the determining factor in nodule location.

33.3   As shown in Table 33.1, a higher proportion of patients considered to have markedly active disease on admission was found among those with nodules, with the reverse true in respect to mild activity. (The relationship here may well depend merely upon definition, since the finding of nodules may be considered a sign of disease activity.) No differences were discovered, however, in regard to the occurrence of "frequent" fever, a history of weight loss, a preceding infection, anemia, or enlargement of lymph nodes or spleen. An acute, severe type of onset was also associated with the development of subcutaneous nodules (Table 33.2). No association was found between nodule formation and either a history of prodromal symptoms or longer disease duration be-

Table 33.1

Disease activity on hospital admission in relation to presence or absence of nodules among patients of present series

Patients	No.	Disease activity*					
		Mild		Moderate		Marked	
		No.	Per cent	No.	Per cent	No.	Per cent
Total	293	59	20.1	175	59.7	59	20.1
With nodules	34	2	5.9	20	58.8	12	35.2
Without nodules	259	57	22.0	155	59.8	47	18.1
Difference in percentages:			16.1 ± 7.4				17.1 ± 7.2
			$\chi^2 = 8.33; p < .02$				

* See definition, par. 4.27.

Table 33.2

Acute onset of arthritis in relation to presence or absence of nodules among patients of present series

Patients	No.	Onset acute No.	Per cent
Total	293	64	21.8
With nodules	34	12	35.3
Without nodules	259	52	20.1
	Difference in percentages:	15.2 ± 7.5	

fore admission. In fact, in 1 patient of the present series a typical nodule was discovered only three weeks after disease onset and in another patient seen at the clinic but not a member of the series, a nodule was found four months after disease onset. The latter was confirmed by biopsy. It should also be noted that the majority of our patients who developed nodules within a year had experienced an acute onset. No differences were found in the frequency of nodule formation among patients whose arthritis began in small or large joints or in a single joint. Similarly, nodules were found with equal frequency among those with unilateral or bilateral distribution of joint involvement at the onset. Not a single nodule was discovered, however, among the 14 patients of the present series whose disease was unilateral at the time of hospital admission, or in a similar group of 13 patients subsequently encountered in our clinic. (It should be mentioned that these patients with unilateral involvement were composed largely of those with mild disease activity and severity.)

33.4 A subcutaneous nodule was found in only 1 spondylitic of the present series—a female who also had peripheral joint involvement. Since the closing of the series we have examined 14 spondylitics with one or more nodules and have obtained confirmatory biopsies in 6 cases. In every one of these patients peripheral joints other than the shoulders and hips were also involved. The absence of nodules in what might be termed the "pure" form of spondylitis has been recorded by others [135] and has constituted one argument for regarding ankylosing spondylitis as a separate entity.

33.5 Contrary opinions have been expressed in the literature as to a relationship between the finding of subcutaneous nodules and arthritis of marked severity. Dawson and Boots [136] believed that nodules

Table 33.3
Presence of nodules among patients of present series in relation to total severity of arthritis on hospital admission

Degree of total severity	No. of patients	Nodules present	
		No.	Per cent
Total	293	34	11.6
Mild	72	2	2.8
Moderate	172	24	14.0
Marked	49	8	16.3

$\chi^2 = 7.58; p<.05$

Table 33.4
Presence of nodules among patients of present series in relation to course of rheumatoid arthritis after discharge

Course after discharge	No. of patients	Nodules present	
		No.	Per cent
Total	293	34	11.6
Improved	133	11	8.3
Unimproved	117	13	11.1
Remainder*	43	10	23.3

* 21 patients were excluded because they had received special forms of therapy and 22 because follow-up studies were inadequate.

were usually observed in severe cases and that their presence indicated an unfavorable prognosis, while McCrae [333] believed that there was no association between disease severity and nodule formation. Neither paper presented figures to confirm the authors' viewpoints. The results shown in Table 33.3 would tend to uphold the opinion of Dawson and Boots [136], since we found nodules almost exclusively in patients with moderate or marked severity* of arthritis on admission. As to the relationship of nodule production to prognosis, Table 33.4 shows that 11 of the 34 patients with nodules improved after discharge from the hospital. One can at least state, then, that the presence of nodules in a given patient does not preclude the possibility of a favorable course of his disease.†

33.6   Nodules entirely similar in histologic appearance to those

* See definition, par. 4.26.
† For a complete list of associations, see Appendix Table 47.

found in the subcutaneous tissues have been identified in the sclera [544] and in the pericardium, pleura, and synovial membrane [35, 38]. In at least one instance, they accompanied extensive subcutaneous nodule formation. It therefore seems likely that nodules were actually in process of formation in some part of the body in many of the patients who were classified in the group without nodules at the time of physical examination. It would then be more accurate to classify the 34 patients mentioned above in "the group with nodules in tissues subject to irritation and trauma near the body surface." Such nodules were not found in patients with joint involvement confined to the spine (with or without arthritis of shoulders and hips), but they were associated with an acute onset and a relatively active and severe type of disease. Surely certain rheumatoid arthritics with multiple nodules, often rapidly growing and reaching a large size, may justifiably be termed "nodule formers" in contrast to those with disease of equal or greater severity but without a single nodule on careful examination. Perhaps rheumatoid activity is more readily precipitated by trauma in some individuals. The situation may be analogous to that mentioned in par. 20.7, in which intercurrent infection seems to play the same role.

SUMMARY

33.7 Subcutaneous nodules were found on hospital admission in 34 patients, or 11.6 per cent, of the present series. No differences were evident between patients with and without nodules in respect to age, sex, duration of disease, and other factors, with the exception that nodule formation was associated with an acute onset of disease and a greater degree of activity and severity of arthritis on admission. No subcutaneous nodules were found in patients with spondylitis (unless peripheral joints other than shoulders or hips were also involved) nor have reports of any been found in the literature. In our experience, patients with arthritis confined to one side of the body did not develop nodules. At least one-third of our patients with nodules showed improvement subsequent to leaving the hospital.

33.8 Objective for further study:

The role of trauma in the formation of nodules, to include further attempts at their experimental production in rheumatoid subjects [522].

34

Joint Examination

PHYSICAL SIGNS

34.1 Detailed descriptions of the physical signs exhibited by the joints in rheumatoid arthritis are readily available in the literature and need not be repeated here. It seems sufficient for the purposes of this analysis to comment briefly on the frequency of the more important articular signs among patients of the present series. As shown in Table 34.1, actual limitation of motion, as distinguished from subjective stiffness, was present in over 90 per cent. Nearly all those without this limitation had relatively mild forms of rheumatoid arthritis. Almost half of them had arthritis of shorter duration (one year or less), and the majority of those with disease of longer duration had enjoyed one or more remissions before the final attack which brought them into the hospital. Over 90 per cent of the patients showed articular swelling. Among those without swelling, 20 had spondylitis—in most instances either confined to the spine or with hips and shoulders the only peripheral joints affected. In the remaining 7 patients without joint swelling, the arthritis was either early and mild or in an advanced atrophic state without detectable swelling. In only 4 patients was neither joint limitation nor swelling evident on hospital admission, but both developed later during follow-up studies. The absence of such objective changes in patients otherwise satisfying the requirements for a diagno-

Table 34.1

Frequency of articular signs among 293 rheumatoid arthritics

Signs	No. of patients	Percentage of patients
Limitation of motion	267	91.1
Swelling	266	90.8
Effusion	112	38.2
Heat	65	22.2
Osseous overgrowth	38	13.0
Redness	31	10.6

sis of rheumatoid arthritis has been mentioned by others [320, 463, 518]. Articular heat was noted in about one-fifth of the patients, but the recording of this finding apparently varied with different observers. Further statistical treatment is therefore omitted in view of the absence of objective measurement of skin temperature. The proportion with joint effusion, 38 per cent, was very close to that of 44 per cent found in a series of 532 patients [320], from whom spondylitics were largely eliminated. Osseous overgrowth was found in a relatively small number of patients and represented hypertrophic changes, either coincidental in older patients or secondary to the underlying rheumatoid arthritis.

34.2   The patients with articular effusion and those with acutely inflamed joints (as evidenced by redness) were considered in more detail. Table 34.2 shows the nature of the association of various factors with these two signs. Fluid accumulation was apparently not related to sex, age on hospital admission, or disease duration before admission. The negative association with spondylitis was to be expected. Nevertheless, when spondylitics without involvement of peripheral joints other than shoulders and hips were excluded from consideration, joint effusion was found as often in patients with spondylitis as in the remainder. The associations found between articular effusion and both lymphadenopathy and fever lead to interesting speculations. On the one hand absorption from joint effusions may result in regional lymphadenopathy, and on the other it may produce an effect on the heat regulating centers. The table also shows positive associations between joint effusion and increased disease activity* and severity.* This result loses significance in the case of activity in that joint effusion was often one of the criteria

---

* See definitions, pars. **4.26** and **4.27**.

Table 34.2
Association of various factors with articular fluid and redness among patients of present series

Factor	Fluid	Redness
Sex	0	0
Prodromal symptoms	0	0
Infection before onset	0	0
Onset acute	0	0
Onset unilateral	0	+
Age on admission	0	0
Duration before admission (longer)	0	—
Intermittent course before admission	0	0
Vasomotor symptoms	0	0
Vasomotor signs	0	0
Muscular atrophy	0	0
Fever	+	0
Lymphadenopathy	+	0
Nodules	0	0
Spondylitis (in males)	—	—
Activity of disease	+	0
Extent of joint involvement	+	—
Total severity (increased)	+	0
Improvement (after discharge)	—	+
Articular redness	0	
Articular fluid		0

Note: + signifies positive association, — negative association, and 0 absence of association.

determining the degree of activity of the disease process. Redness of joints was related to a shorter disease duration before admission and a unilateral onset but not to infection as a precipitant or to an acute, severe type of onset. The lack of antagonism between articular redness and both vasomotor symptoms and signs indicates, as others [343] have observed, that increased vasomotor tone may persist in the presence of acute joint inflammation. A negative association was found between redness of joints and spondylitis, whether or not patients with disease confined to spine, shoulders, and hips were excluded. The somewhat surprising absence of a relationship between increased disease activity and joint redness suggests that the latter factor was not considered important in determining the activity of the arthritis in a given patient. Articular redness, unlike joint effusion, was related to less extensive joint involvement.* In distinction to patients with articular effusion,

* See definition, par. 4.22.

whose course after discharge was less likely to be favorable, those with redness of joints did better than the remainder in follow-up studies. Too much importance should not be assigned to the last association, since it may depend upon a mutual association between improvement and both shorter disease duration and articular redness.

ROENTGENOGRAMS

34.3 In the case of each patient roentgenograms of representative joints were taken and the findings were recorded on the checklists. For the purposes of statistical analysis, the patients were divided into those with and those without bony or cartilaginous changes visible in roentgenograms. Such changes included loss of bony substance, joint narrowing, and lipping or osteophyte formation. Degenerative changes consistent with age and soft tissue swelling or joint effusion were not considered reasons for including a given patient among those with roentgenographic changes. Such changes were not found in 46 patients, or 15.7 per cent of the series. That a reasonably accurate diagnosis of rheumatoid arthritis may be made without evidence of bony or cartilaginous alterations in joint roentgenograms has been noted by several authors [133, 251, 463]. In one Army series [463], where the disease was usually encountered in an early or mild stage, only 25 per cent of those with peripheral joint involvement exhibited roentgenographic changes of the type described. Table 34.3 shows the nature of the associations between the absence of bony or cartilaginous changes and various factors. The positive association with age under forty on hospital admission may be only apparent, since the younger patients tended to have milder forms of disease. The relationship with prodromal symptoms is difficult to explain, unless one assumes that the constitutional aspects of the disease are more prominent than the articular in such patients. In our experience an acute, severe onset, as mentioned before (par. 15.3), has tended to lead to early hospital admission, often before roentgenographic changes have become evident. The distribution of primary joint involvement was apparently not related to the presence or absence of roentgenographic changes. It seems reasonable to expect that disease of mild severity and of relatively short duration would not be accompanied by roentgenographic changes except in the soft tissues. Only 6 patients

Joint Examination

Table 34.3
Association of various factors with negative x-ray findings in respect to bony or cartilaginous changes

Factor	Nature of association
Sex	0
Prodromal symptoms	+
Onset acute	+
Onset in small joints	0
Onset in large joints	0
Onset monarticular	0
Age on admission under 40	+
Duration before admission (longer)	—
Total severity (increased)	—
Improvement (after discharge)	+

Note: + signifies positive association, — negative association, and 0 absence of association.

with disease duration of more than five years failed to display bony or cartilaginous alterations, but all of these had enjoyed at least one period of remission before the attack which led to hospital admission. There was also a relationship between improvement after discharge and absence of roentgenographic changes, since 15 of the 46 patients without roentgenographic changes were in complete remission at the time of follow-up examination.

EXTENT OF INVOLVEMENT

34.4 While the joints involved, as well as the physical signs, were recorded for each patient of the present series, no compilation was made in regard to the frequency with which individual joints were affected at the time of examination. Reference may be made here, for the sake of completeness, to an enumeration of symptomatic joints [320] based on the histories of 532 rheumatoid arthritics. This group was made up of patients with disease duration of five years or less and largely without spondylitis. The percentages, as shown in Table 34.4, approximate the order of frequency listed by Dawson [133], Freund [192], and Monroe [362].

34.5 Each patient was classified by several observers in regard to the extent of articular involvement,* as well as to the degree of activity and the total severity of the arthritis on admission. Three divisions were utilized, with the following results: mild involvement in 111 patients,

* See definition, par. 4.22.

Table 34.4

Specific joints involved according to histories of 532 rheumatoid arthritics studied by Lewis-Faning [320]

Joints	Percentage of patients
Proximal phalangeal	83
Wrists	79
Knees	78
Metacarpo-phalangeal	71
Ankles	68
Shoulders	62
Carpal	53
Elbows	50
Metatarso-phalangeal	46
Tarsal	46
Toes	23
Cervical spine	22
Terminal phalangeal	17
Hips	16
Temporo-mandibular	15
Sternoclavicular	8
Lumbar spine	8
Dorsal spine	5

or 38.5 per cent of the series; moderate involvement in 120 patients, or 40.3 per cent of the series; and marked involvement in 62 patients, or 21.2 per cent of the series. Table 34.5 shows the nature of the association found between various factors and joint involvement. Again, it must be pointed out that an indeterminate number of the recorded associations may merely reflect interrelationships among various factors chosen for tabulation or not yet explored. Definite conclusions therefore cannot be based on the material in this table. However, it seems reasonable that involvement should have been less extensive in patients with disease of shorter duration and hence often relatively young. Apparently, an acute onset did not foretell extensive involvement, nor did initial involvement of one joint or one side of the body necessarily rule out subsequent involvement of multiple joints. Certain systemic manifestations of rheumatoid arthritis were seemingly related to extensive joint involvement. These include atrophy of the skin, muscular wasting, lymphadenopathy, and subcutaneous nodules but not vasomotor symptoms or signs. In

Table 34.5

Association of various factors with increased articular involvement

Factor	Nature of association
Sex	0
Onset acute	0
Onset in small or large joints or monarticular	0
Onset unilateral	0
Age on admission under 40	—
Duration before admission (longer)	+
Intermittent course before admission	0
Vasomotor symptoms	0 (except cyanosis+)
Vasomotor signs	0
Muscular atrophy	+
Lymphadenopathy	+
Atrophy of skin	+
Nodules	+
Articular effusion	+
Joint redness	—
Activity of disease	+
Total severity (increased)	+
Improvement (after discharge)	—

Note: + signifies positive association, — negative association, and 0 absence of association.

general, a parallelism was shown between the degree of disease activity and the extent of the involvement, although in 8 patients, activity was marked and involvement mild or vice versa. The association between involvement and total severity was expected, since the extent of the involvement formed part of the definition of total severity* as applied to the patients of the present series. Finally, more extensive involvement appeared to be related to a less favorable course after discharge from the hospital.

SUMMARY

34.6 All but a few of the patients showed objective evidence of articular disease, most commonly joint swelling and limitation. Joint effusion was recognized in slightly over one-third of the series and was related to "frequent" fever and lymphadenopathy but not to disease duration. The roentgenograms of 15 per cent of the patients who other-

* See definition, par. 4.26.

wise satisfied the diagnosis of rheumatoid arthritis showed no bony or cartilaginous abnormalities. This group was made up of patients with shorter disease duration and milder severity. Articular redness was also associated with shorter disease duration, as well as with unilateral onset and less extensive joint involvement. The extent of joint involvement was regarded as mild or moderate in the majority of the patients but marked in about one-fifth. Extensive involvement was more common in older patients with longer disease duration and was related to skin and muscle atrophy, lymphadenopathy, and the presence of subcutaneous nodules. Articular redness and the absence of roentgenographic changes indicated a more favorable prognosis, and the opposite was true of articular effusion and extensive joint involvement.

35

Gallbladder

35.1 In view of previous indictments of the gallbladder as a possible focus of infection in rheumatoid arthritis [258, 288, 560, 566], most of the patients in the present series were examined by cholecystography. The results, as shown in Table 35.1, reveal that about 15 per cent gave definite or probable evidence of gallbladder disease, by the presence of gallstones or the absence of gallbladder shadows in the cholecystograms or by a history of the surgical removal of a diseased gallbladder. Those whose tests were classified as doubtful showed either a faint shadow or failure to empty the organ after a fatty meal. As would be expected, the majority of the patients with gallbladder disease were female and more than forty years of age on admission to the hospital. No comparable studies on patients with rheumatoid arthritis are available in the literature. However, Judd and Hench [288] found "gallbladder infection" in 5.7 per cent of 124 patients with rheumatoid arthritis, and Hartung and Steinbrocker [243] found a frequency of gallbladder disease in a series of patients with various forms of rheumatism which was equivalent to the prevalence reported for general hospital admissions. Since the frequency of gallstones and cholecystitis in the general population varies according to the age and sex of the patients studied and since the Graham test was not used to evaluate our control group, no conclusions

Table 35.1

Cholecystographic findings for patients of present series who were tested for gallbladder disease

Type of evidence	Patients	
	No.	Per cent
Positive tests and/or cholelithiasis (in 14)	36	13.4
Doubtful tests	18	6.7
Negative tests	209	77.7
Gallbladder previously removed	6	2.2
Total	269	100.0

can be drawn from the findings in the present series in regard to an association of gallbladder disease with rheumatoid arthritis.

35.2   Several authors [258, 288, 566] have advised surgical or medical treatment of gallbladder disease in patients with rheumatoid arthritis and have noted favorable results on the course of the arthritis following such therapy. In the most extensive study thus far reported in detail, Judd and Hench [288] followed 46 patients on whom cholecystectomies had been performed. Complete remission was noted in 5, marked improvement in 11, and moderate improvement in 8. Such figures lack significance when compared with those obtained from follow-up studies of a group receiving simple medical and orthopedic treatment (see Chapter 44). Cholecystectomies were performed on 6 patients of the present series during the course of their arthritis, either before or after hospital admission. In 2, mild postoperative exacerbations were noted, and in the remainder no effect was observed on the state of their joint disease.

SUMMARY

35.3   Roentgenographic evidence of gallbladder disease was found in nearly 15 per cent of our patients. The significance of this percentage is uncertain, since suitable control figures are not available. Although favorable effects on the course of rheumatoid arthritis have been reported following treatment of gallbladder disease, no direct relationship between the two conditions has been established.

36

Colon

36.1 As far back as 1910, a relationship was postulated between chronic arthritis and intestinal stasis [214, 310], especially when accompanied by ptosis of the gastro-intestinal tract. Later roentgenographic studies of the colon by Pemberton [402], Fletcher and Graham [185], and others [242, 489] were interpreted as demonstrating a characteristic appearance of this organ in patients with both rheumatoid and osteoarthritis. The changes upon which stress was laid by these authors included: (1) absent or lessened tone, manifested by dilatation, absence of haustration, and incompetence of the ileocecal valve, (2) redundance along with elongation, folding, or looping, (3) ptosis and (4) hypermobility along with spasms and narrowing. Improvement in the status of the arthritis, with or without therapy directed toward the bowel, was usually accompanied by a return toward normal in the roentgenologic appearance of the large intestine [185, 382, 402].

36.2 In order to test the validity of this concept, the status of most of the patients of the present series was determined by means of a barium enema. The results, as set forth in Table 36.1, demonstrate that changes corresponding to those described by others were demonstrable in only 27.7 per cent. When spasm without other changes was excluded, this figure fell to 22.2 per cent, as compared with 62 to 80 per cent recorded in several previous studies [185, 242, 489]. Others have been unable to

Table 36.1

A. Roentgenographic findings for patients of present series who were examined for colonic abnormalities

Finding	Patients No.	Per cent
Colon normal	177	68.1
Diverticula and/or polyps	9	3.5
Ulcerative colitis	2	0.8
1 or more features of "arthritic pattern"	72	27.7
Total	260	100.1

B. Analysis of roentgenographic findings for patients with "arthritic pattern"

Finding	Changes No.	Per cent
Low position of colon	38	45.8
Spasm	16	19.3
Redundancy	14	16.9
Loss of tone	8	9.6
Loss of haustrations	5	6.0
Ileo-cecal valve incompetency	2	2.4
Total	83	100.0

corroborate the presence of a characteristic roentgenographic appearance of the colon in rheumatoid arthritis. These include Lang [311], Martin [344], and Haft [231], the last of whom noted a corresponding frequency of colonic abnormalities in a control group. In the present study the controls were not examined roentgenographically, but it was the opinion of the radiologists performing the examinations on the patients that similar changes were frequently observed in patients without arthritis.

36.3   No association was found in the present series between an "arthritic pattern" in the colon and either sex or age. Likewise, neither the duration of the disease nor the total severity* appeared to be related to the frequency of the roentgenographic changes in the large intestine. This absence of association was confirmed by one author [242] in contradiction to the findings in two other studies [382, 402]. The low frequency of diverticula among our patients deserves comment, in view of the suggestions raised that diverticulitis, as a focus of infection, may

* See definition, par. 4.26.

Colon 343

sometimes be related to the onset or course of rheumatoid arthritis [*104, 402*]. At the present time the theory that changes in the function or shape of the colon bear an important relationship to the development of rheumatoid arthritis is receiving little attention, except for the observation that idiopathic ulcerative colitis may be accompanied by an arthritis resembling the rheumatoid variety both clinically and pathologically.

36.4   That changes in the colon, as demonstrated by roentgenograms, do occur in rheumatoid arthritis cannot be overlooked. It seems most probable that they represent functional alterations, perhaps secondary to inactivity [*375, 382*] and malnutrition [*185*] or perhaps mediated through the autonomic nervous system in a fashion similar to that of peripheral vasomotor instability [*489*]. Reference has already been made to an increased frequency of constipation and diarrhea among the patients of the present series as compared with the controls (par. 25.2). Gross or histologic evidence of atrophy or other changes in the intestine was absent in the 4 cases studied by Keefer [*289*] at autopsy. We therefore regard this roentgenographic pattern in the colon as an inconstant observation in patients with rheumatoid arthritis rather than a finding peculiar to the disease or likely to be related to its pathogenesis or course.

SUMMARY

36.5   Changes in the roentgenographic appearance of the colon similar to those previously described in rheumatoid arthritis were found in about one-fourth of 260 patients of the present series. At present, evidence is lacking that such colonic abnormalities are in any way specifically related to this form of arthritis.

36.6   Objective for further study:
See par. 25.7, no. 1.

37

Foci of Infection

37.1 The role of foci of infection has long constituted one of the most controversial points in discussions of the pathogenesis of rheumatoid arthritis. Although out of favor at present, perhaps temporarily, the search for focal infections and their removal or treatment if found were assigned an important place in the therapeutics of this disorder from the days of Billings [*40*]. Presentation in detail of the affirmative and negative arguments in the focal infection debate is available in the literature [*429*] and need not be set forth here. This chapter will rather be devoted to our findings in the present series and to a comparison of the results obtained by follow-up studies of patients whose foci were treated and those in whom they were left alone.

37.2 After historical data had been obtained in regard to the presence of focal infection and to previous treatment, each patient was examined according to a set plan. This consisted of a combined clinical, roentgenologic, and laboratory study directed toward the teeth, tonsils, sinuses, prostate, female genital organs, and gallbladder. In each case, roentgenograms were obtained of the teeth, sinuses, and gallbladder and prostatic secretion was examined for evidence of chronic infection. In women, a gynecologist conducted a careful search for infection of the cervix and other possible genital sites. Clinical examination of the teeth was made by a dentist and of the tonsils and sinuses by an otolaryngolo-

Foci of Infection

gist, while the male genito-urinary apparatus was checked by a urologist. Although final decision as to the presence or absence of focal infection was left to the specialist concerned, it should be mentioned that only apical infection was regarded as significant in the case of the teeth and that thickening in the lining membranes of sinuses was not regarded as indicative of localized infection, unless accompanied by other clinical or roentgenographic evidence. As far as the gallbladder was concerned, either a positive Graham test, the presence of calculi, or both were regarded as reasons for classifying this organ as a focus. (In Chapter 35, the relationship of gallbladder disease to rheumatoid arthritis has been considered in detail.) Similar studies were not carried out in the control group.

37.3 The data in regard to focal infections in the present series are summarized in Table 37.1. About two-thirds of our patients were found to have one or more foci on hospital admission, and less than half of this group had already been treated for localized infection, in most instances following the onset of their arthritis. The remaining third showed no evidence of focal infection despite careful study, but in nearly all, one or more foci had been eliminated by therapy, either before their disease had started or during its course. The previous history of the entire series in regard to the management of focal infection may be summarized by the statement that 118 patients, or 40.2 per cent, had already had foci removed or treated during their arthritis, presumably in an

Table 37.1

Status of patients of present series with respect to focal infection

Status of patient	No. of patients	
No evidence of focal infection on hospital admission		95
Foci removed or treated before onset of arthritis	26	
Foci removed or treated after onset	46	
Foci removed or treated before and after onset	12	
Foci not removed or treated before admission	11	
1 or more foci of infection found on hospital admission		198
Partial removal or treatment of foci before admission	85	
No foci removed or treated before admission	113	
Total		293
Patients receiving treatment for focal infection during course of arthritis		118

attempt to exert a favorable influence upon its course. Table 37.2 lists the location of the infected areas found in 198 patients on admission. Tonsils and teeth head the list, with about the same frequency, followed fairly closely by the sinuses, while the genital organs in both sexes were only occasionally believed to harbor foci of infection. The table also demonstrates that over half the patients in this group had more than one focus of infection.

37.4 About 85 per cent of the present series, or 250 patients, were utilized in a previously reported study on the course of rheumatoid arthritis [466], the circumstances and results of which are reviewed in Chapter 44. None of these patients received other than simple medical or orthopedic treatment for their arthritis, and improvement was measured by objective criteria rather than by gains in joint function or the abatement of symptoms. Table 37.3 gives the distribution of patients with and without foci of infection at the time of hospital admission and summarizes our findings with respect to the management of focal infection. This was somewhat inconsistent, partly because the therapeutic viewpoints of the staff changed while the series was being collected and partly because a few patients refused to accept the recommended treatment. As shown in the table, the rate of improvement was approximately the same, irrespective of the presence or management of focal infection. (A single exception was found in the small group of 10 patients who had never been treated for focal infection and in whom no foci were found while in the hospital. All but 2 of these improved, but the numbers are too small for statistical significance.) In order to eliminate the possibility that a preponderance of favorable prognostic factors in one or more of the other groups might have influenced the results, the frequency of males, of patients under forty, of those with disease duration of one year or less, and of those with mild severity was determined in each of the four divisions. No significant differences were observed. It was also found that focal infections occurred and were treated at about the same rates among the patients who were not included in the follow-up study as among those who were.

37.5 Certain reports [97, 150, 427] have stressed the improvement which resulted from the removal of foci of infection in patients with rheumatoid arthritis of the so-called "infectious" type. In such patients the disease usually had an acute onset, frequently followed an acute in-

Foci of Infection

Table 37.2

Location of focal infections found at hospital admission among 293 rheumatoid arthritics

	Patients	
Foci	No.	Per cent
1 or more found on hospital admission (total)	198	67.5
Distribution of foci		
Tonsils	91	31.1
Teeth	90	31.0
Sinuses	62	21.2
Gallbladder	36	12.3
Cervix	17	9.1*
Prostate	16	14.9†

* Based on 186 females.
† Based on 107 males.

Table 37.3

Improvement after discharge in relation to presence or absence of foci of infection (and their management if present) among patients included in 1947 follow-up study (see Chapter 44)

Foci of infection	No. of patients	Improved after discharge	
		No.	Per cent
Total	250	133	53.2
None found on hospital admission	80	42	52.2
None previously treated	10	8	80.0
All removed or treated	48	25	52.1
Partially removed or treated	33	20	60.6
None removed or treated	89	46	51.7

fection, and was often limited to a few joints. When those of our patients with either an acute onset or a preceding infection were considered separately, the results were again the same whether or not foci had been eliminated. Further negative evidence is thus made available in regard to the influence of foci of infection on the course of rheumatoid arthritis, whether or not of the "infectious" variety.

37.6   In presenting these data in regard to focal infections among our patients, the intention has not been to add controversial material to an already overburdened literature. Since the control group was not comparably examined, no statement can be made as to whether foci were more or less common in the patients than in persons without rheumatoid arthritis. Furthermore, by the time that many of our patients had been admitted to the hospital, foci had been completely or partially removed in consequence of the arthritis. The possibility also remains that in certain instances foci present at the time of the onset of the arthritis might have cleared spontaneously, whether or not the appearance of prodromal symptoms is accepted as the real start of the disease. The prevalence of foci of infection in rheumatoid arthritis cannot be determined without a controlled study of patients in an early stage of their disease. Such a study is not yet available, although reports have shown that diseased foci are found as often in non-arthritics as in patients with rheumatoid arthritis of varying duration [*130*]. The figures presented here in regard to the presence of foci and the history of previous treatment thus lack any important significance and merely round out one aspect of a clinical description of rheumatoid arthritis based upon this group of patients. Similarly, the therapeutic worth of elimination of foci is hardly settled by the failure to obtain superior results in the patients whose foci were treated or removed. The time-worn arguments can again be raised in rebuttal—for example, that the wrong focus was removed, that the right focus was not completely removed or removed too late, and that the real focus was never found. More light on the etiology or at least the pathogenesis of rheumatoid arthritis is required before the practicing physician can be relieved of his state of indecision when confronted by a patient with the combination of rheumatoid arthritis and focal infection.

SUMMARY

37.7   Each patient in the present series was carefully studied for the presence of focal infection. Presumptive evidence of such infection was discovered in two-thirds of the patients, most commonly in the teeth, tonsils, and sinuses. In about 40 per cent of our patients foci had been removed or treated before admission at some time during the course of their arthritis. Follow-up studies failed to reveal a significant effect upon the course of the disease by means of treatment or removal of infectious foci.

38

Red-Cell, White-Cell, and Differential Counts

38.1 As part of the systematic study of the patients in the present series, red-cell and white-cell counts and differential leukocyte counts were performed at the time of admission to the hospital. The counts were done according to the usual technique by the members of the house staff who were in charge of the patients. Hemoglobin determinations were also made, but these have been omitted from consideration on account of the inaccuracy of the method employed (Tallqvist). Since the anemia in rheumatoid arthritis is usually hypochromic [*105, 161, 230, 381, 444, 500, 546*], it is evident that milder degrees of anemia may not have been recorded by utilization of the red-cell level alone.

RED-CELL COUNT

38.2 Table 38.1 shows that in slightly more than one-fifth of our patients the red-cell count was below the figures usually considered the lower levels of normal (4.5 million/mm^3 in males and 4.0 million/mm^3 in females). No significant sex difference was found in the frequency of anemia as thus defined, although if the figure 4.0 million had been utilized in both males and females, the anemic group would have been composed, with 1 exception, entirely of women. In another series [*381*] where a similar comparison was made, although hemoglobin instead of red-cell levels were employed, anemia was present with greater frequency in women with rheumatoid arthritis than in men.

Table 38.1

Frequency of anemia among patients of present series, divided according to sex

	No. of patients	Anemia present	
		No.	Per cent
Total	289*	65	22.5
Males†	104	27	26.0
Females**	185	38	20.5
	Difference in percentages:		5.5 ± 5.2

* 2 males with coincidental pernicious anemia, 1 male with nephritis, and 1 female with cirrhosis of the liver (all with severe anemia) were not included.
† Red-cell count below 4.5 million/mm.^{3}
** Red-cell count below 4.0 million/mm.^{3}

38.3 A number of authors [13, 97, 133, 150, 188] have stated that anemia constitutes a common manifestation of rheumatoid arthritis. A recent British study [320] of the hemoglobin levels in 517 patients compared with controls selected both from hospital patients and from the general population, clearly demonstrated association between anemia and this form of joint disease. In three reports [97, 223, 477] where red-cell counts were recorded, the proportion of patients with levels below 4.0 million varied from 16 to 31 per cent. Statements have also appeared that the finding of anemia is related to the activity of the arthritis [381], to the presence of fever [381], or to disease duration[105]. In our series no association was demonstrated between fever and anemia, but a relationship was apparent between anemia and disease activity,* and, as shown in Table 38.2, total severity on admission.† (The last two associations, of course, might be expected by the definitions of activity and severity.) In regard to duration of arthritis, anemia was found more commonly in patients whose onset dated back more than one year but less than five years than in either those with shorter or longer duration (Table 38.3). As pointed out below (par. 40.5), anemia was more frequently recorded for patients with gastric anacidity than for those with hydrochloric acid present. An intermittent compared with a progressive course was apparently unrelated to the presence or absence of anemia on hospital admission, and as far as could be determined from the follow-up of our patients, those with anemia did as well after dis-

* See definition, par. **4.27**.
† See definition, par. **4.26**.

Table 38.2
Anemia in relation to total severity of rheumatoid arthritis on hospital admission among patients of present series

Degree of total severity	No. of patients	Anemia present	
		No.	Per cent
Total	289*	65	22.5
Mild	71	6	8.5
Moderate	169	47	27.8
Marked	49	12	24.5
$\chi^2 = 10.78; p<.01$			

* See note, Table 38.1.

Table 38.3
Anemia in relation to duration of rheumatoid arthritis before hospital admission among patients of present series

Duration before admission	No. of patients	Anemia present	
		No.	Per cent
Total	289*	65	22.5
1 year or less	84	15	17.9
5 years to 1 year	125	43	34.4
More than 5 years	80	7	8.8
$\chi^2 = 19.9; p<.001$			

* See note, Table 38.1.

charge as those without. There was no evidence in our series of relationships between a low red-cell count and fatigue or weakness; increased pulse rate; prodromal symptoms; acute as opposed to gradual onset; or the findings on physical examination of lymphadenopathy, splenomegaly, or subcutaneous nodules. There was also no difference in respect to anemia in patients over or under the age of 40 on admission, and spondylitics were as subject to a lowered red-cell count as patients without spinal involvement.*

38.4 It is generally agreed that the anemia found in rheumatoid arthritis is usually of hypochromic type, but reports are conflicting as to whether it is normocytic [161, 444] or microcytic [381]. Excluding 4 patients with anemia of extraneous cause, we found only 2 patients with red-cell counts below 3.5 million, which bears out the statement

* For a complete list of associations, see Appendix Table 47.

that extreme anemia is rare in rheumatoid arthritis. The causation of anemia in this disease is not clearly understood. Although purpura and gastro-intestinal bleeding are very occasionally encountered, no data are available in support of extravascular blood loss or hemorrhage as important factors. A few patients respond to oral administration of iron, presumably because they have a coincidental iron deficiency anemia [*161, 280*]. On the basis of one study [*280*] it was concluded that the absorption of iron from the intestine was inadequate because iron given orally failed to influence the degree of anemia, while iron administered intravenously was at least temporarily effective. However, direct measurements have failed to show impaired intestinal absorption of iron by rheumatoid patients [*446*]. Furthermore, the utilization of iron given intravenously is often poor [*161*], especially by patients with highly active disease [*444*]. Two recent reports [*148, 201*] have presented evidence that increased plasma volume and reduction in red-cell mass may determine the degree of anemia, as measured by hemoglobin levels and red-cell counts, while a third [*280*] concluded that plasma volumes were normal. Studies on the survival time of red cells in rheumatoid subjects have also demonstrated an increased rate of red-cell destruction, with a resultant anemia due to failure of a compensatory increase in red-cell production [*161, 191a*]. From the information available to date, one must conclude that more than one mechanism may be operative and that the pathogenesis of the anemia of rheumatoid arthritis may differ among individual patients. At any rate, it would be of interest to attempt to confirm by numerical studies the impression that the hemoglobin and red-cell levels constitute in many patients an index of the course of the arthritis. Improvement in these levels seems to occur during remissions and the opposite during exacerbations.

WHITE-CELL COUNT

38.5   White-cell counts within the normal range were recorded for the majority of our patients, but counts of over 10,000 mm^3 were recorded for 73 patients, or 24.9 per cent of the series (Table 38.4). Other investigators [*97, 223, 333, 374, 477, 546*] have found leukocytosis of this degree in frequencies varying from 19.6 to 36 per cent of rheumatoid arthritics. Marked elevations of the white-cell count may be encountered

Red-Cell and White-Cell Counts

Table 38.4
White-cell and differential counts recorded for 293 rheumatoid arthritics

	Patients	
	No.	Per cent
White-cell counts		
Above 10,000/mm³	73	24.9
10,000 to 5,000/mm³	215	73.4
Below 5,000/mm³	5	1.7
Differential counts		
Polymorphonuclears 80 per cent or over	27	9.2
Polymorphonuclears below 50 per cent	12	4.1
Lymphocytes 40 per cent or over	18	6.1
Monocytes 10 per cent or over	26	8.9
Eosinophils 4 per cent or over	37	12.6
"Normal"	197	67.2

on rare occasions—according to McCrae [*333*] in association with "complications" such as pleurisy. Coss and Boots [*121*] believe that marked elevations are unfavorable omens in children. Reports in the literature state that leukocytosis is usually associated with arthritis of short duration [*97, 105, 223*] and a high degree of activity [*133, 251*] and is often concurrent with fever [*176*]. We were unable to corroborate such relationships in patients with white-cell counts above 10,000 (although 5 of the 11 patients with counts over 15,000 were febrile and 4 were suffering from an acute initial attack or an exacerbation). Joint effusion, articular redness, preceding infection, and the presence of lymphadenopathy or subcutaneous nodules were apparently not connected with increased concentration of white cells in the circulating blood. In fact, the only evidence of a relationship between leukocytosis and increased disease activity was its positive association with an acute, severe onset. A ready explanation is lacking for the relatively high frequency of leukocytosis among males.

38.6   That leukocytosis sometimes occurs in rheumatoid arthritis is of little aid in elucidating the pathogenesis of this disease, since an increase in circulating white cells may result from a diversity of processes, ranging from common infections to metabolic disturbances such as diabetic acidosis. Leukocytosis has been attributed to "physiologic" causes such as muscular exercise and pain and even to emotional disturbances. From Menkin's findings [*348, 349*] it follows that leukocytosis-promoting factors may be absorbed into the blood stream from the inflammatory exudates of rheumatoid lesions and may thus act upon the bone marrow, as is believed to be the case when other forms of tissue injury are accompanied by increased white-cell counts. In the same way, the variation in the white-cell count in rheumatoid arthritis may depend upon the balance between Menkin's leukopenia and leukocytosis-producing factors. From a less speculative and more practical viewpoint, it is helpful to realize that a leukocytosis, even of high degree, may be one of the manifestations of rheumatoid arthritis, rather than an indication of intercurrent infection or other complication. Furthermore, when an increased white-cell count is present, other signs of a highly active arthritis, including fever and acutely inflamed articulations, may be absent.

38.7 White-cell counts lower than normal (below $5,000/mm^3$) were found in only 5 of our patients, or 1.7 per cent of the series (Table 38.4). Other authors [223, 333, 477] have found leukopenia of this degree less rarely, in frequencies varying from 4 to 5.9 per cent. There is general agreement that low white-cell counts appear more often in chronic stages of the disease [97, 133, 251]. In our 5 patients with leukopenia the average duration of arthritis was nearly five years, but in 1 individual with a count below 5,000 the disease duration was only eight months. Splenomegaly in association with leukopenia justified application of the term "Felty's syndrome" to only 3 patients. Only 1 of these, however, with an absolute neutrophil count of 1,000, fulfilled Collins' [106] conditions for a pathologic neutropenia. The status of Felty's syndrome as a rare variant of rheumatoid arthritis has already been discussed (see par. 2.29). The possibility still remains that splenic abnormalities may occasionally influence the white-cell level in rheumatoid arthritis, whether or not the splenomegaly is due to an extraneous cause. It may be noted in passing that the spleen was palpable in only 1 of the 73 patients with white-cell counts above 10,000, a frequency significantly lower than that in the remainder of the series.

DIFFERENTIAL WHITE-CELL COUNT

38.8 The differential white-cell count in rheumatoid arthritis is usually within normal limits, but variations sometimes occur (see Table

Red-Cell and White-Cell Counts

38.4). An absolute or relative increase in polymorphonuclears is associated with marked disease activity or with fever according to certain observers [133, 176]. Polymorphonuclears were found in frequencies above 90 per cent in 2 patients of the present series and above 80 per cent in 27 patients, more than half of whom also showed leukocytosis. An increased frequency of these cells apparently occurred irrespective of the activity, severity, or duration of the arthritis or the presence or absence of fever. In 12 patients the polymorphonuclears were decreased below 50 per cent, almost always in association with lymphocytosis, and in 18 patients the lymphocytes rose to 40 per cent or over. Others [106, 374] have reported lymphocytosis of this degree among patients with arthritis of relatively long duration, but such was not the case in the present series, nor was there a relationship between lymphocytosis and marked total disease severity.* Only one author [133] has described an increase in monocytes in rheumatoid arthritis. An increased percentage (10 per cent or over) of these cells was found in the peripheral blood of 26 of our patients, again without relation to the duration or severity of their disease. Of more interest perhaps, is the occasional increase in eosinophils found in rheumatoid arthritis [121, 190, 251, 403], in view of the relationship of adrenocortical function to the number of these cells in the blood. Eosinophil counts of 4 per cent or over were recorded for 37 patients, or 12.6 per cent of the present series. Attempts to differentiate the group with eosinophilia from the remainder of the series were unsuccessful. No differences were evident in respect either to disease duration, activity, or severity or to the presence or absence of fever, lymphadenopathy, splenomegaly, or subcutaneous nodules. The highest eosinophil count recorded for our patients at the time of hospital admission was 16 per cent but later much higher counts (43 per cent for 1 patient) were occasionally recorded. These were comparable with the eosinophil levels found in allergic disease and polyarteritis nodosa.

SUMMARY

38.9 A definite anemia, evidenced by red-cell counts below 4.5 million in males and below 4.0 million in females, was encountered in more than one-fifth of the patients of the present series. Anemia of this

* See definition, par. **4.26**.

degree was related to disease activity and severity and to gastric anacidity, but otherwise no differences were found between those with anemia and the others. The white-cell count was within normal limits in about 75 per cent of the patients; in the remainder leukocytosis of over 10,000 was much more common than leukopenia. Increase in the white-cell count, with or without polynucleosis, appeared irrespective of the duration or state of activity of the disease. Splenomegaly was common in patients with leukopenia but rare in those with leukocytosis. In about two-thirds of the patients, the white-cell differential counts were within normal limits. In those with an abnormal count, the chief alterations were increases in the polymorphonuclears, lymphocytes, monocytes, or eosinophils.

38.10   Objectives for further study:

1. The mechanism and pathogenesis of the anemia in rheumatoid arthritis.

2. Observations on the relationship between anemia and disease activity.

3. The reasons for eosinophilia in certain patients with rheumatoid arthritis.

4. Hypersplenism in rheumatoid arthritis.

39

Urine, Blood Uric Acid, and Blood Non-Protein Nitrogen

39.1 Results in two autopsied series of patients with rheumatoid arthritis have suggested that glomerulitis may be included among the common systemic manifestations of the disease [8, 179]. Of the 61 patients in one series [179], 8 showed this renal lesion at necropsy—glomerulonephritis having been diagnosed in 2 cases before death. Of the 30 patients in the other series [8], 19 patients were found to have glomerulitis—in 6 cases of a more severe degree (grade 2). More than a trace of albumin was found in about one-fourth of the patients in the first series, while albuminuria was a frequent clinical finding in the second. About 10 per cent of the patients in the combined series were found to have renal amyloidosis, but it was believed that in most instances the glomerulitis discovered at necropsy was the underlying cause of the albuminuria. It must be admitted that the suppurative processes which were present before death in many of the patients may have been responsible for the glomerular alterations, but the evidence presented offers some basis for the inclusion of rheumatoid arthritis among connective tissue diseases with renal involvement.

39.2 More than a faint trace of albumin was present in the urine of 21 patients of the present series, or 7.2 per cent (Table 39.1). Those with albuminuria apparently due to pyuria were excluded. No differences were evident in this group in respect to sex, age on hospital ad-

Table 39.1

Urinary, blood non-protein nitrogen, and uric acid findings for 293 rheumatoid arthritics

	Patients	
	No.	Per cent
Albuminuria (more than faint trace)	21	7.2
Casts	34	11.6
Albuminuria and/or casts	52	17.7
Blood non-protein nitrogen over 40 mg/100 cc.	5	1.7
Blood uric acid over 4 mg/100 cc.	10	3.6*

* Figured on 278 patients.

mission, total disease severity* or the presence or absence of fever. Casts were found in the urinary sediment of 34 patients, or 11.6 per cent of the series. In this instance, an association was demonstrated between cylindruria and age over forty on admission. Urinalysis revealed both albumin and casts in only 3 patients, so that a total of 52 individuals showed either albuminuria or cylindruria or both. Significant differences existed between this group of patients and the remainder of the series due to larger proportions of females and patients over forty, as well as of those with fever and those with greater disease severity,* in the group with urinary findings. In one of these patients, whose urine consistently showed large amounts of albumin and many casts, the diagnosis of chronic nephritis was later confirmed by findings of hypertension, retinal arteriosclerosis, cardiac enlargement, cardiac failure, and nitrogen retention. In the rest, both clinical evidence of nephritis and azotemia were absent.

39.3   Systematic examination of the urine in a sizable series of rheumatoid arthritics was undertaken by two other observers. In both of these studies, as in the present study, the absence of data on controls comparable in regard to age and sex lessened the significance of the results. The figures of Eaton and Cocheu [160] were quite similar to ours, in that albuminuria was noted in 12 per cent of 170 patients, cylindruria in 13 per cent, and either one or the other in 21.2 per cent. Again, a very small number (7 in all) showed both, and the females were more prone to urinary abnormalities than the males. In McCrae's [333] series of

* See definition, par. 4.26.

Urine, Blood Uric Acid, and NPN

319 patients 20 per cent had albuminuria (degree not specified), "more than half" with casts. With these exceptions, little attention has been paid to the possibility that a renal lesion furnishes additional evidence of the systemic nature of rheumatoid arthritis. To establish this concept more firmly, further study should be directed toward autopsy material from patients dying without infection or amyloidosis. In addition, quantitative methods should be used in measuring the excretion of albumin, cellular elements, and casts; and modern techniques used in evaluating renal function.

39.4 In order to exclude those with gouty arthritis, 278 patients, or nearly 95 per cent of the series, were tested for uric acid—the determinations being made on whole blood. Simultaneous determinations of the blood non-protein nitrogen levels were also made, in an effort to rule out depressed renal function as a factor if hyperuricemia were present. (The blood non-protein nitrogen was slightly elevated in an insignificant number—only 5 patients, none of whom had hyperuricemia.) With the upper limit of normal set at 4.0 mg. per 100 cc., 10 patients, or 3.6 per cent of the series, were found to have hyperuricemia (Table 39.1). In 3 of these, subsequent determinations of the serum uric acid levels showed a persistent elevation. In the remaining 7, tests were made on single specimens only. Chemical and roentgenologic findings suggested a diagnosis of gouty arthritis for only 1 of the 10 patients with hyperuricemia, 8 of whom were males. This patient had "punched out" areas which somewhat resembled those seen in advanced gouty arthritis, but his clinical course was that of rheumatoid arthritis and a synovial tissue biopsy failed to reveal urate deposits. The infrequency of an elevated serum uric acid in rheumatoid arthritis has recently been emphasized by a study of 412 patients [320], only 2.7 per cent of whom had concentrations above 5.5 mg. per 100 cc. and only 1.6 per cent had concentrations above 6.0 mg. In fact, comparison of these findings with a larger group of unmatched controls suggested that serum uric acid levels in rheumatoid arthritis may be even lower than normal. In the control group employed [495], consisting of 927 hospital patients without evidence of renal insufficiency or gouty arthritis, the frequency of hyperuricemia (above 5.9 mg. per 100 cc.) was 6.4 per cent—a figure slightly higher than that obtained in the present series. It seems fair, then, to conclude that the frequency of hyperuricemia is no greater among rheumatoid arthritics than among controls.

SUMMARY

39.5   Albuminuria, cylindruria, or both were recorded for nearly one-sixth of our patients, in only 1 of whom a clinical nephritis was recognized. In two other large series of rheumatoid arthritics, a corresponding frequency of urinary abnormalities has been reported. These findings, taken in conjunction with autopsy studies, suggest the possibility that a renal lesion may be one of the systemic manifestations of rheumatoid arthritis. Elevation of the blood uric acid was present in 3.6 per cent of our patients, a percentage slightly lower than that observed in a control group.

39.6   Objectives for further study:

1. Histologic observations on the kidney in rheumatoid arthritis derived from autopsy and biopsy material.

2. Quantitative measurements of the excretion of albumin, cellular elements, and casts in this disease along with tests of renal function by modern techniques.

3. Investigations of the co-existence of gout and rheumatoid arthritis in the same patient or within a family (see par. 2.3).

40

Gastric Acidity

40.1 Previous studies on gastric acidity in rheumatoid arthritis may be divided into two groups. In the first, much larger, group which has been reviewed and tabulated by Hartung and Steinbrocker [244] histamine was not employed. The relatively high frequency of a decreased or absent secretion of hydrochloric acid encountered in these studies thus lacks significance. To form a second group, in which histamine was utilized, only two papers could be found [164, 360], but both of these reported an increased frequency of anacidity in rheumatoid arthritis. In an attempt to evaluate this finding, gastric analysis was included in our program of clinical and laboratory studies.

40.2 Gastric analyses were performed on 270 of the 293 patients in the series. As for the remainder, either the patient was unwilling to have the test made or the state of his disease rendered the procedure too difficult or painful. All tests were performed, in the morning after a twelve-hour fast, by members of the resident staff. A nasal tube was first passed into the stomach and the fasting contents aspirated. Histamine phosphate in a dosage of 0.5 mg. was then injected subcutaneously, and the patient was given a test meal by tube of 50 or 100 cc. of 7 per cent alcohol. Aspirations were made after thirty and sixty minutes. Free and combined hydrochloric acid were determined by the usual methods in each of the three samples, with the results expressed in cubic centimeters of N/10 hydrochloric acid. Only the amounts of free acid were used in this study. No tests were performed on the controls, but reports of two numerical studies of tests made on individuals without gastro-intestinal disease or disorders likely to affect gastric acidity are available in the literature. The first was carried out in this hospital by Lerman, Pierce, and Brogan [*316*], who tested 200 patients selected for the absence of gastro-intestinal disease. Their methods were exactly the same as ours. In the second study, 654 patients found to have no significant disease on diagnostic examination were tested by Polland [*412*], who also employed histamine but did not give a test meal.

40.3 Table 40.1 shows the frequency of anacidity among patients and controls divided according to sex and to age below and above forty. No significant differences were apparent in the subgroups between the patients and the first control series. When the second series of controls (Polland [*412*]) was compared with the arthritics, a significantly higher frequency of anacidity was found among the patients under forty than among controls of the same age group. Otherwise the distribution of anacidity was essentially the same. In addition, the figures for the two control series show very close agreement. It may be noted in the table that the frequency of anacidity shows a definite increase with advancing age in the two control series, while the difference in this respect between those under and above the age of forty is slight among the rheumatoid arthritis patients. In Table 40.2 the patients have been divided into ten-year groups according to age on hospital admission. The lack of variation with increasing age in those with arthritis can be seen in more detail in this table, as well as the steadily mounting frequency of anacidity with advancing age among Polland's [*412*] controls. The suggestion thus arises that younger individuals with rheumatoid arthritis may be more prone to show anacidity than controls. Except for this possibility, the data presented above fail to show an increased frequency of gastric anacidity in rheumatoid arthritis.

40.4 It has been mentioned above that only two studies were encountered in the literature in which the gastric acidity in rheumatoid arthritis has been studied with the aid of histamine. The first, by Moltke and Ohlsen [*360*], appeared in 1936. Among 30 patients with "true rheumatoid arthritis" the frequency of anacidity was 30 per cent. Among

Table 40.1

Frequency of anacidity among rheumatoid arthritics—patients of present series who were tested for anacidity compared by sex and age at hospital admission with representative series from the literature

	Present series			Lerman et al. [316]			Polland [412]		
		Anacidity present			Anacidity present			Anacidity present	
	No. of patients	No.	Per cent	No. of patients	No.	Per cent	No. of patients	No.	Per cent
Males									
Under 40	56	4	7.1	31	1	3.2	163	5	3.1
40 or more	41	3	7.3	59	8	13.6	221	36	16.3
Females									
Under 40	77	13	16.9	37	5	13.5	113	7	6.2
40 or more	96	19	19.8	73	12	16.4	157	31	19.7
All patients									
Under 40	133	17	12.8	68	6	8.8	276	12	4.3
40 or more	137	22	16.1	132	20	15.2	378	67	17.7
All males	97	7	7.2	90	9	10.0	384	41	10.7
All females	173	32	18.5	110	17	15.5	270	38	14.1
Total	270	39	14.4	200	26	13.0	654	79	12.1

Note: No significant differences were found between our series and that reported by Lerman et al. [316]. With respect to all patients under age 40 one significant difference (8.5 ± 2.7) was found between our series and that reported by Polland [412].

Table 40.2

Frequency of anacidity among rheumatoid arthritics—patients of present series who were tested for anacidity compared by age at hospital admission with Polland's series [*412*] of 654 patients

Age on hospital admission	Present series			Polland's series [*412*] Percentage with anacidity
	No. of patients	With anacidity		
		No.	Per cent	
Total	270	39	14.4	12.1
10–19	20	3	15.0	0.0
20–29	57	4	7.0	3.5
30–39	56	10	17.9	5.2
40–49	44	8	18.2	14.3
50–59	71	12	16.9	15.7
60 or more	22	2	9.1	28.4

the 31 additional patients with "proliferative arthritis," all but 2 had a diagnosis of multiple infective arthritis. The proportion with anacidity in this group was 16.1 per cent. If modern nomenclature were employed, it is probable that nearly all patients in both groups would be included under the diagnosis of rheumatoid arthritis. In this case, the frequency of anacidity among the 61 patients would be 23 per cent. This figure is distinctly higher than that obtained in our series of rheumatoid arthritics (14.5 per cent) or in either of the control series (13.0 per cent and 12.1 per cent respectively), but, owing to the small number of patients studied by Moltke and Ohlsen [*360*], the differences are not statistically significant. Furthermore, the patients tested by these authors belonged to a distinctly older group, 80 per cent of whom were forty or over when examined. The second report appeared in 1939 under the authorship of Edström [*164*]. In this series of 432 patients with "typical chronic rheumatoid infective (atrophic) arthritis," the frequency of histamine-refractory anacidity was 12.8 per cent among patients aged forty or less and 28.6 per cent among those over forty. In Edström's younger age group the frequency of anacidity was the same as it was in our younger age group but greater than it was in the comparable age group of either control series (although significantly so only when compared with Polland's series). Among Edström's older patients the frequency was greater than it was among patients over forty in our series and in both control series. Thus the findings from our data are only in partial agree-

Gastric Acidity

ment with those of Edström in that they suggest an association of gastric anacidity and rheumatoid arthritis in patients under forty.

40.5 In the patients of the present series a higher frequency of anacidity was recorded for females than for males. This finding was not confirmed by Edström [164], who noted a slight but not significant excess of males with achlorhydria. That gastric acidity is generally higher in males and anacidity less common has been pointed out in several reports on large groups of normal individuals [316, 412, 543], so that this sex difference should not be considered an attribute of rheumatoid arthritis. As already stated, our findings differed from Edström's [164] and from findings among normal individuals [316, 412, 543] with respect to an increase in the frequency of anacidity with advancing age. Our findings also differed from Edström's in that anacidity was not associated with arthritis of marked severity. They were in agreement with Edström's [164] in respect to the absence of a relationship between disease duration and the frequency of anacidity. As shown in Table 40.3, anemia was more commonly recorded for patients with anacidity than for those with free hydrochloric acid present. Although this association was confirmed by Collins [105] (who did not, however, employ histamine), the authors of two studies on rheumatoid arthritics [164, 381] and two on normal individuals [316, 411] came to the opposite conclusion. Since anacidity interferes with the absorption of iron [350], absence of free hydrochloric acid may well be a contributory factor in the development of anemia, but it remains doubtful that this mechanism is consistently operative in the development of anemia in rheumatoid arthritis (par. **38.4**).

Table 40.3

Frequency of anemia among patients of present series who were tested for gastric anacidity

Anacidity	No. of patients	Anemia present*	
		No.	Per cent
Total	270	32	11.9
Present	39	9	23.1
Absent	231	23	10.0
	Difference in percentages:	13.1 ± 5.6	

* Red-cell count under 4.5 million/mm^3 in males and under 4.0 million/mm^3 in females.

40.6   No relationship was found in our series between anacidity and gastro-intestinal symptoms (including anorexia, nausea, vomiting, constipation, and diarrhea) or with evidence of gallbladder disease from either a history of cholecystectomy, the presence of stones, or a positive Graham test. Cold and moist extremities were noted less often in patients with anacidity than in those without, but vasomotor symptoms occurred equally often in both groups. One positive association—that between anacidity and splenomegaly—is difficult to explain, but may actually depend upon chance or mutual relationships with other factors. Anacidity was also less frequent in patients with a unilateral onset. Otherwise, no differences were observed between the patients with anacidity and the rest of the series; the factors tested included an acute onset, an intermittent course before hospital admission, spinal involvement, muscular wasting, prodromal symptoms, and a family history of rheumatoid arthritis.*

SUMMARY

40.7   Gastric analyses utilizing histamine injections and a test meal of 7 per cent alcohol were performed upon 270 of the patients of the present series. The results differed from those obtained in comparable control series to the extent that patients under forty showed a tendency toward an increased frequency of anacidity. Contrary to the findings in another study of 432 patients with rheumatoid arthritis, the findings in patients over forty were similar to those in controls.

40.8   Objective for further study:

Further observations on the gastric acidity of patients with Sjögren's syndrome [259].

* For a complete list of associations, see Appendix Table 47.

41

*Basal Metabolism
and the Thyroid*

41.1 The first paper reporting abnormal basal metabolism rates in a large series of carefully diagnosed patients with rheumatoid arthritis was published by Swaim and Spear in 1927 [*516*]. Since then Swaim [*515*] has confirmed their findings by tests of additional patients, and three other studies have appeared [*164, 233, 425*]. Rates below the lower level of normal (minus 10 per cent) were recorded for about 25 per cent of the patients of each series, and elevated rates (above plus 10 per cent) for a smaller proportion. It therefore seemed worthwhile to us to study the basal metabolism rates of our patients. The results were approximately the same as those reported by previous observers.

41.2 Basal metabolism tests were performed on 259 patients of the present series during their hospital stay. The rate was determined by the Benedict-Roth spirometer, calculations being made by means of the Aub-Dubois standards. Additional tests were performed on 177 patients, or 68 per cent of those tested, and the lowest reading was adopted. As shown in Table 41.1, rates lower than minus 10 were recorded for 29.4 per cent of our patients (compared with 3.2 per cent of the normal series) and rates higher than plus 11 for 8.1 per cent of our patients (compared with 4.7 per cent of the normal series). In the latter instance the difference between the proportions was not significant. It should be noted, however, that Boothby and Sandiford's [*46*] series was more

Table 41.1

Basal metabolism rates in rheumatoid arthritis—patients of present series who were tested for thyroid activity compared with 127 nonarthritic individuals tested by Boothby and Sandiford [46]

Basal metabolism rate	Present series				Nonarthritic series
	Lowest test		First test		
	No.	Per cent	No.	Per cent	Per cent
Below —20	14	5.4	7	2.7	0.0
—20 to —15	17	6.6	12	4.6	0.0
—15 to —10	45	17.4	31	12.0	3.2
—10 to +11	162	62.5	172	66.4	92.1
+11 to +16	14	5.4	15	5.8	4.0
Above +15	7	2.7	22	8.5	0.7
Total	259	100.0	259	100.0	100.0
Below —10	76	29.4	50	19.3	3.2
Above +10	21	8.1	37	14.3	4.7

heavily weighted than ours with males and with individuals over forty years of age and especially that only 18 out of 127 subjects were tested on different days. To offset the effect of the last-mentioned variable, we made an additional tabulation, which utilizes only the data recorded on the first tests of our patients. In regard to the rates above and below normal significant differences resulted from this tabulation. (The metabolic rates of all but one individual in the normal series fell between minus and plus 15 per cent. As shown in Table 41.1, the rates of an appreciably smaller number of patients were found outside these limits than when minus and plus 10 per cent were employed.) In Table 41.2 the findings in the present series are compared with those in four similar series of rheumatoid arthritics. In all but one of these [425] multiple tests were performed and the lowest or last rate was utilized. As approximately the same results were obtained in regard to lower than normal rates, one is justified in concluding that low basal metabolism may be expected in about 25 per cent of rheumatoid arthritics.

41.3 We next considered as a group the 76 patients with low basal metabolism rates in an attempt to find features differentiating them from the remainder with normal or elevated rates. Only a few differences were observed. While a higher proportion of females was found among the patients with low rates, this difference in sex ratio may be

Basal Metabolism and the Thyroid

Table 41.2

Basal metabolism rates in rheumatoid arthritis—patients of present series who were tested for thyroid activity compared with representative series from the literature

	No. of patients in each series					
	Swaim [515]	Hall and Monroe [233]	Rawls et al. [425]	Edström [164]	Present series (lowest test)	Combined series
	240	106	284	369	259	1,258
Basal metabolism rate		Percentage of patients				
Less than −10	25.0	36.0	23.9	24.0	29.4	26.2
−10 to +11	61.3	53.0	57.8	70.0	62.5	62.1
More than +10	13.7	11.0	18.3	6.0	8.1	11.7

only apparent since the majority of the 34 untested patients were males. Swaim [515] noted that high, low, and normal rates were equally distributed between the two sexes in his series. Our finding of a positive association between a low rate and the constitutional symptoms weakness and anorexia may actually depend on the preponderance of females in both groups. Patients over forty were found in a significantly higher frequency among the group with low rates. One author [233] agreed with this finding, while another [515] did not. Although low basal metabolism was found as often among patients with disease duration of one year or less as in the remainder of our series, analysis of the data showed a positive association between a low rate and duration of more than five years. Without presenting figures, Rawls and others [425] made the statement that a low basal metabolism was more common in patients with long-standing joint disease, while Swaim [515] concluded that after ten years the low rates tended to return to normal. However, in approximately half of our patients with disease duration of more than ten years the rate was below minus 10; in this group the total disease severity* approximated that of the remainder of the series.

41.4   In other respects no essential differences were made out between the group with low rate and the other patients. In that marked total disease severity* did not predominate in the group with low rates,

* See definition, par. 4.26.

we were unable to confirm Edström's [164] finding that low basal metabolism accompanied a "malignant" type of arthritis. We were also unable to find evidence in support of the theory that low basal metabolism is related to malnutrition. Analysis of our data revealed no positive associations between a low rate and any of the following: a history of weight loss, a subnormal weight on hospital admission, or muscular atrophy. Pemberton [402] has been the chief exponent of another explanation of the lowered rates in rheumatoid arthritics—that it may be dependent upon diminished tissue uptake of oxygen due to a decrease in peripheral blood flow. In this event, a concurrence of low rates and vasomotor symptoms and signs would be expected, but no relationship between these factors was found in our series. A number of other factors were tested for an association with a low basal metabolism, with negative results. These included: prodromal symptoms, an acute onset, an intermittent rather than a progressive course before admission, nervousness or emotional upsets, spondylitis, subcutaneous nodules, lymphadenopathy, anemia, and gastric anacidity.* Finally, there should be mentioned the group of 14 patients with unusually low metabolic rates, ranging from minus 21 per cent to minus 29 per cent. None of these patients gave a history of thyroidectomy or showed signs or symptoms of myxedema. All were females and in all but 3 the disease had been present for more than a year. While 10 out of 14 gave a history of weight loss, the majority were either overweight or normal at the time of hospital admission and vasomotor symptoms and signs were recorded in frequencies approximating those found in the remainder of the series.

41.5   As stated above, a disproportionate number of basal metabolism rates higher than plus 10 was encountered in our series only when we analyzed the results of the first tests rather than the lowest. (On 29 of the 37 patients with higher than normal rates, more than one test was performed.) As shown in Table 41.2, the frequency of high basal metabolism rates surpassed expectancy in three of the series collected from the literature but not in one. This discrepancy is not dependent upon whether the readings were obtained from single or multiple tests. While the available data thus suggest the occurrence of basal metabolism rates higher than normal in a small proportion of rheumatoid arthritics,

* For a complete list of associations, see Appendix Table 47.

Basal Metabolism and the Thyroid

the possibility remains that a coincidental, undiagnosed hyperthyroidism or fever due to the arthritis may account for some of the increased rates. In our series no differences were made out between the 21 patients with basal metabolism rates above plus 10 per cent (persisting if more than one test was performed) and the remainder in respect to age and sex distribution, weight loss, tachycardia, or gastric anacidity. No relationship was found between basal metabolism rates above normal and increased disease activity,* as stated in one paper [233]. Although vasomotor symptoms were present in the expected frequency among patients with high rates, only 3 had cold and moist extremities at the time of examination. Although 7 patients had rates above plus 15, extraneous factors may have been responsible in 4 cases. These included coincidental thyrotoxicosis, active bronchiectasis, cardiac failure, and spondylitis with markedly diminished chest expansion. Only one test was performed in 2 other cases.

41.6   It is true that many of the symptoms and signs of hyperthyroidism may be duplicated in patients with rheumatoid arthritis. These include weight loss, vasomotor instability, tachycardia, sweating, and exophthalmos. As a rule the two conditions can be readily differentiated except in the not infrequent instances when they co-exist in the same individual. Jones [286] was one of the first to point out this combination in 14 patients. More recently, Monroe [361] found that 3.4 per cent of a series of 414 patients with thyrotoxicosis had had attacks of rheumatoid arthritis but "were not suffering from it at the time of their treatment for hyperthyroidism." As shown in Table 41.3, hyperthyroidism was found in 5 patients, or 1.7 per cent of our series—a frequency approximated in reports by two other authors [150, 187]. Although the true prevalence of neither rheumatoid arthritis nor hyperthyroidism is known, the two diseases apparently resemble each other in sex and age distribution. Further investigation of an association seems warranted. Monroe [361] found 3 cases of rheumatoid arthritis among a series of 98 patients with myxedema, but did not state whether the myxedema was spontaneous or acquired in these instances. We found no patients with myxedema in the present series but encountered 2 patients with arthritis and myxedema after the series was completed (par.

* See definition, par. 4.27.

Table 41.3

Frequency of thyroid abnormalities among rheumatoid arthritics—patients of present series compared with controls

Abnormality*	Patients		Controls		Difference in percentages
	No.	Per cent	No.	Per cent	
Colloid goiter	15	5.1	6	2.0	
Thyroiditis	2	0.7	0	0.0	
Nontoxic adenoma	5	1.7	1	0.3	
Thyrotoxicosis past or present	5	1.7	1	0.3	
None present	266	90.8	285	97.3	6.5 ± 2.0
Total	293	100.0	293	99.9	
$\chi^2 = 11.84; p < .01$					

* With the exception of 3 colloid goiters in patients and 2 in controls, the abnormalities found in the present series were confined to females.

10.7). The frequency of colloid goiter (Table 41.3) was higher in the present series than in the control group and certainly much higher than in the population of an essentially nongoiterous state like Massachusetts [347]. (No data are available as to how many of our patients came to Massachusetts from goiterous areas.) Coates and Delicati [97] reported a frequency of 20 per cent among 100 patients with rheumatoid arthritis but gave no information about the patients' geographical background. The apparently higher frequency of rheumatoid arthritis in regions where simple goiter is prevalent has been discussed by Jones [286]. As shown in Table 41.3, we found a statistically significant difference between patients and controls with respect to the presence of thyroid abnormalities. Sufficient evidence is thus at hand to suggest a relationship, of a type as yet undetermined, between rheumatoid arthritis and thyroid disorders.

41.7 In discussing the origin of hypometabolism, which has been found in over 25 per cent of the rheumatoid patients studied, consideration will first be given to extrathyroid causes. Malnutrition may be a factor, but as already pointed out, low basal metabolism rates may be obtained from well-nourished subjects. Decreased oxygen utilization resulting from diminished blood supply to the periphery has already been mentioned as a possibility (par. 41.4), and diminished blood flow to the thyroid itself should also be considered. Hypofunction of the anterior

Basal Metabolism and the Thyroid

pituitary or of the adrenal cortex, both of which may result in a low basal metabolism, has yet to be established in rheumatoid arthritis. Only 1 of our patients (whose metabolic status was not tested) had glomerulonephritis and none had amyloid nephrosis. It is generally recognized that hypometabolism is occasionally found in otherwise normal individuals but not in a frequency as high as 25 per cent. The role of the nervous system cannot be dismissed, since patients with neuroses or psychoses as well as those with intracranial lesions, sometimes have low basal metabolism rates. It should also be mentioned that comparable frequencies of hypometabolism were found in two series of patients with osteo-arthritis [425, 515], while in more than 40 per cent of 166 patients with "low-grade chronic illnesses" studied by Stiles [503] the basal metabolism rate was minus 10 or below. No one reasonable extrathyroid cause of the hypometabolism of rheumatoid arthritis has thus far been discovered. However, recent studies by Wolfson and others [568] strongly suggest that a true hypothyroidism is often present in this disease. During investigations of corticogenic hypothyroidism, these authors determined the thyroid status in rheumatoid subjects before treatments with cortisone or ACTH. As in other studies, hypometabolism (below minus 10 per cent) was found in about one-fourth, while the serum protein-bound iodine level and the radio-iodine uptake were depressed in about one-half of the determinations. In no instance, however, was the serum cholesterol elevated. It was noted that the hypothyroidism was not accompanied by clinical evidence of this disorder and was not related to greater disease activity, malnutrition, or prior administration of gold. (Anatomic evidence of thyroid hypofunction was not observed in one series of 30 autopsies on rheumatoid patients [8].) If these studies can be confirmed, a possible explanation of hypometabolism in rheumatoid arthritis is at hand, but, as the authors point out, our lack of knowledge of thyroid function in comparable chronic diseases rules out the conclusion that hypothyroidism may be a specific manifestation of rheumatoid arthritis.

SUMMARY

41.8 The consensus of our study and four others reported in the literature is that the basal metabolism is lower than normal in about 25 per cent of patients with rheumatoid arthritis. In our series no differences were found between the patients with low basal metabolism and the remainder in regard to disease severity or evidence of malnutrition. Recently published studies suggest that a true hypothyroidism rather than extrathyroid factors may be responsible for the metabolic findings. The basal metabolism was elevated in about 8 per cent of our patients. From the available evidence it seems likely that a relationship exists between rheumatoid arthritis and thyroid disorders.

41.9 Objectives for further study:

1. Additional observations on the serum protein-bound iodine level and radio-iodine uptake in rheumatoid subjects.

2. Further histopathologic investigation of the thyroid in patients with rheumatoid arthritis [8].

3. The relationship between thyroid disorders and the development of rheumatoid arthritis.

42

Spondylitis

42.1 In a previous section (pars. **2.14** and **2.15**) we have stated the rationale which has led many to classify rheumatoid spondylitis as a separate disease entity and have also given our reasons (par. **2.16**) for including patients with rheumatoid spondylitis in the present series, whether or not the peripheral joints were also affected. The following paragraphs summarize the similarities and differences between the 252 patients with little or no spinal involvement and the 41 patients who were classified as spondylitics at the time of hospital admission.

42.2 No patient was thus classified unless either or both of two conditions was fulfilled: (1) persistent objective finding of spinal arthritis, chiefly in the form of limitation of motion not due to other forms of spinal disease and (2) characteristic roentgenographic changes, usually in the sacro-iliac joints. In most cases the diagnosis of spondylitis resulted from both clinical and roentgenographic examination, but in a few it was dependent on one or the other type of evidence. Table 42.1 shows the distribution of the 41 spondylitics in three groups, according to the type of involvement: 8 patients with spinal or sacro-iliac involvement alone; 8 with additional involvement of the hips and/or shoulders; and 25 with additional involvement of other peripheral joints. Although more than half fell into the last group, they did not differ markedly from the rest in regard to sex and age distribution. An additional 44 pa-

Table 42.1
Description of patients with spondylitis and of those with minor spinal involvement

Involvement			No. of patients	Percentage of males
Total (with spondylitis)			41	80.5
Spinal joints alone			8	87.5
Spine plus hips and/or shoulders			8	100.0
Spine plus other peripheral joints			25*	72.0
Minor, of spine			44	18.2

			Diagnosis evident by	
Involvement	Median age at onset	Median age on hospital admission	Phys. exam. (per cent)	X-ray exam. (per cent)
Total (with spondylitis)	24	28	85.4	85.4†
Spinal joints alone	20	27	100.0	100.0
Spine plus hips and/or shoulders	28	35	100.0	87.5
Spine plus other peripheral joints	24	28	76.0	80.0
Minor, of spine	41	49	0.0	0.0

* Peripheral involvement preceded in 16 patients (see par. 16.8).
† Ligamentous calcification in 9 patients.

tients of the series had symptoms referred to the spine, but without persistent signs warranting a diagnosis of spondylitis. In each such instance roentgenographic examination failed to reveal changes characteristic of spondylitis. As shown in Table 42.1, less than 20 per cent were males, a direct reversal of the sex ratio in the spondylitic group. The group with minor spinal involvement was also mainly composed of older individuals, and it is possible that some of their symptoms may have been due to degenerative joint disease. Lewis-Faning [320], in a study of 532 patients with rheumatoid arthritis from which those with spondylitis had been excluded, recorded physical signs of spinal involvement in 11.9 per cent—a proportion which may be compared with the 17.5 per cent of the non-spondylitics in the present series who had spinal symptoms or signs. It should finally be mentioned that in the course of the follow-up of the patients of the present series, 7 additional patients were classified as spondylitics who had insufficient clinical or roentgenographic evidence for this diagnosis at the time of hospital admission.

Spondylitis

42.3 As shown in Table 42.1, 80.5 per cent of the spondylitics in our series were males. Reference has already been made (par. 5.2) to this finding, which is generally agreed to in the literature [152, 413, 470] and which constitutes one of the major differences between the spondylitics and the remaining patients in the series. Another important difference which is generally accepted is the age at onset. In the present series, the median age at onset in male spondylitics was twenty-four, compared with thirty-five in the remaining males. In addition, the majority of the 1,018 patients with rheumatoid spondylitis reported by Polley and Slocumb [413] experienced onset in the third decade and less than 10 per cent experienced onset after forty years of age. On the other hand, 11 patients in a recently reported series of 200 spondylitics [470] and 2 patients in the present series experienced onset after the age of fifty. Table 42.2 lists the chief factors studied in the series analysis by degree of

Table 42.2
Association of various factors with spondylitis among male patients of present series

1. *Positive*	3. *Absence of association*
Age at onset under 40	Family history of rheumatoid arthritis
Duration before admission (longer)	Prodromal symptoms
Anorexia	Strain before onset
Nervousness and/or emotional upsets	Infection before onset
	Onset acute
	Intermittent course before admission
2. *Negative*	Fatigue
Cyanosis	Weight loss
Nodules	Cold extremities
Atrophy of skin	Paresthesias
Improvement (after discharge)	Vascular spasm
	Vasomotor signs
	Neurologic symptoms
	Exaggerated reflexes
	Muscular atrophy
	Fever
	Tachycardia
	Lymphadenopathy
	Splenomegaly
	Anemia
	Gastric anacidity
	Low basal metabolism
	Total severity (increased)

association with spondylitis. Because the spondylitic group was so heavily weighted with males, in each case the comparison is limited to males with and without spondylitis. As shown in the table, duration before admission was apparently longer among spondylitics. The reasons for this are obscure but may relate to a slow progression of symptoms before a degree of disease severity is reached which requires hospital admission. Among constitutional symptoms, anorexia, but not fatigue or weight loss, was more common among the male spondylitics. A history of nervousness and/or emotional upsets was also associated with spondylitis, but neither mental nor physical strain was more common in this group as a precipitating factor. Among vasomotor symptoms, only cyanosis was less frequent among the spondylitics. The relative infrequency of nodules has been referred to in a previous chapter (par. 33.4), as well as the fact that, in the absence of involvement of peripheral joints other than shoulders or hips, we have encountered no spondylitics with nodules, either in our own experience or in the literature. Skin atrophy was also associated with a peripheral rather than a spinal distribution of arthritis (par. 31.2). A final important difference is shown in Table 42.3, which indicates that a distinctly less favorable subsequent course was evidenced by the male spondylitics, with total severity* on admission and duration of follow-up essentially the same in the two groups.

42.4   The third column of Table 42.2, which lists factors without positive or negative association with spondylitis, is by far the longest. A family history of rheumatoid arthritis (either spinal or peripheral) was recorded in the spondylitics as often as in the remainder (par. 8.7). Prodromal symptoms and precipitating factors, including surgical operations, exposure, and trauma as well as strain and infection, occurred with approximately equal frequency in the two groups. An acute, severe type of onset was experienced by 14 per cent of a series of 1,035 spondylitics [*413*]—a proportion corresponding to that noted in our series. However, "exacerbations and remissions were a characteristic feature of the course" of 72 per cent of the patients in this same large series, whereas a progressive course before admission was followed by nearly 80 per cent of the spondylitics in the present series. The discrepancy probably

* See definition, par. **4.26**.

Spondylitis

Table 42.3

Frequency of improvement among males of present series with and without spondylitis

Spondylitis	No. of males	Improved No.	Per cent
Total	94*	54	57.4
Present	30	11	36.7
Absent	64	43	67.2
Difference in percentages:		30.5 ± 11.5	

* Excludes 13 males who received "specific" therapy or whose follow-up data were inadequate.

rests upon utilization of differing criteria for an intermittent type of course. In regard to factors apparently altering the course, those with spondylitis were affected by strain, infection, and cold or moisture as often as the remainder. With minor exceptions, constitutional, vasomotor, and neurologic manifestations appeared with equal frequency among patients with spinal involvement and those with peripheral involvement alone, as did the laboratory factors tested, including anemia, gastric anacidity, and low basal metabolism. Among physical signs, fever, tachycardia, lymphadenopathy, and splenomegaly were found in equal proportions in the two groups, but, as mentioned above, nodules and skin atrophy, were less common among spondylitics. For completeness it should be mentioned that two additional physical findings are apparently more prevalent among spondylitics—iritis (par. 29.4) and the form of valvular heart disease, usually aortic, considered to be a systemic manifestation of rheumatoid arthritis [89]. The present study also confirmed the absence of ligamentous calcification about peripheral joints whether or not the spine was also involved.

42.5 Certain important and generally accepted differences between patients with rheumatoid spondylitis and those with peripheral arthritis have been confirmed in the present series. These include sex and age distribution and absence of subcutaneous nodules except where peripheral joints other than shoulders and hips were involved. Otherwise, numerical study of the two groups has shown them to be essentially similar as far as the clinical and laboratory features listed in Table 42.2 are concerned. No data are available from this study in regard to other points of difference which have been cited in the literature. These include the relative infrequency among spondylitics of inflammatory foci in muscles, cited in four reports [*142, 193, 296, 470*] but not confirmed in a fifth [*485*], and of positive serologic reactions—such as agglutination of streptococci [*47, 133*] or of sensitized sheep erythrocytes [*576*]. The favorable effects of roentgenotherapy [*482*] but not of gold [*468*] and the greater frequency of spinal fluid abnormalities [*330*] in patients with spondylitis have also been mentioned as differences. Until knowledge of the etiology or pathogenesis of rheumatoid arthritis is available, the question of whether or not rheumatoid spondylitis constitutes a separate disease entity must remain an open one and a matter of opinion. At any rate, the authors thus far see no justification in excluding those with spinal involvement, who constitute one-seventh of the entire group, from a numerical study of patients with rheumatoid arthritis. It is their belief that such an exclusion would render the series less rather than more representative of rheumatoid arthritis severe enough to warrant hospitalization.

42.6 If it is assumed that rheumatoid spondylitis represents merely the spinal localization of rheumatoid arthritis, the dividing line between the patients with spondylitis and those with purely peripheral involvement must be determined arbitrarily, as has been done in the present series (par. 42.2). It is probable that if routine spinal roentgenograms had been taken of each patient, a larger number would have been found with roentgenographic evidence of spondylitis but without sufficiently definite clinical findings to make this diagnosis. According to a recently published study [*417*] of 61 children with rheumatoid arthritis, roentgenographic evidence of spondylitis was found in over half the series. Nearly one-third of the present series, or 92 patients, either had spondylitis or definite symptoms referred to the spine at the time of hospital admission or developed spondylitis in the course of follow-up. Future descriptions of rheumatoid arthritis in adults should include serial roentgenograms of the spine as well as careful clinical observation in regard to spinal localization of the disease.

SUMMARY

42.7 On the basis of persistent spinal limitation and/or characteristic roentgenographic changes, 41 patients, or 14 per cent of the series, were considered to have spondylitis. In more than half of these 41 patients the involvement included other peripheral joints besides the shoulders and/or hips. In addition, 44 patients had minor spinal symptoms or signs, and 7 patients developed spondylitis during the follow-up period. The majority of those with spondylitis were males of the younger age group, and females past the age of forty predominated in the group with minor spinal involvement. A numerical comparison between male spondylitics and the remaining males revealed important differences only in regard to age distribution and, among the spondylitics, the relative infrequency of nodules and of a favorable subsequent course. The results of this study favor the conception of rheumatoid spondylitis as the spinal localization of rheumatoid arthritis rather than a separate disease entity.

42.8   Objectives for further study:

1. The frequency of spinal involvement among patients with rheumatoid arthritis apparently confined to peripheral joints.

2. The frequency of inflammatory foci in muscles and nerves in rheumatoid spondylitis.

3. Whether or not rheumatoid spondylitis constitutes a distinct disease entity.

43

Total Disease Severity and Disease Activity on Hospital Admission

43.1 When the present study was planned, it was decided at the onset that it would be helpful to have two or more observers classify the patients according to the extent of articular involvement, the total disease severity, and the degree of disease activity on admission. As defined in this study,* these are not mutually exclusive categories, since the estimation of total severity took into consideration both involvement and activity, as well as the degree to which each constitutional symptom and sign was present, the speed at which the disease progressed, and the amount of disability. The extent of articular involvement has already been considered (par. 34.5), and the nature of the associations between the three types of involvement and various factors has been analyzed (Table 34.5). A close association between involvement and total severity was found, as would be expected from the definition of severity just given.

43.2 A second major component of the definition of severity was the examiners' opinion of the activity of the disease process, with both articular and extra-articular manifestations taken into account. While disease activity was estimated for each patient, the relationship of activity to other factors was determined only in the comparatively few instances that seemed of particular interest. The results obtained

---
* See pars. 4.22, 4.26, and 4.27.

Disease Severity and Disease Activity

have been mentioned in previous chapters, but will be summarized here. Disease activity was not related to either an older age on admission or a longer duration of arthritis (pars. 18.2 and 18.5), while extent of involvement and total severity were associated with both. Such results might be expected in a group of patients who were hospitalized primarily for the study and treatment of their arthritis rather than for rehabilitation or orthopedic measures. Contrary to statements in the literature, lymphadenopathy and splenomegaly were not related to a higher degree of disease activity as estimated in this study (pars. 30.4 and 30.6). The finding of subcutaneous nodules (par. 33.3), joint effusions (par. 34.2), or anemia (par. 38.3), each of which was associated with increased disease activity, was probably taken into account in the observers' formulation of the degree of activity present. Rather surprisingly, joint redness (par. 34.2) was apparently not thus taken into account and furthermore was not accompanied by other factors connoting increased activity (Table 34.2). Findings which were not related to the degree of disease activity were a leukocytosis (par. 38.5), a polynucleosis (par. 38.8), an eosinophilia (par. 38.8), and a high basal metabolism (par. 41.5).

43.3 The results of the classification of the series patients according to activity, involvement, and severity are listed in Table 43.1. The proportions under the three headings are quite similar except for a higher percentage of patients with mild involvement and a smaller number with moderate involvement than in the other two categories. These differences imply that, in certain patients, the degree of disease

Table 43.1

Disease activity, articular involvement, and total severity of rheumatoid arthritis on hospital admission among patients of present series

Degree	Activity		Involvement		Severity	
	No.	Per cent	No.	Per cent	No.	Per cent
Mild	59	20.1	111	37.9	72	24.6
Moderate	175	59.7	120	41.0	172	58.7
Marked	59	20.1	62	21.1	49	16.7
Total	293	99.9	293	100.0	293	100.0

activity and other elements in the definition of severity outweighed the relatively mild or localized joint involvement in the estimation of total disease severity.

43.4 Table 43.2 sets forth the nature of the association of various factors with increased severity on admission. The list is divided into two groups: the first, Group A, includes those factors likely to have been taken into account when the observer decided upon the degree of total severity according to its definition; and the second, Group B, those apparently unrelated to the points mentioned in the definition. It may be seen at a glance that a much greater proportion of positive associations occurred among the factors related by definition to increased severity than in those unrelated. However, a considerable number of factors in Group A showed absence of association. Although the speed of progression formed part of the definition of total disease severity, the type of onset, whether acute and severe or gradual, and the course before admission, whether intermittent or progressive, turned out to bear no relation to the degree of severity at the time of hospitalization. However, relatively long duration of arthritis before hospital admission was associated with increased severity on admission. The reason for this may lie partially in the fact that duration was measured from the beginning of the first attack and not, in those with a remittent or partially remittent course, from the onset of the attack which resulted in hospitalization. In addition, longer duration was associated with more extensive articular involvement (see Table 34.5) and would be expected to result in greater disability. Constitutional and neurologic symptoms were in general associated with increased total severity on admission, but three of the four vasomotor symptoms considered, along with vasomotor signs, were not. Among the extra-articular findings, fever, subcutaneous nodules, anemia, atrophy of muscles, and atrophy of skin or nails were related to increased severity, but tachycardia and enlargement of spleen or lymph nodes were not. Finally, as mentioned before and as would have been expected by definition, estimations of disease activity and extent of articular involvement ran closely parallel to total severity.

43.5 Our findings in regard to the factors not included in the definition of total disease severity* were of greater interest and importance.

* See definition, par. 4.26.

Table 43.2

Association of various factors with increased total severity of rheumatoid arthritis on hospital admission

GROUP A: RELATED TO DEFINITION OF SEVERITY	
Positive association	*Absence of association*
	Type of onset: acute or gradual
	Course before hospital admission: intermittent or progressive
Constitutional symptoms: anorexia, weight loss	Constitutional symptoms: weakness
Vasomotor symptoms: cold extremities	Vasomotor symptoms: paresthesias, cyanosis, vascular spasm
Neurologic symptoms: tremor, twitching	Neurologic symptoms: vertigo, nervousness
Findings on hospital admission: muscular atrophy, atrophy of skin or nails, fever, nodules, articular effusion, x-ray changes	Findings on admission: vasomotor signs, tachycardia, lymphadenopathy, splenomegaly, articular redness
Laboratory tests: anemia	
Increased disease activity or more extensive joint involvement	

GROUP B: UNRELATED TO DEFINITION OF SEVERITY	
	Family history of rheumatoid arthritis
	History of previous serious illness, operation, or injury
	Prodromal symptoms
	Precipitating factors: strain, infection, exposure, operation, trauma
Onset bilateral	Onset: before or after age 40, within 2 years of menopause, joints first involved, occupation at time
Course before hospital admission: longer, unaffected by strain	Course before admission: unaffected by infection or by cold and moisture
Age on hospital admission 40 or more	Findings on admission: exaggerated reflexes, spondylitis (in males), presence of foci, "arthritic" pattern in colon
Laboratory tests: albuminuria and/or cylindruria	Laboratory tests: abnormal differential counts, gastric anacidity, low basal metabolism
No improvement (after discharge)	

These are listed in Table 43.2 under Group B. The relationships between total severity on admission and the apparent effect on the preceding course of cold and dampness, strain, and intercurrent infection have been discussed in par. 20.6. The association between greater age on admission and increased severity may depend on a mutual relationship with longer duration of disease. The relationship between severity on admission to the subsequent course will be referred to in the next chapter. A more severe disease on admission was not found in patients with a family history of rheumatoid arthritis, nor a less severe disease in those whose past medical history was uneventful. Total disease severity on admission was also unrelated to a history of either prodromal symptoms or precipitating factors; to age or occupation at onset; and to closeness of the menopause to onset. A bilateral distribution of joint involvement at onset was associated with increased severity on admission, but no difference in this regard was evident whether the arthritis began in small or large joints, in a single joint, or in the spine. From the nature of the factors in Group B listed under the headings "Findings on admission" and "Laboratory tests," one might expect in most an absence of association with disease severity as defined in this study. One exception, age past forty on admission, has already been referred to in this paragraph. With respect to the other exception, albuminuria and/or cylindruria, the mutual association should be noted between this factor and both a greater age and to increased severity on admission. The lack of relationship between either gastric anacidity or a low basal metabolism and more severe disease runs counter to the results in a previously reported study [164] of these aspects of rheumatoid arthritis.

SUMMARY

43.6 In the case of each patient the degree of disease activity, the extent of articular involvement, and the total disease severity,* as of the time of hospitalization, were estimated by two or more observers. With respect to total severity, in addition to constitutional manifestations, speed of progression, and degree of disability, both activity and involvement were taken into consideration. The proportions classified as mild, moderate, or marked in each of the three categories were quite

* See definition, par. 4.26.

Disease Severity and Disease Activity

similar except for a higher percentage with mild involvement and a lower percentage with moderate involvement than in either of the other two categories (Table 43.1). Thus, in certain cases, the degree of activity and other factors related to disease severity apparently outweighed the relatively mild articular involvement in the observers' estimation of disease severity. A longer duration of arthritis and hence usually a greater age on hospital admission were related to more extensive involvement and to increased severity but not to the degree of disease activity.

43.7   When the relationships were studied numerically, factors likely to have been taken into account by definition in the estimation of total disease severity* were generally found in association with severity of a more marked degree (Table 43.2, Group A). Of greater interest and of possible prognostic importance were the relationships between the degree of total severity and certain of the factors which were not included in the definition of severity (Table 43.2, Group B). These factors were chiefly concerned with the onset of the arthritis or with events preceding onset. For example, bilateral involvement from the start was related to increased severity on admission, but the degree of severity was not related to age or occupation at onset or to the proximity of menopause to onset.

43.8   Objective for further study:

Anthropometric comparison between rheumatoid arthritics with mild disease severity and those with marked severity.

* See definition, par. 4.26.

44

Subsequent Course of Disease

44.1 To supplement the clinical and laboratory data recorded at the time of hospital admission for the 293 patients of the present study three tabulations have been made of the changes in status which occurred after each patient's discharge. The first part of this chapter will review the results of the 1947 follow-up study which have been previously reported [466] and will discuss the prognostic value of certain factors which were found to be associated with favorable or unfavorable course. The second part of the chapter will present a comparison of the shifts in status which occurred between 1937 and 1954. As the series was collected between 1930 and 1936, patients will be included in this comparison who were followed in some instances for nearly twenty years.

FOLLOW-UP STUDY OF 1947

44.2 The aim of the 1947 study was to evaluate the course of rheumatoid arthritis in patients who had received simple medical and orthopedic therapy. In selecting patients for tabulation, 22 patients were excluded because of inadequate follow-up data and 21 were eliminated because they had received special forms of therapy—either vitamin D in massive dosage or gold salts. Of the 293 patients in the series, 250 therefore remained. The majority of these 250 patients had been hospitalized for no more than two or three weeks for trial of and instruction

Subsequent Course of Disease 389

in conservative therapy that could be continued at home—bed rest, applications of heat to affected joints, analgesics (chiefly aspirin), adequate diets supplemented by vitamins, corrective exercises, and nonoperative orthopedic procedures if needed. To round out the picture, it must be added that 16 patients also received blood transfusions, 52 received fever therapy, in which we were interested at the time [465], and 75 received medical or surgical treatment for foci of infection. But since the rate of improvement in each of these groups approximated that obtained in the remainder of the series, such patients were not excluded from the study group. Thirty-eight patients were rehospitalized for three months or more during their illness. As might have been expected, they tended to follow a progressive course, and only 29 per cent had improved when last seen. While the conservative routine outlined above is generally believed to be helpful, there is no evidence that it alters the natural course of the disease. In a limited sense, then, the 250 patients of the 1947 study may be considered a control series, and the findings tabulated here may be used for comparison with other groups of rheumatoid arthritics who have received special forms of therapy over similar periods.

44.3 The original plan for the follow-up study was to examine each patient at least once or twice a year. But regularity of attendance at the clinic naturally depended upon their need or willingness to return or, in the case of patients living at a distance or markedly disabled, their ability to make the trip. Certain patients were thus unavoidably seen at irregular intervals. We were aided in obtaining reports on the absentees and in getting them back to the clinic by trained follow-up workers and by nurses attached to the departments of public health in Massachusetts and other New England states. We kept in touch by letter with the small number who had left New England, but accepted none as improved unless the evidence was definite and classified none as in remission without examination at the clinic. When the data were compiled in 1947, the length of observation ranged from six months to sixteen years (Table 44.1). The average for the group was nine and one-half years, but 200 patients, or 80 per cent, had been followed for more than five years.

44.4 The status of the 250 patients according to the most recent

Table 44.1

Duration of observation for group of rheumatoid arthritics included in 1947 follow-up study

Duration of observation	Patients	
	No.	Per cent
1 year or less	14	5.6
3 to 1 years	9	3.6
5 to 3 years	27	10.8
10 to 5 years	80	32.0
15 to 10 years	114	45.6
More than 15 years	6	2.4
	250*	100.0

* Includes 25 patients who were last seen in 1937 or earlier and 11 patients who returned to observation after 1937.

information available up to April 1947 is expressed in Table 44.2. They are divided into three main groups, the base line in all cases being the patients' condition on admission to the hospital. The first group has also been subdivided according to the degree of improvement exhibited. On each return visit to the clinic a detailed examination was made of the patient's articular system, and objective and subjective findings pertinent to the clinical course were carefully recorded. Complete physical examinations were also made at frequent intervals, and sedimentation rates were determined on nearly every return visit. The patients of the group labeled "in remission" in Table 44.2 were asymptomatic and showed no evidence of disease other than residual deformity, which was noted in a few cases. In each case the sedimentation rate (Rourke-Ernstene) was normal or only slightly increased. The next group, with moderate improvement, showed noteworthy subjective and objective gains but could not justly be called in remission. Those judged slightly improved showed definite objective changes of a favorable nature. Patients were not classified as improved because of gains in joint function due to conservative or operative orthopedic procedures or because of increased capacity for work or self-care. The patients of the stationary group were essentially the same when last seen, but at least half had previously pursued a fluctuating course, with periods of both exacerbation and improvement. Those with minor variations in symptomatology and joint findings were also included

Table 44.2
Disease status of group of rheumatoid arthritics included in 1947 follow-up study

Disease status	Patients	
	No.	Per cent
Improved	133	53.2
In remission	38	15.2
Moderately improved	43	17.2
Slightly improved	52	20.8
Stationary	32	12.8
Worse	85	34.0
Total	250*	100.0

* See note, Table 44.1.

under this designation. The classification "worse" requires little explanation. It included some patients who were subjectively better and even less disabled, but the disease had progressed as determined by physical examination and, in a few instances, by roentgenograms. Conversely, 4 patients who showed marked lessening of disease activity, but no functional changes in their joints or even decreased motion in some, were put into the slightly improved group.

44.5 The 1947 follow-up study was based upon 94 males and 156 females. Table 44.3 demonstrates that the difference in outcome between the two sexes was not significant, although the males did slightly better. However, it was noted that a much larger proportion of the males had spondylitis. On the basis of the evidence presented in Table 42.3, which shows a much higher frequency of improvement among

Table 44.3
Improvement in relation to sex distribution of group of rheumatoid arthritics in 1947 follow-up study

Sex	No. of patients	Improved	
		No.	Per cent
Total	250*	133	53.2
Males	94	55	58.4
Females	156	78	50.0

Difference in percentages: 8.4 ± 6.5
Males: average length of observation, 9.0 years
Females: average length of observation, 10.1 years

* See note, Table 44.1.

male patients without spinal involvement, it was decided to exclude spondylitics from consideration. Table 44.4 indicates that the remaining 64 males improved at a significantly higher rate than the remaining 149 females. The suggestion is thus raised that, in peripheral rheumatoid arthritis, males do better than females. A similar difference in outcome was recorded by Duthie and others [154] in a comparable series of 282 patients followed for periods ranging from one to four years.

44.6   Most authors expressing an opinion regarding the influence of the patient's age on the course of rheumatoid arthritis believe that older persons tend to do better [75, 81, 333, 362]. The one exception that we have encountered is Schnell [452], who states that the prognosis is much worse in cases starting after the age of fifty-five. In the present series, patients who were admitted to the hospital before the age of forty showed a higher rate of improvement than the remainder (Table 44.5). However, the younger age group contained a relatively large proportion of males and of patients with mild disease severity. Both these factors were associated with a more favorable course. When the analysis was based on age at onset, the rate of improvement was about the same—a finding confirmed by Duthie and others [154]. In the absence of corroborative evidence from other series only tentative conclusions can be drawn regarding age and improvement.

44.7   Of the various factors under consideration, disease duration before hospital admission was found to have the most important bearing on prognosis. Nearly 75 per cent of the 81 patients with disease duration of one year or less (Table 44.6) and an even higher percentage of those with duration of six months or less (Table 44.7) showed some improvement. Moreover, 37 per cent of those with duration of one year or less before admission were in remission in 1947, compared with 4.7 per cent of the remainder. Table 44.7 also shows that among patients whose onset dated back more than one year the prognosis was essentially the same irrespective of disease duration. That the results are better in patients seen shortly after onset has frequently been stated without evidence derived from numerical studies [61, 75, 191, 286, 356, 362], but the point has also been subjected to statistical analysis. From investigation of a series of 254 patients with peripheral rheumatoid arthritis, Lewis-Faning and Fletcher [321] concluded that a higher percentage

Table 44.4

Improvement in relation to sex distribution of group of rheumatoid arthritics in 1947 follow-up study, exclusive of 37 spondylitics

Sex	No. of patients	Improved No.	Per cent
Total	213*	117	54.8
Males	64	43	67.2
Females	149	74	49.7

Difference in percentages: 17.5 ± 7.5
Males: average duration of observation, 9.1 years
Females: average duration of observation, 10.0 years

* See note, Table 44.1.

Table 44.5

Improvement in relation to age on hospital admission among rheumatoid arthritics included in 1947 follow-up study

Age on admission	No. of patients	Improved No.	Per cent
Total	250*	133	53.2
Less than 40	133	80	60.2
40 or more	117	53	45.3

Difference in percentages: 14.9 ± 6.2
Younger group: average length of observation, 9.8 years
Older group: average length of observation, 9.1 years

* See note, Table 44.1.

Table 44.6

Improvement in relation to short and long disease duration before hospital admission among rheumatoid arthritics included in 1947 follow-up study

Duration before admission	No. of patients	Improved No.	Per cent
Total	250*	133	53.2
1 year or less	81	60	74.1
More than 1 year	169	73	43.2

Difference in percentages: 30.9 ± 6.8
Short duration: average length of observation, 9.9 years
Long duration: average length of observation, 9.3 years

* See note, Table 44.1.

Table 44.7

Improvement in relation to disease duration before hospital admission among rheumatoid arthritics included in 1947 follow-up study

		Improved	
Disease duration	No. of patients	No.	Per cent
Total	250*	133	53.2
6 months or less	53	43	81.1
1 year to 6 months	28	17	60.6
3 years to 1 year	64	29	45.3
5 years to 3 years	35	12	34.3
10 years to 5 years	39	19	48.7
More than 10 years	31	13	41.9

* See note, Table 44.1.

of success was obtained when the duration of the disease was less than one year. In 1926 Cecil and Archer [78] reported that 82 per cent of the patients whom they saw within six months of onset either completely recovered or greatly improved—a rate comparable to that presented in Table 44.7. More recently, our findings in regard to the relationship between disease duration and prognosis have been confirmed by Duthie and others [154] in a follow-up study of 282 patients receiving simple medical and orthopedic treatment. Although frequently neglected, the implications of this study should always be taken into consideration in the evaluation of methods of therapy. However, they constitute insufficient evidence for a conclusion that early treatment increases the likelihood of improvement or remission and may merely reflect a higher rate of spontaneous remissions in the first year of the disease.

44.8 Table 44.8 summarizes the factors which appear to influence (1) the course pursued before hospital admission, whether intermittent or progressive, (2) the severity of the disease on admission to the hospital, and (3) the subsequent course. It is evident that only factors preceding or associated with the onset could possibly influence the type of course before admission. As shown in the table, onset in multiple small joints was unfavorable, whereas monarticular onset, acute onset, and onset before age forty were favorable (i.e., usually foretelling an intermittent course). The sex of the patient and the presence or absence of prodromal symptoms or precipitating factors apparently did not influence the course before admission. As pointed out in the discussion of Table

Subsequent Course of Disease

Table 44.8
Factors of possible prognostic assistance in rheumatoid arthritis because of association with course before hospital admission, total disease severity on admission, and subsequent course

	FAVORABLE	
1. *Course before admission*	2. *Total severity on admission*	3. *Subsequent course*
Age at onset under 40	Onset unilateral	Sex, male (spondylitics excluded)
Onset acute	Age on admission under 40	Age on admission under 40
Onset monarticular	Duration before admission (shorter)	Duration before admission (shorter)
	Absence of articular effusion	Absence of articular effusion
	Absence of x-ray changes	Absence of x-ray changes
	Activity of disease milder	Activity of disease milder
	Articular involvement less extensive	Articular involvement less extensive
		Total severity (decreased)
	UNFAVORABLE	
Onset in small joints	Anorexia	Onset after menopause
	Weight loss	Tremor (subjective)
	Cold extremities	Exaggerated reflexes
	Twitching	Atrophy: muscle, skin, nails
	Tremor (subjective)	Spondylitis (in males)
	Fever	
	Atrophy: muscle, skin, nails	
	Nodules	
	Anemia	

43.2, most of the factors associated with the degree of disease severity on admission bear a relationship to severity by definition and hence are of dubious value in prognosis. The only exceptions among those listed in Table 44.8 are a unilateral onset, a shorter duration of disease, and admission before age forty—all of which were favorable. Factors unrelated to severity by either definition or association are listed in Table 43.2 and include a family history of rheumatoid arthritis, prodromal symptoms, and precipitating factors.

44.9 Most of the factors related either favorably or unfavorably to the patients' subsequent course have been mentioned in the appropriate chapter, while the influence of sex, age on hospital admission, spondylitis, and duration have been referred to in preceding paragraphs of this chapter. It is of interest that tremor and exaggerated reflexes apparently foretold an unfavorable course in the present series, but the relationship cannot be accepted as prognostic without confirmation in other series. That atrophy of muscles, skin, and nails should connote a more severe form of disease (and absence of joint effusions and x-ray changes the opposite) was to be expected. With evidence derived from the present study, one might assemble, as follows, a composite hospitalized patient who would be likely to do well: a man, under forty years of age, without spondylitis, with disease of less than a year's duration, with mild joint involvement, slight disease activity, and mild total severity.*

44.10 The 1947 follow-up study of our series [466] was believed at the time to represent an improvement in method over previous studies. Defects in these were listed and certain principles that seemed important to follow in the selection and analysis of patients under observation were presented. Subsequent experience has led to the recognition of the serious limitations of this, as well as other studies of the underlying course of rheumatoid arthritis. These limitations have been outlined elsewhere [431] along with a suggested scheme for the collection of better data on the course of the disease. This scheme, which will not be repeated here in detail, is based on the principle that the proportion of patients improved or in remission on a given date or when last observed is of less interest than the length of time spent in remission or in leading a relatively normal life. In addition, it seems preferable to classify patients according to their absolute status at the time of each examination, rather than by their change in status relative to previous examinations. It is hoped that methods of this type will yield a more accurate description of the course of rheumatoid arthritis than is available at present.

FOLLOW-UP STUDY OF 1954

44.11 By 1954, when a third follow-up study was made, only 174 patients were available for tabulation—59 having died before additional observation was possible and 17 having failed to return for observation. As might have been expected, most of those who died were in the older

* See definition, par. 4.26.

Subsequent Course of Disease

age group; these have been utilized in a recently published report [99] on life expectancy and the causes of death in rheumatoid arthritis. The average period of observation for the 174 patients in the 1954 study was 14.4 years; 29 patients had been under observation for over twenty years. Table 44.9 compares the results of the studies made in 1937, 1947, and 1954. In order to avoid duplication of patients under 1937 and 1947, only the patients actually examined after 1937 were included in the 1947 column. Since the total was thus reduced from 250 to 225, the numbers and percentages differ somewhat from those given in Table 44.2. According to Table 44.9 about the same proportion of patients was in remission in 1947 as in 1937, but the same patients are represented only in part. About half of those in remission in 1937 had left this status in 1947, but their loss was made up for by recruits from patients with lesser degrees of improvement or even no improvement in 1937. Between 1937 and 1947 a significant increase was found in the worse group and a similar decrease in the stationary group. During the seven years from 1947 to 1954 the percentage of those considered improved dropped from 54.7 to 35.0, largely at the expense of the slightly improved group. In only 4 patients was the disease still considered station-

Table 44.9

Results of 1954 follow-up study—patients of present series who were available for observation in 1937, 1947, and 1954 evaluated with respect to disease status

Status of disease	1937		1947		1954	
	No.	Per cent	No.	Per cent	No.	Per cent
In remission	41	17.2	38	16.9	23	13.2
Moderately improved	30	12.6	35	15.6	23	13.2
Slightly improved	58	24.3	50	22.2	15	8.6
Stationary	64	26.8	26	11.6	4	2.3
Worse	46	19.2	76	33.8	109**	62.6
Total	239*	100.1	225†	100.1	174††	99.9
Total improved	129	54.0	123	54.7	61	35.0

* This total is smaller than that in Tables 44.1–7, because 11 patients who met the criteria of the follow-up program returned for observation after 1937.
† This total is smaller than that in Tables 44.1–7, because the 1947 analysis included 25 patients last seen in 1937 or before.
** 1 patient in this group received cortisone.
†† This total is smaller than that in Tables 44.1–7, because 17 patients failed to return for observation and 59 had died before further observation was possible.

ary, and the percentage considered worse rose from 33.8 to 62.6. Whereas about one-fourth of 110 patients classified as stationary or worse in 1937 attained partial improvement by 1947, such a gain was made by only 1 of 102 patients between 1947 and 1954. On the whole, the results in Table 44.9 indicate a gradual deterioration, but a substantial proportion of the patients showing improvement early in the course of the follow-up study were able to maintain this status. The data also point out the unlikelihood of improvement after ten or more years of failure to demonstrate a favorable course. The follow-up program is continuing and further tabulations of results will be presented at a later date, along with a tabulation of the causes of death among patients of the present series.

44.12 There are few reports in the literature based on the continued observation for one or more years of comparable series of patients with rheumatoid arthritis. Three may be cited briefly: 77 cases studied by Pemberton and Peirce [*403*]; 274 by Thompson, Wyatt, and Hicks [*531*]; and 254 by Lewis-Faning and Fletcher [*321*]. In the first series of patients, 90.9 per cent evidenced some degree of improvement, and 22 per cent were considered to be in remission. The figures were, respectively, 87.2 and 6 per cent in the second series and 64.4 and 24.6 per cent in the third. There is thus a wide variation in the percentages given for improvement but a general agreement with the present study that a small minority of patients are likely to enter upon a sustained remission. In addition, Sashin, Spanbock, and Kling [*450*] stated that 15 per cent of their 120 patients "improved markedly"—a proportion that happens to coincide almost exactly with the proportion found in remission in 1947 in our series (Table 44.9). One series of patients that should be mentioned in greater detail was studied by Ragan [*423*] and reported on in 1949. This included 374 patients who had been followed for more than five years, with an average duration of follow-up of eleven years. Of these, 201 had received gold salts and the remaining 173 patients had received either no therapy or one or more of the simple medical and orthopedic procedures which were utilized for our patients. Since the outcome was essentially the same in both groups, the gold therapy was not considered to have influenced the patients' final status. Only a general comparison is possible between Ragan's results and those

Subsequent Course of Disease

obtained in the present series, since no information is available as to age, sex, severity, and other factors of possible prognostic importance in his patients. Also the end results were taken at one point in time, as in the present series, but the patients were classified according to their absolute status rather than according to their condition at the time they came under observation. The group with "good end result" made up 48 per cent of Ragan's patients, with over half of these, 26 per cent of the series, showing no signs of arthritis. These figures approximate the 54.7 per cent improved and 16.9 per cent in remission found between 1937 and 1947 in our series, while Ragan's 52 per cent with "poor end result" corresponds quite closely to the 45.4 per cent who remained stationary or worse in our series (Table 44.9). In spite of the different criteria employed, the results from both studies are in general agreement and may be useful for comparative purposes in the evaluation of long-term forms of therapy in rheumatoid arthritis.

SUMMARY

44.13   The patients of the present series first came under observation on their admission to the hospital between 1930 and 1936. Tabulations of their status relative to their condition at hospital entrance were made in 1937, 1947, and 1954, based on patients with adequate follow-up who received only simple medical and orthopedic treatment. The results of the 1947 study, which indicated that 53.2 per cent had improved and 15.2 per cent were in remission when last seen (Table 44.2), were utilized in an attempt to obtain information of possible prognostic importance. In this way, the following factors were associated with subsequent improvement: male sex (among those without spondylitis), age on hospital admission under forty, disease duration of one year or less before admission, absence of spondylitis (among males), and mild disease severity* on admission.

44.14   The results obtained in the 1947 study approximated those obtained in the 1937 study in regard to the proportions improved or in remission, but relatively more patients were considered worse in 1947 and fewer patients stationary. In 1954, with an average follow-up period of over fourteen years, the percentage deemed improved had fallen to

* See definition, par. **4.26**.

35 per cent and of those considered worse had risen to 62.6 per cent. However, a substantial proportion of those who improved early in the course of their disease were able to maintain this status. The data also showed the unlikelihood of improvement after ten or more years of failure to demonstrate a favorable course.

44.15 The results in the present follow-up study as tabulated in 1947 are in essential agreement with those obtained by Ragan [*423*] in a study of 374 patients followed for an average of eleven years. On this account they may be helpful for comparison with the outcome of groups of patients receiving special forms of therapy and followed for similar periods of time, although the authors are aware of the serious limitations of this method of studying the course of rheumatoid arthritis.

44.16 Objectives for further study:

1. Better methods for studying the course of rheumatoid arthritis.

2. Additional observations on factors which might permit prediction of future remissions or exacerbations.

45

Summary

45.1 Rheumatoid arthritis is a chronic inflammatory disease of unknown etiology and pathogenesis which is systemic in nature and characterized by the manner in which it involves joints. It has been the authors' purpose to present a clinical description of this disease based upon a numerical study of hospitalized patients. The series utilized was drawn from 300 consecutive patients who were admitted to the medical wards of the Massachusetts General Hospital between 1930 and 1936 and in whom the diagnosis of rheumatoid arthritis was supported by extensive clinical and laboratory study. Diagnostic re-appraisal was carried out by five observers in 1938, two years after the required number had been obtained, with the resultant removal of 7 patients and reduction of the series to 293. While it is believed that the patients selected were representative of rheumatoid arthritics more than twelve years of age who might be referred to a general hospital in New England, there is no present way of ascertaining the extent to which they might depart from the characteristics of a random sample of rheumatoid arthritics drawn from New England communities. Information of this type, which is greatly needed, awaits epidemiologic investigation of suitable population groups.

45.2 Early in the course of the study, the need became evident for a clear and unequivocal statement of the diagnostic criteria employed and for a definition of rheumatoid arthritis (one which, to be sure, must be regarded as provisional until more complete knowledge is obtained of the etiology or pathogenesis of the disease). To insure proper orientation, an account has been given of the development of the concept of rheumatoid arthritis as a disease entity. This process has involved the separation of other, unrelated forms of joint disease and the restoration of conditions which probably represent clinical variants rather than separate entities. In regard to the first, patients with gouty arthritis were carefully excluded, as were those with degenerative joint disease unless the latter was associated with rheumatoid arthritis either coincidentally or in a secondary role. In accordance with our present knowledge, it would appear that one form of so-called menopausal arthritis should be included under degenerative joint disease, while another seemingly consists in musculo-skeletal symptoms accompanying the climateric. For the purposes of the study, rheumatoid arthritis and rheumatic fever were regarded as separate entities, in spite of border-line cases and the finding of valvular heart disease in a certain number of patients who otherwise satisfied the diagnosis of rheumatoid arthritis and were therefore included in the series. Arthritis due to specific infection, either with organisms present in the joints or in association with a disease known to be of infectious origin, forms an admittedly distinct group from rheumatoid arthritis. The weight of evidence is also against the existence of "tuberculous rheumatism" (par. 2.72) and of a chronic, progressive arthritis due to the gonococcus, to brucellosis, or to syphilis. It has been pointed out, however, that a disease of infectious origin may be present along with rheumatoid arthritis and may at times apparently precipitate an attack or exacerbation of the latter disease. While fibrositis, in the sense of inflammatory changes in extra-articular fibrous structures, is a frequent manifestation of rheumatoid arthritis, patients with "primary fibrositis" were carefully distinguished from those with rheumatoid arthritis in a mild or early stage, whether or not the "fibrositis" was considered to be of psychogenic origin. Patients with Reiter's syndrome were also excluded from the series, although some of its features, including the occasional development of a chronic, progressive arthritis, have given rise to the suggestion that it may be a variant of rheumatoid arthritis. Finally, in spite of the recognition that both clinical and patho-

Summary

logic relationships exist between rheumatoid arthritis and other connective tissue diseases, it seemed best to regard this group as made up of distinct diseases. Patients were thus eliminated who were at first thought to have rheumatoid arthritis and later developed features of another connective tissue disease.

45.3   Syndromes which merit restoration to their proper classification as variants of rheumatoid arthritis include Still's disease (both juvenile and adult) and Felty's syndrome. Consequently, no reason was found to exclude patients with disease onset in childhood or with varying combinations of lymphadenopathy, splenomegaly, or leukopenia. Women with rheumatoid arthritis starting at the menopause were included, as were patients with intermittent hydrarthrosis forming merely one stage in the clinical course of a disease syndrome otherwise consistent with rheumatoid arthritis. It was decided to include in the series 3 patients with ulcerative colitis, in view of the insufficient data available at present for the recognition of an independent type of joint disease in patients with ulcerative colitis and an accompanying arthritis. The same may be said of the combination of psoriasis and arthritis, with the possible exception of a destructive arthritis confined to the terminal interphalangeal joints and associated with psoriatic nails [22]. The series therefore included 10 patients with psoriasis in conjunction with arthritis. The evidence has also been outlined against the partition of rheumatoid arthritis into primary and "infectious" types, although a so-called infectious stage resembling an arthritis due to a specific infection may sometimes be recognized, most often early in the disease course. Opinion is still divided as to whether rheumatoid spondylitis should be regarded as a variant of rheumatoid arthritis or a disease *sui generis*. Nevertheless, it was decided to include patients with spinal arthritis either with or without involvement of peripheral joints, since it was believed that the exclusion of patients with spondylitis would render the series less rather than more representative of rheumatoid arthritis requiring hospitalization.

45.4   The last two paragraphs were not intended to leave the reader with the impression that the diagnosis of rheumatoid arthritis is made chiefly by exclusion. On the contrary, as set forth in the text, patients with well-marked rheumatoid arthritis manifest characteristic symptoms, physical signs, articular roentgenograms, and histopathologic changes, at least in the subcutaneous nodule and synovial membrane. Proof of the identity of rheumatoid arthritis on etiologic grounds is of course lacking. Until this advance is made, it remains possible that the disease may represent one type of response to a single agent or disease mechanism shared by other disorders or that multiple causes or mechanisms are responsible for the varied and at times seemingly unrelated clinical pictures included under a single diagnostic heading. Medical opinion is thus far generally in favor of the independent status of this disease. The authors are willing to commit themselves, with reservations, to the opinion of the majority and to consider rheumatoid arthritis an independent disease of unitary though unknown etiology.*

45.5 The present numerical study of hospitalized patients with rheumatoid arthritis may be divided into two parts. The first is a cross-sectional description—which includes information in regard to factors preceding and associated with the onset, as well as to the type of course pursued before hospital admission—and the second, a long-term follow-up study of patients with this disease who were treated with simple medical and orthopedic measures. To facilitate the collection of data for the cross-sectional description, a plan of observation was prepared before the study began and a check-list of the factors to be statistically analyzed was prepared in advance. An equal number of non-arthritic persons, corresponding to the patients in sex and age distribution, provided a control group for the evaluation of certain signs and symptoms noted in the patients. For the follow-up study, a clinic was organized for continued observation and management of the patients, and an effort was made to obtain data on each patient at least once a year. Those unable to return were visited in the home by trained follow-up workers or public health nurses.

45.6 In the numerical comparisons made between the patients of the present series and the control group or among subgroups of the patients, a difference was termed significant when expected by chance

---

* Our current speculations in regard to the etiology of this chronic inflammatory disease of systemic nature are in favor of the initiation of the inflammatory process by a micro-organism (virus or pleuropneumonia-like organism) or by a hitherto undescribed form of antigen-antibody reaction.

Summary

less than 5 per cent of the time. The results of comparison between the patients and controls are summarized in Table 46, but each finding has also been presented in the appropriate chapter. For comparisons among the patients, all were classified according to the presence or absence of thirty-nine clinical or laboratory attributes and all possible pairs of these attributes were then examined systematically for the presence of association. The results are expressed in Table 47, but those of particular interest or importance have been put into separate tables or referred to in the text. Sources of difficulty in the interpretation of the data have been set forth in Chapter 3. These include the comparability of patients and controls, the retrospective nature of the observations, the influence of hidden factors on associations between variables, and finally the fact that the information was obtained from a series of hospitalized patients.

45.7   The remainder of this summarizing chapter will be devoted to a résumé of the results obtained in the numerical study and of references, where appropriate, to the findings of others. In the first place, there is fairly general agreement that about twice as many females as males seek clinic or hospital admission for rheumatoid arthritis. The reason for this is unknown, but a number of other diseases of equally obscure origin show a predilection for one sex. There is also agreement that women are more susceptible to rheumatoid arthritis in the fifth and six decades than at other ages, a finding which suggests an influence of the menopause. However, no close temporal relationship was demonstrated between disease onset and time of menopause, when the cessation of menstruation was used as a reference point. Our finding that males of all ages above fifteen were equally susceptible has not been confirmed in other series. Since studies of this type depend on the assumption that the patients chosen are representative of rheumatoid arthritics in the general population, better information should be obtainable from epidemiologic studies of population groups. The relative frequency of rheumatoid arthritis among races or in different geographic locations remains as yet undetermined. Similarly, present evidence is insufficient to suggest a relationship between type of occupation and the onset or development of the disease.

45.8   A higher frequency of serious illness other than arthritis was recorded for the patients than for the controls, but not of injury or operation. With the exception of psoriasis, ulcerative colitis, and thyroid disorders, no association or antagonism between rheumatoid arthritis and other diseases has been demonstrated in the patients of our series or in others reported in the literature. In particular, no analogy can be drawn between rheumatoid arthritis and diseases of recognized allergic origin on the basis of an increased frequency of asthma, hay fever, or urticaria in rheumatoid subjects or their families. While the familial nature of rheumatoid arthritis seems to be established, the evidence is insufficient to determine the etiologic importance of environment, contagion, or heredity. In addition to rheumatoid arthritis, rheumatic fever was present more frequently in the families of patients than in the families of controls.

45.9 The onset of the actual arthritis may be preceded by prodromal symptoms, which may rightly mark the beginning of the disease. Over one-half of the series patients gave a history of one or more potentially disturbing events preceding the onset of a persistent arthritis. Strain was noted most commonly, with infection, exposure, operation, trauma, and childbirth following in this order. The significance of such "precipitating" factors is still undecided, since similar results were obtained in one study when control subjects were questioned in regard to a reference point in time fixed to correspond with disease onset in the patients. In any case, if it is assumed that the prodromal symptoms mark the disease onset, our data suggest that precipitating factors merely determine a more disabling phase with articular localization of the process.

45.10 A severe, acute onset was recorded in about one-fifth of the patients. This type of onset was associated with both a preceding infection and early hospital admission. It was also more common in patients experiencing at least one remission before hospital entry and hence may be of prognostic importance. In the present series, the arthritis first affected large and small joints with about equal frequency. Small joints, especially of the hands, were initially attacked more commonly in females than in males and in those who ran a progressive rather than an intermittent course before admission. Contrary to opinions expressed in the literature, joints of the legs were more frequently affected in the beginning than those of the upper extremities. In about one-sixth of the series, the onset was monarticular and when persistent this type of in-

Summary

volvement sometimes occasioned difficulty in formulating the correct diagnosis. In about one-half of those with spondylitis on admission, the disease began in peripheral joints, almost invariably those of the lower extremities. The concept of an atypical "infectious" form of rheumatoid arthritis initially involving one or a few joints (par. 2.101) has not been established by testing for associations among the criteria usually assigned to what is more likely merely a stage of the disease. The arthritis was unilateral in about one-third of the patients, at first, but it had become bilateral in nearly all by the time of admission. A unilateral onset was more common in males, in patients with onset before the age of forty, and in those with mild disease severity* on admission. The involvement of corresponding joints on opposite sides of the body constitutes an unexplained, but outstanding, clinical feature of rheumatoid arthritis.

45.11   When the ages of the patients on admission to the hospital are compared with the age distribution of the Massachusetts population, the results approximate those obtained in regard to the age of onset, with a marked increase in females admitted between the ages of fifty and sixty. Age forty or over on admission was associated with a more severe disease and a less favorable subsequent course. The duration of arthritis before hospital admission showed a wide range of variation among the patients. Shorter duration was related to less severe disease, and improvement following discharge was observed in three-quarters of those admitted within a year of onset. Slightly over one-fourth of the patients experienced one or more complete or nearly complete remissions before admission. In a large majority of these patients, the attacks were of one year's duration or less, with remissions of varying length. Attacks lasting more than one year were much less likely to be followed by remissions. About twice as much time was spent in remission as in exacerbation by this group of 80 patients. Remissions occurred throughout the year, but exacerbations were more frequent during the colder months, a distribution corresponding to the season of onset of rheumatoid arthritis. Possible reasons for this seasonal distribution, other than climatic changes, have been listed.

45.12   According to the patients' impressions, arthritic symptoms

* See definition, par. 4.26.

were more frequently affected by strain and climatic conditions than by intercurrent infections. In the last instance, patients with infection as a precipitating factor seemed more prone to subsequent exacerbation associated with intercurrent infectious illnesses. About half the patients experienced a worsening of symptoms with cold and moisture and an improvement with heat. Some additional evidence is supplied by our data in favor of the concept that cold, heat, and dampness exert their effects through alterations in vasomotor tone.

45.13   With the aid of the controls, fatigue, anorexia, and weight loss were shown to be characteristic constitutional symptoms of rheumatoid arthritis. At least half the patients were of normal or more than normal weight on admission. Such individuals were thus as liable to the development of the disease as those who were undernourished. Evidence of vasomotor instability, both subjective and objective and including paresthesias, was encountered with significantly greater frequency in the patients than in the controls. Among the patients, younger females and older males were more likely to display vasomotor instability. These age and sex differences may merely reflect a similar distribution of susceptibility to peripheral circulatory disorders in the population at large. The finding, corroborated elsewhere by quantitative studies, that in about one-fourth of the patients no evidence of a vasomotor defect was present constitutes an important argument against regarding vasomotor changes as essential to the development of rheumatoid arthritis. That neurologic manifestations form an integral part of the disease picture was confirmed in the present study. Three neurologic symptoms, twitching, vertigo, and tremor were found with greater frequency in patients than controls, and, to a lesser degree, a history of nervousness or emotional upsets. Tendon reflexes were increased in about one-third of the patients. Muscular atrophy, present in a majority of the series, was related to marked disease severity on admission and to an unfavorable subsequent course.

45.14   Pleurisy, presumably a disease manifestation, was diagnosed in 5 patients and was accompanied by an effusion in 1 patient. Pulmonary tuberculosis was found in 9 patients (either on hospital admission or later) and bronchiectasis in 4. No clinical or roentgenographic evidence was obtained of pulmonary lesions as systemic manifestations of rheumatoid arthritis. The frequency of valvular and other types of heart disease was essentially the same in patients and controls. Among gastrointestinal symptoms, vomiting, constipation, and diarrhea were recorded with greater frequency for patients than for controls. The evidence thus far available suggests that peptic ulcer occurs in rheumatoid arthritics at least as often as in the population at large.

45.15 During hospital observation, fever of inconsistent pattern was encountered in about one-third of the patients. No essential differences were found between those with fever and the remainder. For a small proportion of the patients, pulse rates over 90 were recorded in the absence of fever. That hypotension constitutes a characteristic clinical attribute of rheumatoid arthritis was not supported in the present study nor in a recently reported study in which controls were also employed. An abnormally low arterial tension was found in certain patients, and a clinical impression was obtained that severe degrees of essential hypertension are unusually rare in association with rheumatoid arthritis.

45.16 Inflammatory eye lesions, most commonly involving the uveal tract, may be regarded as systemic manifestations of rheumatoid arthritis. (In the case of scleromalacia perforans, study of the scleral nodules reveals a microscopic picture identical with that of the subcutaneous rheumatoid nodule.) An association between iritis and spondylitis was suggested by our data, but was not confirmed in a study done elsewhere. Lymph node enlargement and splenic enlargement were noted more frequently in patients than controls, but no support was obtained for the creation of separate syndromes on the basis of these findings. Liver enlargement was equally frequent in both groups. Atrophy of the skin was recorded for nearly one-third of the patients and atrophic changes in the nails for about one-sixth, and both findings were more common in patients with relatively long-standing and severe arthritis. Psoriasis was present in 3.4 per cent of the patients, a frequency significantly higher than that in the controls and suggesting more than a chance association between the two conditions. Edema not due to an extraneous cause was found in about 5 per cent of the patients, in nearly all instances associated with an active arthritis in the underlying joints rather than with disuse and dependency.

45.17 Subcutaneous nodules were recorded on admission for slightly more than one-tenth of the patients. Nodule formation was associated with an acute, severe onset and a more severe and active disease on admission. Thus far, subcutaneous nodules have not been found in patients with spondylitis, unless peripheral joints other than shoulders or hips were also involved. They have also failed to appear, in our experience, in patients with arthritis confined to one side of the body. All but a few of the patients showed objective evidence of articular disease on admission, and the remainder developed joint swelling or limitation during subsequent observation. An association was found between joint effusions, recognized in over one-third of the patients, and fever, as well as lymph node enlargement and an unfavorable subsequent course. Roentgenographic changes indicative of bony or cartilaginous abnormalities were absent in about one-seventh of the patients otherwise satisfying the diagnosis of rheumatoid arthritis.

45.18 Roentgenographic evidence of gallbladder disease was found in about one-seventh of the patients, but no relationship between this condition and rheumatoid arthritis was established. Changes in the roentgenographic appearance of the colon similar to those previously described in rheumatoid arthritis were found in about one-fourth of the series. There is no reason to believe that such abnormalities are in any way specifically related to the disease. Presumptive evidence of focal infection was discovered in two-thirds of the patients, most commonly in the teeth, tonsils, and sinuses, although foci had been removed or treated before admission in about 40 per cent of the series. Follow-up studies failed to reveal that the course of the arthritis was affected by treatment or removal of infectious foci during hospitalization.

45.19 A definite anemia, measured by the red-cell count, was encountered in more than one-fifth of the patients. Anemia was related to greater disease activity and severity and to gastric anacidity. The white-cell count was within normal limits in 75 per cent of the series, and leukocytosis was much more frequent than leukopenia in the remainder. Splenomegaly was common in patients with leukopenia but rare in those with leukocytosis. Albuminuria, cylindruria, or both were recorded for nearly one-sixth of the patients. This finding, taken in conjunction with autopsy studies, suggests the presence of a renal lesion

Summary

among the systemic manifestations of rheumatoid arthritis. Elevation of the blood uric acid was found in about the same frequency as in control groups. The results obtained from gastric analyses differed from those in comparable control series to the extent that patients under forty years of age showed a tendency toward an increased frequency of anacidity. Contrary to the results in another study, our findings in patients over forty years of age were similar to those in controls. In agreement with previous studies, the basal metabolism rate was found to be below normal in one-fourth of the patients. Recent observations elsewhere have suggested that a true hypothyroidism is responsible for this condition. In our series, as well as in some reported by the literature, an association was apparent between rheumatoid arthritis and thyroid disorders.

45.20   A diagnosis of rheumatoid spondylitis was made in 14 per cent of the series on the basis of either persistent spinal limitation or characteristic roentgenographic changes, or, in most instances, both. In over half of these patients, peripheral joints distal to the hips and shoulders were involved. Minor spinal symptoms or signs were noted in 44 additional patients. This group was composed largely of females over forty years of age, in contrast to the group with spondylitis which was composed chiefly of younger males. A numerical comparison between the male spondylitics and the remaining males revealed important differences only in regard to age distribution and, among the spondylitics, a less favorable subsequent course and the infrequency of nodules. These results favor the concept of rheumatoid spondylitis as the spinal localization of rheumatoid arthritis rather than a separate disease entity.

45.21   In each patient of our series, the degree of disease activity, the extent of articular involvement, and the total disease severity* at the time of hospitalization were estimated by several observers. A longer duration of arthritis and hence usually a greater age on admission were related to more marked involvement and severity but not to the degree of disease activity. Bilateral distribution of joint involvement from the start was also related to increased severity but no association was found between severity on admission and age or occupation at onset or, in women, onset in proximity to the menopause.

45.22   In an attempt to obtain information of possible prognostic

* See definition, par. 4.26.

importance, tabulations were made of the patients' disease status in 1937, 1947, and 1954 relative to their condition on hospital admission between 1930 and 1936. Patients were excluded from the tabulations if they were unavailable for follow-up or if they had received special therapy. The 1947 study was based on 250 patients who had received only simple medical and orthopedic treatment, and all but 11 of these had been included in the 1937 study. The rate of improvement—53.2 per cent—was approximately the same as it had been in 1937, and the following factors were associated with improvement: male sex (among those without spondylitis); age under forty on admission; duration of arthritis for one year or less before admission; absence of spondylitis (among males); and mild disease severity on admission. By 1954, with an average follow-up period of fourteen years, the percentage deemed improved had fallen to 35 per cent. Although a substantial proportion of those who had improved early in the course of their disease were able to maintain this status, improvement rarely followed failure to demonstrate a favorable course over a period of ten years or more. The results of the 1947 study agree essentially with those of a study reported in 1949 [423] of a similar series of patients. While we are now aware of the limitations of some of the methods used to evaluate the course of rheumatoid arthritis, we believe that the outcome is useful for comparison with series of patients receiving special forms of therapy over similar periods of time.

45.23   Although it was our original intention to provide a complete cross-sectional and longitudinal description of rheumatoid arthritis, it is evident that our goal was not accomplished. It is hoped, however, that this study will stimulate others to devise means of reaching the original objective. Only in this way shall we obtain much-needed information about the nature of rheumatoid arthritis and other chronic diseases of unknown causation and of great economic and social significance.

Appendix

Table 46

Summary of historical and physical findings for patients of present series and corresponding controls

	Patients		Controls		Difference in percentages*
	No.	Per cent	No.	Per cent	
Family history:					
Cardio-vascular-renal disease	120	41.0	128	43.7	2.7
Cancer	52	17.8	63	21.5	3.7
Diabetes mellitus	28	9.6	28	9.6	0.0
Migraine	10	3.4	12	4.1	0.7
Allergic disease	47	16.0	47	16.0	0.0
Degenerative joint disease	17	5.8	15	5.1	0.7
Rheumatoid arthritis	35	11.9	15	5.1	6.8 ± 2.3
Rheumatic fever	34	11.6	10	3.4	8.2 ± 2.2
"Undetermined and other" forms of rheumatism	68	23.2	37	12.6	10.6 ± 3.2
Total with rheumatic disease	124	42.3	71	24.2	18.1 ± 3.9
Past or present allergic disease:					
Asthma	5	1.7	9	3.1	1.4
Hay fever	10	3.4	13	4.4	1.0
Urticaria	31	10.6	20	6.8	3.8
1 or more of above	39	13.3	40	13.7	0.4
History of:					
Serious illness	170	58.0	126	43.0	15.0 ± 4.1
Serious operation	115	39.2	101	34.5	4.7
Severe injury	42	14.3	37	12.6	1.7
Menopause:					
Artificial	15	8.1	11	5.9	2.2
Natural	73	39.2	70	37.6	1.6
Prodromal symptoms:					
Fatigue	137	46.8	62	21.2	25.6 ± 3.9
Skeletal pain	86	29.4	82	28.0	1.4
Appetite loss	50	17.1	28	9.6	7.5 ± 2.8
Sensory symptoms	37	12.6	27	9.2	3.4
Symptoms intensified by weather	32	10.9	27	9.2	1.7
None	119	40.6	151	51.5	10.9 ± 4.1

* Shown with standard error when significant.

Table 46 (cont.)

	Patients		Controls		Difference in percentages*
	No.	Per cent	No.	Per cent	
Constitutional symptoms:					
Weakness or fatigue	234	79.9	62	21.2	58.7 ± 4.1
Anorexia	153	52.2	22	7.5	44.7 ± 3.8
Weight loss	228	77.8	43	14.7	63.1 ± 4.1
Headache	72	24.6	67	27.7†	3.1
Vasomotor symptoms:					
Cold extremities	161	54.9	44	15.0	39.9 ± 3.9
Paresthesias	102	34.8	27	9.2	25.6 ± 3.4
Cyanosis	61	20.8	11	3.8	17.0 ± 2.6
Vascular spasm	33	11.3	8	2.7	8.6 ± 2.1
Vasomotor signs	97	33.1	27	9.2	23.9 ± 3.4
Neurologic symptoms:					
Twitching	83	28.4	24	8.2	20.2 ± 3.2
Vertigo	61	20.9	36	12.3	8.6 ± 3.1
Tremor	64	21.9	22	7.5	14.4 ± 2.9
Tinnitus	48	16.4	37	12.7	3.7
Nervousness and/or emotional upsets	177	60.6	142	48.6	12.0 ± 4.1
Neurologic signs:					
Tremor	22	7.5	19	6.5	1.0
Exaggerated reflexes	96	32.8	50	17.1	15.7 ± 3.3
Valvular heart disease	6	2.0	4	1.4	0.6
Abnormal pulmonary signs:					
Consolidation	11	3.8	4	1.4	2.4
Emphysema	10	3.4	13	4.5	1.1
Rales (without consolidation)	34	11.6	17	5.8	5.8 ± 2.3
Pleurisy	5	1.7	3	1.0	0.7
Gastro-intestinal symptoms:					
Nausea (total)	44	15.0	29	9.9	5.1
Nausea with vomiting	33	11.3	19	6.5	4.8 ± 2.4
Abdominal pain	28	9.6	28	9.6	0.0
Flatulence	62	21.2	66	22.5	1.3
Constipation	113	38.6	43	14.7	23.9 ± 3.7
Diarrhea (ulcerative colitis excluded)	8	2.7	1	0.3	2.4 ± 1.0

* Shown with standard error when significant.
† Figured on 242 controls, since 51 with eye disease were excluded.

Table 46 (cont.)

	Patients		Controls		Difference in percentages*
	No.	Per cent	No.	Per cent	
Systolic blood pressure:					
Less than 110	40	13.7	15	5.1	8.6 ± 2.4
110 to 140	209	71.3	193	65.9	5.4
Greater than 140	44	15.0	85	29.0	14.0 ± 3.3
Ocular abnormalities:					
Arcus senilis	22	7.5	17	5.8	1.7
Pupillary	19	6.5	16	5.5	1.0
Arteriosclerosis of fundi	49	16.7	64	21.8	5.1
Enlargement of:					
Lymph nodes	86	29.4	26	8.9	20.5 ± 3.4
Spleen	19	6.5	6	2.0	4.5 ± 1.7
Liver	22	7.5	26	8.9	1.4
Skin atrophy	92	31.4	18	6.1	25.3 ± 3.2
Skin disease:					
Psoriasis	10	3.4	2	0.7	2.7 ± 1.2
Acne	8	2.7	13	4.4	1.7
Eczema	6	2.0	7	2.4	0.4
Herpes zoster (by history)	4	1.4	8	2.7	1.3
Vitiligo	3	1.0	2	0.7	0.3
Carotinemia	2	0.7	0	0.0	0.7
Keratoses	2	0.7	1	0.3	0.4
Edema:					
Total	28	9.6	16	5.5	4.1
Not due to extraneous causes	14	4.8	2	0.7	4.1 ± 1.3
Varicosities	24	8.2	43	14.7	6.5 ± 2.6
Subcutaneous nodules	34	11.6	2	0.7	10.9 ± 2.0

* Shown with standard error when significant.

Note: For **Table 47**, showing list of associations, see inside the back cover.

Bibliography

Bibliography

1. à Court, A. H., The treatment of chronic arthritis, *M. J. Australia* 2:415–418, Sept. 1936
2. Adams, R., *Illustrations of the Effects of Rheumatic Gout, or Chronic Rheumatic Arthritis, on All the Articulations; with Descriptive and Explanatory Statements.* 31 pp. John Churchill, London, 1857
3. Allen, E. V., Relationship of sex to disease, *Ann. Int. Med.* 7:1000–1012, Feb. 1934
4. Allison, N., and Ghormley, R. K., *Diagnosis in Joint Disease: a Clinical and Pathological Study of Arthritis.* 196 pp. William Wood, New York, 1931
5. Aronoff, A., Bywaters, E. G. L., and Fearnley, G. R., Lung lesions in rheumatoid arthritis, *Brit. M. J.* 2:228–232, July 1955
6. Bach, F., "Chronic arthritis and its possible relation with the function of the thyroid and parathyroid glands," in C. W. Buckley (ed.), *Reports on Chronic Rheumatic Diseases*, pp. 133–137, H. K. Lewis, London, 1935
7. Baggenstoss, A. H., and Rosenberg, E. F., Cardiac lesions associated with chronic infectious arthritis, *Arch. Int. Med.* 67:241–258, Feb. 1941
8. Baggenstoss, A. H., and Rosenberg, E. F., Visceral lesions associated with chronic infectious (rheumatoid) arthritis, *Arch. Path.* 35:503–516, April 1943
9. Baker, B. M., Jr., Undulant fever presenting the clinical syndrome of intermittent hydrarthrosis, *Arch. Int. Med.* 44:128–141, July 1929
10. Balboni, V. G., and Kydd, D. M., "The status of the two types of arthritis following gonorrhea, with a report of eighty-nine cases resembling rheuma-

toid arthritis," in C. H. Slocumb (ed.), *Rheumatic Diseases*, pp. 77–81. Saunders, Philadelphia, 1952

11. Ball, J., Rheumatoid arthritis and polyarteritis nodosa, *Ann. Rheumat. Dis.* 13:277–290, Dec. 1954

12. Balzer, F., and Burnier, Psoriasis et arthropathies, *Bull. Soc. franç. de dermat. et syph.* 22:179–190, May 1911

13. Bannatyne, G. A., *Rheumatoid Arthritis, Its Pathology, Morbid Anatomy, and Treatment* Second edition. 182 pp. John Wright, Bristol, 1898

14. Barber, H. W., Acrodermatitis continua vel perstans (dermatitis repens) and psoriasis pustulosa, *Brit. J. Dermat.* 42:500–518, Nov. 1930

15. Bargen, J. A., Complications and sequelae of chronic ulcerative colitis, *Ann. Int. Med.* 3:335–352, Oct. 1929

16. Bargen, J. A., *The Management of Colitis* (M. Fishbein [ed.], National Medical Monographs). 234 pp. National Medical Book Company, 1935

17. Bargen, J. A., Jackman, R. J., and Kerr, J. G., Studies on the life histories of patients with chronic ulcerative colitis (thrombo-ulcerative colitis) with some suggestions for treatment, *Ann. Int. Med.* 12:339–352, Sept. 1938

18. Barker, L. F., Differentiation of the diseases included under chronic arthritis, *Am. J. M. Sc.* 174:1–29, Jan. 1914

19. Barter, R. W., Familial incidence of rheumatoid arthritis and acute rheumatism in 100 rheumatoid arthritics, *Ann. Rheumat. Dis.* 11:39–46, March 1952

20. Bauer, J., Der sogenannte Rheumatismus. 142 pp. Steinkopff, Leipzig, 1929

21. Bauer, J., and Vogl, A., Psoriasis und Gelenkleiden; zugleich ein Beitrag zur Kenntnis des hereditären Hydrops articulorum intermittens, *Klin. Wchnschr.* 10:1700–1705, Sept. 1931

22. Bauer, W., Bennett, G. A., and Zeller, J. W., Pathology of joint lesions in patients with psoriasis and arthritis, *Tr. A. Am. Physicians* 56:349–352, 1941

23. Bauer, W., and Clark, W. S., The systemic manifestations of rheumatoid arthritis, *Tr. A. Am. Physicians* 61:339–342, 1948

24. Bauer, W., and Engleman, E. P., A syndrome of unknown etiology characterized by urethritis, conjunctivitis, and arthritis (so-called Reiter's disease), *Tr. A. Am. Physicians* 57:307–313, 1942

25. Bauer, W., Giansiracusa, J. E., and Kulka, J. P., "The protean nature of the connective tissue diseases," in C. H. Slocumb (ed.), *Rheumatic Diseases*, pp. 391–400. Saunders, Philadelphia, 1952

26. Bayles, T. B., Rheumatoid arthritis and rheumatic heart disease in autopsied cases, *Am. J. M. Sc.* 205:42–48, Jan. 1943

Bibliography

27. Bayles, T. B., Palmer, R. J., Massod, M. F., and Judd, E. H., Vitamin B excretion studies in patients with rheumatoid arthritis, *New England J. Med.* 242:249–252, Feb. 1950

28. Bayliss, R. A., Acute rheumatoid arthritis, *Edinburgh M. J.* n.s. 6:160–164, 1899

29. Beattie, J. W., and Woodmansey, A., Effects of ACTH on the peripheral blood flow in rheumatoid arthritis, *Ann. Rheumat. Dis.* 12:43–45, March 1953

30. Bennett, G. A., Medical criteria which govern relations of trauma to joint disease, *Clinics* 1:1448–1475, April 1943

31. Bennett, G. A., Comparison of the pathology of rheumatic fever and rheumatoid arthritis, *Ann. Int. Med.* 19:111–113, July 1943. Proc.

32. Bennett, G. A., Discussion of paper by D. H. Collins in C. H. Slocumb (ed.), *Rheumatic Diseases,* pp. 317–318. Saunders, Philadelphia, 1952

33. Bennett, G. A., Personal communication

34. Bennett, G. A., Waine, H., and Bauer, W., *Changes in the Knee Joint at Various Ages; with Particular Reference to the Nature and Development of Degenerative Joint Disease.* 97 pp. Commonwealth Fund, New York, 1942

35. Bennett, G. A., Zeller, J. W., and Bauer, W., Subcutaneous nodules of rheumatoid arthritis and rheumatic fever: pathologic study, *Arch. Path.* 30:70–89, July 1940

36. Berens, C., Rothbard, S., and Angevine, D. M., Cultural studies on patients with uveitis and other eye diseases, *Am. J. Ophth.* 25:295–301, March 1942

37. Berger, H., Intermittent hydrarthrosis with an allergic basis, *J.A.M.A.* 112:2402–2405, June 1939

37a. Berkson, J., Limitations of the application of fourfold table analysis to hospital data, *Biometrics Bull.* 2:47–53, June 1946

38. Bevans, M., Nadell, J., Demartini, F., and Ragan, C., The systemic lesions of malignant rheumatoid arthritis, *Am. J. Med.* 16:197–211, Feb. 1954

39. Biering, W. L., Intermittent hydrarthrosis, *J.A.M.A.* 77:785–789, Sept. 1921

40. Billings, F., Chronic focal infections and their etiologic relations to arthritis and nephritis, *Arch. Int. Med.* 9:484–498, 1912

41. Bloom, J., and Rubin, J. H., Transient pulmonary manifestations in rheumatoid arthritis, *Canad. M. A. J.* 63:355–357, Oct. 1950

42. Blumer, G., "Gonococcic infections," Chapter III in H. A. Christian (ed.), *Oxford Medicine,* vol. 5, pp. 39–70. Oxford University Press, New York, 1939

43. Boger, W. P., Pneumococcic arthritis: report of a case of so-called primary pneumococcic arthritis, *J.A.M.A.* **126**:1062–1065, Dec. 1944
44. Boland, E. W., and Corr, W. P., Psychogenic rheumatism, *J.A.M.A.* **123**: 805–809, Nov. 1943
45. Boland, E. W., and Headley, N. E., Treatment of so-called palindromic rheumatism with gold compounds, *Ann. Rheumat. Dis.* **8**:64–69, March 1949
46. Boothby, W. M., and Sandiford, I., Summary of basal metabolism data on 8,614 subjects with special reference to normal standards for estimation of the basal metabolic rate, *J. Biol. Chem.* **54**:783–803, Dec. 1922
47. Boots, R. H., Lipman, M. O., Coss, J. A., Jr., and Ragan, C., "Immunologic reactions in rheumatoid arthritis," in C. H. Slocumb (ed.), *Rheumatic Diseases*, pp. 336–342. Saunders, Philadelphia, 1952
48. Boots, R. H., and McCollom, R. L., Relationship of upper respiratory infections to chronic arthritis, *Bull. New York Acad. Med.* **18**:347–355, May 1942
49. Bourdillon, C., *Psoriasis et arthropathies*. 257 pp. Thèse de Paris, No. 328, 1888
50. Bourgeois, Lorain, and Féréol, Sur les accidents rhumatismaux dans le cours de la blennorrhagie, *Union Méd.* n.s. **32**:611–622, 1866
51. Boyd, C. S., Arthritis of scarlet fever, *M. Clin. North America* **21**:1741–1746, Nov. 1937
52. Brabazon, A. B., Analysis of 100 cases of rheumatoid arthritis treated in the Royal Mineral Water Hospital, Bath, *Brit. M. J.* **1**:723–724, March 1896
53. Brandt, G., and Weihe, F. A., *Ztschr. f. mensch. Vererb. u. Konst.-lehre* **23**: 169–188, 1939. As cited by R. R. Gates in *Human Genetics*, vol. 1, p. 1264. Macmillan, New York, 1946
54. Brav, E. A., and Hench, P. S., Tuberculous rheumatism: a résumé, *J. Bone & Joint Surg.* **16**:839–866, Oct. 1934
55. Bridges, M. A., *Dietetics for the Clinician*, pp. 726–727. Second edition. Lea & Febiger, Philadelphia, 1935
56. British Medical Association Committee on Arthritis, Causation and treatment of arthritis and allied conditions, *Brit. M. J.* **1**:1033–1052, June 1933
57. Brocq, L., Quelques réflexions sur l'étiologie du psoriasis à propos des récentes publications américaines, *Ann. de dermat. et syph.*, series 5, **1**:156–183, 1910
58. Buckley, C. W. (ed.), *Reports on Chronic Rheumatic Diseases, being the Annual Report of the British Committee on Chronic Rheumatic Diseases Appointed by the Royal College of Physicians*, vol. 1, 159 pp. H. K. Lewis, London, 1935

59. Buckley, C. W., "Ankylosing spondylitis," in C. W. Buckley (ed.), *Reports on Chronic Rheumatic Diseases*, vol. 1, pp. 77–89. H. K. Lewis, London, 1935
60. Buckley, C. W., Rheumatism in industry, *J. State Med.* **43**:587–595, Oct. 1935
61. Buckley, C. W., Prognosis in arthritis, *Lancet* **1**:1023–1025; 1081–1082, May 1936
62. Budd, W., On diseases which affect corresponding parts of the body in a symmetrical manner, *Medico-Chir. Tr.*, series 2, **7**:100–166, published by the Royal Medical and Chirurgical Society, London, 1842
63. Bulkley, K., Pneumococcic arthritis, *Ann. Surg.* **59**:71–100, Jan. 1914
64. Bunim, J. J., Sokoloff, L., Williams, R. R., and Black, R. L., Rheumatoid arthritis: a review of recent advances in our knowledge concerning pathology, diagnosis, and treatment, *J. Chronic Dis.* **1**:168–210, Feb. 1955
65. Burks, J. W., and Montgomery, H., Histopathologic study of psoriasis, *Arch. Dermat. & Syph.* **48**:479–493, Nov. 1943
66. Burt, J. B., Discussion on climacteric arthritis, *Proc. Roy. Soc. Med.* (Sect. Balneol. and Climatol.) **20**:513–516, Jan. 1927
67. Burt, J. B., Gordon, R. G., and Brown, A. R., "The autonomic nervous system in rheumatoid arthritis," in *A Survey of Chronic Rheumatic Diseases*, pp. 137–147. Oxford University Press, London, 1938
68. Byfield, A. H., Arthritis deformans, Chapter 166 in I. A. Abt (ed.), *Pediatrics*, vol. 6, pp. 693–715. Saunders, Philadelphia, 1925
69. Bywaters, E. G. L., A variant of rheumatoid arthritis characterized by recurrent digital pad nodules and palmar fasciitis closely resembling palindromic rheumatism, *Ann. Rheumat. Dis.* **8**:1–30, March 1949
70. Bywaters, E. G. L., Relation between heart and joint disease including "rheumatoid heart disease" and chronic post-rheumatic arthritis (type Jaccoud), *Brit. Heart J.* **12**:101–131, April 1950
71. Carroll, J. H., and Nelson, R. L., Still's disease with amyloidosis: case, *Arch. Pediat.* **44**:187–190, March 1927
72. Catchpole, B. N., Jepson, R. P., and Kellgren, J. H., Peripheral vascular effect of cortisone in rheumatoid arthritis, scleroderma, and other related conditions, *Ann. Rheumat. Dis.* **13**:302–306, Dec. 1954
73. Cecil, R. L., Influential factors in recovery from rheumatoid arthritis, *Ann. Int. Med.* **8**:315–326, Sept. 1934
74. Cecil, R. L., *The Diagnosis and Treatment of Arthritis*. (H. A. Christian [ed.], Oxford Monographs on Diagnosis and Treatment, vol. 6.) 263 pp. Oxford University Press, New York, 1936

75. Cecil, R. L., Arthritis—curable disease? *J. Michigan M. Soc.* 41:311–315, April 1952
76. Cecil, R. L., and Angevine, D. M., Clinical and experimental observations on focal infection, with an analysis of 200 cases of rheumatoid arthritis, *Ann. Int. Med.* 12:577–584, Nov. 1938
77. Cecil, R. L., and Archer, B. H., Arthritis of the menopause: a study of fifty cases, *J.A.M.A.* 84:75–79, Jan. 1925
78. Cecil, R. L., and Archer, B. H., Classification and treatment of chronic arthritis, *J.A.M.A.* 87:741–746, Sept. 1926
79. Cecil, R. L., Nicholls, E. E., and Stainsby, W. J., Bacteriology of blood and joints in chronic infectious arthritis, *Arch. Int. Med.* 43:571–605, May 1929
80. Charcot, J. M., *Études pour servir à l'histoire de l'affection décrite sous les noms de goutte asthénique primitive, nodosités des jointures, rhumatisme articulaire chronique (forme primitive), etc.* 58 pp. Thèse de Paris, No. 44, 1853
81. Charcot, J. M., *Clinical Lectures on Senile and Chronic Diseases.* Translated by William S. Tuke. 307 pp. The New Sydenham Society, London, 1881
82. Charcot, J. M., Cited by A. E. Garrod in *A Treatise on Rheumatism and Rheumatoid Arthritis,* p. 270. Charles Griffin, London, 1890
83. Chauffard, A., and Ramond, F., Des adénopathies dans le rhumatisme chronique infectieux, *Rev. de méd., Paris* 16:345–359, May 1896
84. Chesney, A. M., Kemp, J. E., and Baetjer, F. H., An experimental study of the synovial fluid of patients with arthritis and syphilis, *J. Clin. Invest.* 3:131–148, Oct. 1926
85. Chesney, A. M., Kemp, J. E., and Resnik, W. H., Syphilitic arthritis with eosinophilia: recovery of *T. pallidum* from the synovial fluid, *Bull. Johns Hopkins Hosp.* 35:235–239, Aug. 1924
86. Chevais, T. L. M., *Des réflexes tendineux dans le rhumatisme chronique.* 75 pp. Thèse de Paris, no. 599, 1897
87. Ciocco, A., Sex differences in morbidity and mortality, *Quart. Rev. Biol.* 15:59–73; 192–210, March and June 1940
88. Civatte, A., Psoriasis and seborrheic eczema: pathological anatomy and diagnostic histology of the two dermatoses, *Brit. J. Dermat. & Syph.* 36:461–476, Nov. 1924
89. Clark, W. S., and Bauer, W., Cardiac changes in rheumatoid arthritis, *Ann. Rheumat. Dis.* 7:39–40, March 1948. Proc.
90. Clark, K. S., Rheumatoid arthritis; its etiology, clinical symptoms, and pathology, *Scottish Med. & Surg. J.* 22:121–136, Feb. 1908

91. Clemmesen, S., and Arnsø, E., "A statistical analysis of 1000 cases of rheumatoid arthritis in relation to insidious and acute onset, menopause, pregnancy, psoriasis, ankylosing spondylitis and Still's disease," in C. H. Slocumb (ed.), *Rheumatic Diseases*, pp. 54–66. Saunders, Philadelphia, 1952
92. Clinch, T. A., The arthropathic dystrophies, *Brit. M. J.* 2:1925–1927, Dec. 1898
93. Clutton, H. H., Symmetrical synovitis of the knee in hereditary syphilis, *Lancet* 1:391–393, Feb. 1886
94. Coates, V., Clinical types of so-called multiple infective arthritis, *Proc. Roy. Soc. Med.* (Sect. Balneol. and Climatol.) 18:13–18, Jan. 1925
95. Coates, V., Discussion on Climacteric Arthritis, *Proc. Roy. Soc. Med.* (Sect. Balneol. and Climatol.) 20:521–522, Jan. 1927
96. Coates, V., Relation of orthodox rheumatic infection to multiple infective arthritis, *Brit. M. J.* 1:67–68, Jan. 1930
97. Coates, V., and Delicati, L., *Rheumatoid Arthritis and Its Treatment. Studies from the Royal Mineral Water Hospital, Bath.* 114 pp. H. K. Lewis, London, 1931
98. Coates, V., and Delicati, L., The correlation between certain rheumatic disorders and occupation, *Acta rheumatol.* 4:28–32, Dec. 1932
99. Cobb, S., Anderson, F., and Bauer, W., Length of life and cause of death in rheumatoid arthritis, *New England J. Med.* 249:553–556, Oct. 1953
100. Cobb, S., Bauer, W., and Whiting, I., Environmental factors in rheumatoid arthritis: study of the relationship between onset and exacerbations of arthritis and emotional or environmental factors, *J.A.M.A.* 113:668–670, Aug. 1939
101. Coggeshall, H. C., and Bauer, W., Unpublished data
102. Coggeshall, H. C., Bennett, G. A., Warren, C. F., and Bauer, W., Synovial fluid and synovial membrane abnormalities resulting from varying grades of systemic infection and edema, *Am. J. M. Sc.* 202:486–502, Oct. 1941; and also correction on p. 916, Dec. 1941
103. Cole, R., "Gonococcus Infections," Chapter 20 in W. Osler and T. McCrae (ed.), *Modern Medicine, Its Theory and Practice*, vol. 1, pp. 743–765. Second edition. Lea & Febiger, Philadelphia, 1913
104. Coleman, G. H., and Capps, J. A., Diverticulitis of the colon: preliminary report of a study of its potential rôle as a focus of infection in systemic disease, *Arch. Path.* 26:207–209, July 1938
105. Collins, D. H., Observations on anaemia in chronic rheumatic diseases, *Lancet* 2:548–550, Sept. 1935

106. Collins, D. H., "Neutrophil leucopenia, with enlargement of liver and spleen in rheumatoid arthritis; with a note on the leucocytic blood picture in chronic rheumatism," in C. W. Buckley (ed.), *Reports on Chronic Rheumatic Diseases*, vol. 3, pp. 49-58. Macmillan, New York, 1937
107. Collins, D. H., The subcutaneous nodule of rheumatoid arthritis, *J. Path. & Bact.* 45:97-115, July 1937
108. Collins, D. H., *The Pathology of Articular and Spinal Diseases*. 331 pp. Williams & Wilkins, Baltimore, 1950
109. Collins, D. H., "The range of pathologic reactions which can be displayed by human synovial tissues—a contribution to the study of specific lesions," in C. H. Slocumb (ed.), *Rheumatic Diseases*, pp. 317-318. Saunders, Philadelphia, 1952
110. Collins, D. H., and Cameron, C., Multiple arthritis in presumably tuberculous subjects: difficulties in diagnosis and treatment, *Brit. J. Surg.* 24:272-291, Oct. 1936
111. Collins, S. D., Trantham, K. S., and Lehmann, J. L., *Sickness Experience in Selected Areas of the United States* (Public Health Monograph no. 25; issued concurrently with the Jan. 1955 issue of *Pub. Health Reports*, vol. 70, no. 1). 96 pp.
112. Colver, T., Prognosis in rheumatoid arthritis in childhood, *Arch. Dis. Childhood* 12:253-260, Aug. 1937
113. Comroe, B. I., *Arthritis and Allied Conditions*. Third edition. 1359 pp. Lea & Febiger, Philadelphia, 1944
114. Cooperman, M. B., End results of gonorrheal arthritis: review of 70 cases, *Am. J. Surg.* 5:241-251, Sept. 1928
115. Cooperman, M. B., Chronic tuberculous polyarthritis, *Ann. Surg.* 96:1065-1077, Dec. 1932
116. Copeman, W. S. C., "On a tuberculous factor in the aetiology of certain cases of rheumatoid (atrophic) arthritis (Mayo Foundation lecture, abridged)," in C. W. Buckley (ed.), *Reports on Chronic Rheumatic Diseases*, vol. 2, pp. 24-55. Macmillan, New York, 1936
117. Copeman, W. S. C., "The 'rheumatoid syndrome' and the pre-arthritic stage," in *A Survey of Chronic Rheumatic Diseases*, pp. 127-136. Oxford University Press, London, 1938
118. Copeman, W. S. C., and Clay, R. D., Rheumatoid arthritis believed to be of tuberculous origin: report of 2 cases, *Lancet* 2:1460-1461, Dec. 1935
119. Cornil, M. V., Mémoire sur les coincidences pathologiques du rhumatisme articulaire chronique, *Mémoires lus à la Société de biologie*, series 4, 3:3-25, 1864

Bibliography

120. Corscaden, J. A., Arthritis and radiotherapeutic menopause, *Am. J. Roentgenol.* **19**:321-323, April 1928
121. Coss, J. A., Jr., and Boots, R. H., Juvenile rheumatoid arthritis: a study of 56 cases with a note on skeletal changes, *J. Pediat.* **29**:143-156, Aug. 1946
122. Cousin, C., *De Quelques Symptômes communs au rhumatisme chronique et aux affections nerveuses*, 96 pp. Thèse de Paris, no. 382, 1890
123. Craven, E. B., Jr., Splenectomy in chronic arthritis associated with splenomegaly and leukopenia (Felty's syndrome), *J.A.M.A.* **102**:823-826, March 1934
124. Crowe, H. W., Chronic rheumatic arthritis, *The Medical Press and Circular* **194**:426-428, May 1927
125. Curtis, A. C., and Pollard, H. M., Felty's syndrome; its several features, including tissue changes, compared with other forms of rheumatoid arthritis, *Ann. Int. Med.* **13**:2265-2284, June 1940
126. Dahlberg, G., and Sundelin, F., Rheumatoid arthritis and the function of joints, *Acta med. Scandinav.* **135**:40-46, 1949
127. Dameshek, W., and Estren, S., Symposium on specific methods of treatment; hypersplenism, *M. Clin. North America* **34**:1271-1289, Sept. 1950
128. Dance, M., Observations sur une espèce de tétanos intermittent, *Arch. gén. de méd.* **26**:190-205, June 1831
129. Darley, W., and Gordon, R. W., Brucella sensitization: a clinical evaluation, *Ann. Int. Med.* **26**:528-541, April 1947
130. Davidson, L. S. P., Duthie, J. J. R., and Sugar, M., Focal infection in rheumatoid arthritis: a comparison of the incidence of foci of infections in the upper respiratory tract in one hundred cases of rheumatoid arthritis and one hundred controls, *Ann. Rheumat. Dis.* **8**:205-208, Sept. 1949
131. Davidson, L. S. P., and Goldie, W., "Chronic infective arthritis," in C. W. Buckley (ed.), *Reports on Chronic Rheumatic Diseases*, vol. 2, pp. 1-23. Macmillan, New York, 1936
132. Davis, E., Purpura of the skin: a review of 500 cases, *Lancet* **2**:160-161, Aug. 1943
133. Dawson, M. H., "Chronic arthritis," Chapter 29 in *Nelson New Loose-Leaf Medicine*, pp. 605-644. Thomas Nelson & Sons, New York, 1935
134. Dawson, M. H., The rôle of the streptococcus in chronic arthritis, *M. Clin. North America* **21**:1663-1670, Nov. 1937
135. Dawson, M. H., Personal communication
136. Dawson, M. H., and Boots, R. H., Subcutaneous nodules in rheumatoid (chronic infectious) arthritis, *J.A.M.A.* **95**:1894-1896, Dec. 1930

137. Dawson, M. H., Olmstead, M., and Boots, R. H., Agglutination reactions in rheumatoid arthritis; agglutination reactions with Streptococcus hemolyticus, *J. Immunol.* **23**:187–204, Sept. 1932

138. Dawson, M. H., and Tyson, T. L., Relationship between rheumatic fever and rheumatoid arthritis, *J. Lab. & Clin. Med.* **21**:575–587, March 1936

139. Dawson, M. H., and Tyson, T. L., Psoriasis arthropathica, with observations on certain features common to psoriasis and rheumatoid arthritis, *Tr. A. Am. Physicians* **53**:303–309, 1938

140. de Baillou, G., "Liber de Rheumatismo," in *Opera Omnia*, book IV. Paris, 1642. Cited by R. Stockman in *Rheumatism and Arthritis*, p. 4. W. Green & Son, Edinburgh, 1920

141. Delcourt, A., Rhumatisme articulaire noueux chez les enfants, *Rev. mensuelle des maladies de l'enfance* **16**:329–347, July 1898

142. Desmarais, M. H. L., Gibson, H. J., and Kersley, G. D., Muscle histology in rheumatic and control cases: a study of one hundred and nineteen biopsy specimens, *Ann. Rheumat. Dis.* **7**:132–142, Sept. 1948

143. De Wolf, H. F., Pustular psoriasis with arthritis of the fingers, *Arch. Dermat. & Syph.* **26**:587, Sept. 1932. Trans.

144. Dexter, L., "Vascular hypotension," in R. L. Cecil and R. F. Loeb (ed.), *A Textbook of Medicine*, pp. 1079–1080. Eighth edition. Saunders, Philadelphia, 1951

145. Diamentberger, S., *Rhumatisme noueux chez les enfants*, 1891. As cited by R. L. Jones in *Arthritis Deformans*, etc., p. 353. William Wood, New York, 1909

146. Dickson, F. D., Differential diagnosis of tuberculosis arthritis, *J. Lab. & Clin. Med.* **22**:35–43, Oct. 1936

147. Dixon, A. St. J., Kahn, D. S., and Bauer, W. To be published

148. Dixon, A. St. J., Ramcharan, S., and Ropes, M. W., Rheumatoid arthritis: dye retention studies and comparison of dye and radioactively labelled red cell methods for measurement of blood volume, *Ann. Rheumat. Dis.* **14**:51–62, March 1955

149. Doupe, J., Cullen, C. H., and Chance, G. Q., Post-traumatic pain and the causalgic syndrome, *J. Neurol. Neurosurg. & Psychiat.* n.s. **7**:33–48, Jan.–April 1944

150. Douthwaite, A. H., *The Treatment of Rheumatoid Arthritis and Sciatica*. Second edition. 131 pp. H. K. Lewis, London, 1933

151. Duckworth, D., On the nosological relations of chronic rheumatic (rheumatoid) arthritis, *Brit. M. J.* **2**:263–270, Aug. 1884

152. Dunham, C. L., and Kautz, F. G., Spondylarthritis ankylopoietica: review and report of 20 cases, *Am. J. M. Sc.* **201**:232–250, Feb. 1941

153. Dustan, H. P., Taylor, R. D., Corcoran, A. C., and Page, I. H., Rheumatic and febrile syndrome during prolonged hydralazine treatment, *J.A.M.A.* 154:23–29, Jan. 1954

154. Duthie, J. J. R., Thompson, M., Weir, M. M., and Fletcher, W. B., Medical and social aspects of the treatment of rheumatoid arthritis with special reference to factors affecting prognosis, *Ann. Rheumat. Dis.* 14:133–149, June 1955

155. Eaton, E. R., Chronic arthritis, a report based on the study of the blood-cell count in 250 cases, *J. Am. Inst. Homeop.* 25:125–136, Feb. 1932

156. Eaton, E. R., Chronic arthritis: a consideration of the etiologic factors, *J. Am. Inst. Homeop.* 25:379–406, April 1932

157. Eaton, E. R., Chronic arthritis: a study of the symptomatology; systemic manifestations, *J. Am. Inst. Homeop.* 25:612–641, June 1932

158. Eaton, E. R., Chronic arthritis: a study of the symptomatology; local joint manifestations, *J. Am. Inst. Homeop.* 26:321–332, May 1933

159. Eaton, E. R., Chronic arthritis: a study of the habits of five hundred patients, *J. Am. Inst. Homeop.* 26:568–572, August 1933

160. Eaton, E. R., and Cocheu, L. F., Chronic arthritis: original biochemical studies with a review of the literature, *J. Am. Inst. Homeop.* 25:485–528, May 1932

161. Ebaugh, F. G., Peterson, R. E., Rodnan, G. P., and Bunim, J. J. The anemia of rheumatoid arthritis, *M. Clin. North America* 39:489–498, March 1955

162. Ebert, M. H., Psoriasiform eruption with pustular exacerbations, *Arch. Dermat. & Syph.* 27:933–950, June 1933

163. Edström, G., *Febris rheumatica: eine Studie in ihrer Epidemiologie, Klinik, und Prognose; mit besonderer Berücksichtigung des Verhältnissen in Schweden.* 317 pp. Berlingska Boktryckeriet, Lund, 1935

164. Edström, G., Magensekretion und Grundumsatz bei den chronischen rheumatischen Arthritiden, *Acta med. Scandinav.* 99:228–256, 1939

165. Edström, G., Klinische Studien über den chronischen Gelenkrheumatismus —I. Das Erbbild, *Acta med. Scandinav.* 108:398–413, 1941

166. Edström, G., Klinische Studien über den chronischen Gelenkrheumatismus —II. Die variierende Jahreszeitenfrequenz, *Acta med. Scandinav.* 108:414–420, 1941

167. Edström, G., Rheumatoid arthritis and trauma, *Acta med. Scandinav.* 142:11–30, 1952

168. Edström, G., Lundin, G., and Wramner, T., Investigations into the effect of hot, dry microclimate on peripheral circulation, etc., in arthritic patients, *Ann. Rheumat. Dis.* 7:76–82, June 1948

169. Ehlertsen, C. F., The late prognosis in rheumatic fever, *Acta med. Scandinav.* 112:353–392, 1942

170. Ellman, P., and Ball, R. E., "Rheumatoid disease" with joint and pulmonary manifestations, *Brit. M. J.* 2:816–820, Nov. 1948

171. Ellman, P., and Mitchell, S. D., "The psychological aspects of chronic rheumatic joint disease," in C. W. Buckley (ed.), *Reports on Chronic Rheumatic Diseases*, vol. 2, pp. 109–119. Macmillan, New York, 1936

172. Engleman, E., Differential diagnosis of adult rheumatic fever and rheumatoid arthritis, *California Med.* 66:227–230, April 1947

173. Fagge, C. H., Pneumococcal arthritis, *Guy's Hosp. Rep.* 83:444–451, Oct. 1933

174. Fagge, C. H., and Pye-Smith, P. H., "General diseases affecting the joints," in their *Text-Book of the Principles and Practice of Medicine*, vol. 2, pp. 669–732. Third edition. J. & A. Churchill, London, 1891

175. Falk, A., Psoriasis arthropathica (einschlieszlich der sog. "hyperkeratotischen Exantheme") bei gonorrhoischen Gelenkerkrankungen, *Arch. Dermat. & Syph.* 129:299–331, 1921. As cited by G. Nordin, in *Acta dermat.-venereol.* 15:221–242, June 1934

176. Farrar, G. E., Jr., and Rayburn, F. W., The blood in arthritis, *M. Clin. North America* 24:1633–1645, Nov. 1940

177. Faulkner, J. M., Place, E. H., and Ohler, W. R., Effect of scarlet fever upon the heart, *Am. J. M. Sc.* 189:352–358, March 1935

178. Felty, A. R., Chronic arthritis in the adult, associated with splenomegaly and leucopenia: a report of five cases of an unusual clinical syndrome, *Bull. Johns Hopkins Hosp.* 35:16–20, Jan. 1924

179. Fingerman, D. L., and Andrus, F. C., Visceral lesions associated with rheumatoid arthritis, *Ann. Rheumat. Dis.* 3:168–181, May 1943

180. Finney, J. O., Boland, E. W., and Hench, P. S., Precipitating and predisposing factors in rheumatoid arthritis, *Ann. Rheumat. Dis.* 6:91–94, June 1947

181. Fischel, *Inaug. Dissertat.*, Berlin 1897. As cited by F. Balzer and Burnier in *Bull. Soc. franç. de dermat. et syph.* 22:182, May 1911

182. Fischer, A., *Rheumatismus und Grenzgebiete: Fachbücher für Ärzte, herausgegeben von der Schriftleitung der klinischen Wochenschrift*, vol. 15. 223 pp. Springer, Berlin, 1933

183. Fisher, A. G. T., *Chronic (Non-tuberculous) Arthritis: Pathology and Principles of Modern Treatment*. 232 pp. H. K. Lewis, London, 1929

184. Fisher, A. G. T., Classification of rheumatic diseases, *J. State Med.* 44:497–507, Sept. 1936

Bibliography

185. Fletcher, A. A., and Graham, D., The large bowel in chronic arthritis, *Am. J. M. Sc.* **179**:91–93, Jan. 1930
186. Fletcher, E., *Medical Disorders of the Locomotor System Including the Rheumatic Diseases.* Second edition. 884 pp. E. and S. Livingstone, Edinburgh, 1951
187. Fletcher, E., and Lewis-Faning, E., The chronic rheumatic diseases, with special reference to chronic arthritis; a survey based on 1,000 cases, *Postgrad. M. J.* **21**:1–13; 54–63, Jan. and Feb. 1945
188. Forsbrook, W. H. R., *A Dissertation on Osteo-arthritis.* 144 pp. H. K. Lewis, London, 1893
189. Fox, R. F., *Arthritis in Women (A Clinical Survey) with Notes and Statistics from Representatives of Committees on Rheumatism in Various Countries and a Statement on the "Campaign Against Rheumatism, Retrospect and Outlook" (1935); also a Suggestion for Setting up Rest Houses for Rheumatoid Arthritis* (Founded on a lecture delivered at the Institute of Hygiene, London, April 1936). 35 pp. H. K. Lewis, London, 1936
190. Fox, R. F., and van Breemen, J., *Chronic Rheumatism: Causation and Treatment.* 364 pp. J. & A. Churchill, 1934
191. Fraser, T. N., Gold treatment in rheumatoid arthritis, *Ann. Rheumat. Dis.* **4**:71–75, June 1945
191a. Freireich, E. J., Ross, J. F., Bayles, T. B., Emerson, C. P., and Finch, S. C., Mechanism of anemia associated with rheumatoid arthritis, *Ann. Rheumat. Dis.* **13**:365–366, March 1954. Proc.
192. Freund, E., *Gelenkerkrankungen. Einführung in die Pathologie und Therapie.* 497 pp. Urban & Schwarzenberg, Berlin, 1929
193. Freund, H. A., Discussion of *Histologic and Chemical Changes in Skeletal Muscle of Patients with Rheumatic and Nonrheumatic Diseases,* by J. J. Bunim, L. Sokoloff, E. J. Bien, S. L. Wilens, M. Ziff, and C. McEwen, in C. H. Slocumb (ed.), *Rheumatic Diseases,* pp. 302–303. Saunders, Philadelphia, 1952
194. Fridenburg, A. H., A rare form of vaso-motor disease: a contribution to the study of *hydrops intermittens articulorum, M. Rec.* **33**:657–663, June 1888
195. Fuller, H. W., *On Rheumatism, Rheumatic Gout, and Sciatica, Their Pathology, Symptoms, and Treatment.* Third edition. 489 pp. John Churchill, London, 1860
196. Garrod, A., and Evans, G., Arthropathica psoriatica, *Quart. J. Med.* **17**:171–178, Jan. 1924
197. Garrod, A. B., *The Nature and Treatment of Gout and Rheumatic Gout.* 601 pp. Walton & Maberly, London, 1859

198. Garrod, A. B., Cited by A. E. Garrod in *A Treatise on Rheumatism and Rheumatoid Arthritis*, pp. 269–270. Charles Griffin, London, 1890

199. Garrod, A. E., *A Treatise on Rheumatism and Rheumatoid Arthritis*. 342 pp. Charles Griffin, London, 1890

200. Garrod, A. E., Concerning intermittent hydrarthrosis, *Quart. J. Med.* 3:207–220, Jan. 1910

201. Garry, M. W., Use of red cell mass in rheumatoid disease, *Am. J. M. Sc.* 223:642–647, June 1952

202. Ghormley, R. K., and Bateman, J. G., "Synovial membrane in osteoarthritis," in C. H. Slocumb (ed.), *Rheumatic Diseases*, pp. 273–279. Saunders, Philadelphia, 1952

203. Ghormley, R. K., and Brav, E. A., Resected knee joints, *Arch. Surg.* 26:465–484, March 1933

204. Ghormley, R. K., and Deacon, A. E., Synovial membranes in various types of arthritis; study by differential stains, *Am. J. Roentgenol.* 35:740–746, June 1936

205. Ghrist, D. G., and Hench, P. S., Course and prognosis in chronic infectious arthritis; study of relapses, *M. Clin. North America* 13:1499–1518, May 1930

206. Gillet, P. Le rhumatisme chronique endocrinien, *Bull méd., Paris* 43:807–811, July 1929

207. Glover, J. A., *The Incidence of Rheumatic Diseases* (Ministry of Health Reports on Public Health and Medical Subjects, no. 23). 97 pp. H. M. Stationery Office, London, 1924

208. Glover, J. A., *A Report on Chronic Arthritis with Special Reference to the Provision of Treatment* (Ministry of Health Reports on Public Health and Medical Subjects, no. 52). 103 pp. H. M. Stationery Office, London, 1928

209. Goldfain, E., Chronic, atrophic type of brucellosal arthritis, *J. Lab. & Clin. Med.* 27:168–172, Nov. 1941

210. Goldstein, W., Stillisches Krankheitsbild beim Erwachsenen, *Med. Klin.* 22:1527–1529, Oct. 1926

211. Goldthwait, J. E., Infectious arthritis, *Boston Med. & Surg. J.* 150:363–371, April 1904

212. Goldthwait, J. E., The differential diagnosis and treatment of the so-called rheumatoid diseases, *Boston Med. & Surg. J.* 151:529–534, Nov. 1904

213. Goldthwait, J. E., Arthritis: general considerations, *Am. Med.* n.s. 25:589–592, Oct. 1930

Bibliography

214. Goldthwait, J. E., and Brown, L. T., The cause of gastroptosis and enteroptosis, with their possible importance as a causative factor in the rheumatoid diseases, *Boston Med. & Surg. J.* 162:695–703, May 1910
215. Goldthwait, J. E., Painter, C. F., and Osgood, R. B., *Diseases of the Bones and Joints: Clinical Studies.* 685 pp. D. C. Heath, Boston, 1909
216. Gordon, R. G., Osteo-arthritis and its concomitants, *Brit. M. J.* 2:1083–1087, Dec. 1935
217. Gowers, W. R., Lumbago, its lessons and analogues, *Brit. M. J.* 1:117–121, Jan. 1904
218. Graef, I., Hickey, D. V., and Altman, V., Cardiac lesions in rheumatoid arthritis, *Am. Heart J.* 37:635, April 1949. Abstract
219. Graham, T. N., Generalized pustular psoriasis: report of a case, *Arch. Dermat. & Syph.* 32:208–217, Aug. 1935
220. Graham, W., The fibrositis syndrome, *Bull. Rheumat. Dis.* 3:51–52, April 1953
221. Granit, R., Leksell, L., and Skoglund, C. R., Fibre interaction in injured or compressed region of nerve, *Brain* 67:125–140, June 1944
222. Graves, R. J., *A System of Clinical Medicine.* 937 pp. Longman, London, 1843
223. Gray, J. W., Bernhard, W. G., and Gowen, C. H., Clinical pathology of rheumatoid arthritis, *Am. J. Clin. Path.* 5:489–503, Nov. 1935
224. Green, M. E., and Freyberg, R. H., Incidence of brucellosis in patients with rheumatic disease, *Am. J. M. Sc.* 201:495–504, April 1941
225. Green, W. T., Mono-articular and pauciarticular arthritis in children, *J.A.M.A.* 115:2023–2024, Dec. 1940. Abstract
226. Greenblatt, R. B., and Kupperman, H. S., Menopausal arthritis, *M. Clin. North America* 30:576–583, May 1946
227. Gruenwald, P., Visceral lesions in a case of rheumatoid arthritis, *Arch. Path.* 46:59–67, July 1948
228. Gurling, K. J., Association of Sjögren's and Felty's syndromes, *Ann. Rheumat. Dis.* 12:212–216, Sept. 1953
229. Guszman, J., Pathology and symptoms of arthropathic psoriasis; question of common etiology, *Orvosi hetil.* 79:1331–1335, Dec. 1935
230. Haden, R. L., Blood changes in arthritis and rheumatism, *Clinics* 1:531–536, Oct. 1942
231. Haft, H. H., The colon changes in chronic arthritis compared with other chronic diseases, *Am. J. M. Sc.* 185:811–815, June 1933
232. Hall, F. C., Menopause arthralgia: study of 71 women at artificial menopause, *New England J. Med.* 219:1015–1026, Dec. 1938

233. Hall, F. C., and Monroe, R. T., Thyroid gland deficiency in chronic arthritis, *J. Lab. & Clin. Med.* 18:439–457, Feb. 1933
234. Halliday, J. L., Psychological factors in rheumatism; preliminary study, *Brit. M. J.* 1:213;264, Jan. and Feb. 1937
235. Halliday, J. L., Concept of psychosomatic rheumatism, *Ann. Int. Med.* 15: 666–677, Oct. 1941
236. Halliday, J. L., Psychological aspects of rheumatoid arthritis, *Proc. Roy. Soc. Med.* (Sect. Phys. Med.) 35:455–457, May 1942
237. Hamilton, M., Pickering, G. W., Fraser Roberts, J. A., and Sowry, G. S. C., The aetiology of essential hypertension—I. The arterial pressure in the general population, *Clin. Sc.* 13:11–35, Feb. 1954
238. Hanrahan, E. M., Jr., and Miller, S. R., Effect of splenectomy in Felty's syndrome, *J.A.M.A.* 99:1247–1249, Oct. 1932
239. Harkavy, J., and Hebald, S., Association of infectious asthma and arthritis from the point of view of bacterial allergy, *Arch. Int. Med.* 49:698–708, April 1932
240. Hart, F. D., and Maclagan, N. F., Ankylosing spondylitis: a review of 184 cases, *Ann. Rheumat. Dis.* 14:77–83, March 1955
241. Hartfall, S. J., Garland, H. G., and Goldie, W., Gold treatment of arthritis: a review of 900 cases, *Lancet* 2:784–788, Oct. 1937
242. Hartsock, C., Gastro-intestinal tract in chronic atrophic (rheumatoid) arthritis, *M. Clin. North America* 17:917–922, Jan. 1934
243. Hartung, E. F., and Steinbrocker, O., Gall bladder infection and arthritis, *Am. J. M. Sc.* 184:711–716, Nov. 1932
244. Hartung, E. F., and Steinbrocker, O., Gastric acidity in chronic arthritis, *Ann. Int. Med.* 9:252–257, Sept. 1935
245. Hatch, F. N., Atrophic arthritis associated with splenomegaly and leukopenia, *Ann. Int. Med.* 23:201–220, Aug. 1945
246. Hawthorne, C. O., *Rheumatism, Rheumatoid Arthritis, and Subcutaneous Nodules*, 53 pp. J. & A. Churchill, London, 1900
247. Haygarth, J., *A Clinical History of Diseases—Part First: Being 1. A Clinical History of the Acute Rheumatism, 2. A Clinical History of the Nodosity of the Joints.* 168 pp. Cadell & Davies, London, 1805
248. Heller, G., Jacobson, A. S., Kolodny, M. H., and Kammerer, W. H., The hemagglutination test for rheumatoid arthritis—II. The influence of human plasma fraction II (gamma globulin) on the reaction, *J. Immunol.* 72:66–78, Jan. 1954
249. Hench, P. S., The systemic nature of chronic infectious arthritis, *Atlantic M. J.* 28:425–436, April 1925

Bibliography

250. Hench, P. S., Arthropathica psoriatica: presentation of a case, *Proc. Staff Meet., Mayo Clin.* 2:89–90, April 1927. Discussion by P. A. O'Leary, *ibid.*, p. 90

251. Hench, P. S., "Acute and chronic arthritis," in R. K. Ghormley (ed.), *Orthopedic Surgery*, pp. 108–190. Thomas Nelson & Sons, New York, 1938

252. Hench, P. S., "Chronic Arthritis: Chronic infectious arthritis; chronic senescent arthritis; gout," in D. P. Barr (ed.), *Modern Medical Therapy in General Practice*, pp. 3298–3397. Williams & Wilkins, Baltimore, 1940

253. Hench, P. S., An oft recurring disease of joints (arthritis, peri-arthritis, para-arthritis) apparently producing no articular residues, *J.A.M.A.* 115: 2207–2208, Dec. 1940

254. Hench, P. S., Therapeutic "Information Please": arthritis, *J.A.M.A.* 132: 974–979, Dec. 1946

255. Hench, P. S., The potential reversibility of rheumatoid arthritis, *Ann. Rheumat. Dis.* 8:90–96, June 1949

256. Hench, P. S., and Boland, E., Management of chronic arthritis and other rheumatic diseases among soldiers of the United States Army, *Ann. Int. Med.* 24:808–825, May 1946

257. Hench, P. S., and Rosenberg, E. F., Palindromic rheumatism: a "new," oft recurring disease of joints (arthritis, peri-arthritis, para-arthritis) apparently producing no articular residues—report of thirty-four cases; its relation to "angioneural arthrosis," "allergic rheumatism," and rheumatoid arthritis, *Arch. Int. Med.* 73:293–321, April 1944

258. Heyd, C. G., Infection of the gallbladder as a factor in arthritis, *M. Clin. North America* 21:1705–1707, Nov. 1937

259. Holm, S., Keratoconjunctivitis sicca and the sicca syndrome, *Acta ophth.*, suppl. 33, p. 73, 1949

260. Holmes, G., Menopausal arthritis, *Clin. J.* 66:366–373, Sept. 1937

261. Holmes, O. W., as quoted by B. D. Senturia, The role of infection in chronic nonspecific arthritis, *J. Missouri M. A.* 31:229–231, June 1934

262. Holt, L. E., Jr., and McIntosh, R., "Chronic polyarthritis (chronic infectious arthritis; rheumatoid arthritis; Still's disease)," Chapter 78 in *Holt's Diseases of Infancy and Childhood: a Textbook for the Use of Students and Practitioners*, pp. 634–636, Tenth edition, revised by L. E. Holt, Jr., and R. McIntosh. D. Appleton-Century, New York, 1936

263. Holt, R. C., Two graphs by Dr. R. Fortescue Fox. From statistics kindly supplied by Dr. R. C. Holt, Sept. 1932, *Acta rheumatol.* 4:34–35, Dec. 1932

264. Homolle, G., Rhumatisme, *N. dict. de méd. et chir. prat.* 31:548–750. Paris 1882

265. Howard, C. P., Pneumococcic arthritis, *Johns Hopkins Hosp. Rep.* 15:229–245, 1910
266. Hunt, E., Two cases of pustular psoriasis with arthritis, *Proc. Roy. Soc. Med.* 25:1034–1037, May 1932
267. Hunt, E., Psoriasis and rheumatism: comparison, *Lancet* 2:351–352, Aug. 1933
268. Hutchinson, H. E., and Alexander, W. D., Splenic neutropenia in the Felty syndrome, *Blood*, 9:986–998, Oct. 1954
269. Hutchinson, J., *The Pedigree of Disease; Being Six Lectures on Temperament, Idiosyncrasy, and Diathesis Delivered in the Theatre of the Royal College of Surgeons in the Session of 1881.* 142 pp. J. & A. Churchill, London, 1884
270. Hutt, M. S. R., Richardson, J. S., and Staffurth, J. S., Felty's syndrome: report of 4 cases treated by splenectomy, *Quart. J. Med.* 20:57–73, Jan. 1951
271. Hyde, S., *The Causes and Treatment of Rheumatoid Arthritis.* 83 pp. John Bale & Sons, London, 1896
272. Ingram, J. T., The significance and management of psoriasis, *Brit. M. J.* 2:823–828, Oct. 1954
273. Ivy, A. C., Grossman, M. I., and Bachrach, W. H., *Peptic Ulcer.* 1144 pp. Blakiston, Philadelphia, 1950
274. Jacoby, A., Wishergrad, M., and Koopman, J., Evaluation of complement fixation test for gonorrhea, *Am. J. Syph.* 22:32–38, Jan. 1938
275. Jankelson, I. R., McClure, C. W., and Sweetsir, F. N., Chronic ulcerative colitis; complications outside the digestive tract, *Rev. Gastroenterol.* 9:99–104, March–April 1942
276. Järvinen, K. A. J., Investigations on the relations of rheumatoid arthritis and rheumatic fever to allergy, *Ann. med. int. Fenniae* 39:1–99 (suppl. 5), 1950
277. Järvinen, K. A. J., A study of the interrelations of rheumatoid arthritis and diabetes mellitus, *Ann. Rheumat. Dis.* 9:226–230, Sept. 1950
278. Järvinen, K. A. J., Factors aggravating symptoms of rheumatoid arthritis, *Rheumatism* 7:33–37, July 1951
279. Järvinen, K. A. J., Rheumatic arthritis and arterial pressure, *Acta rheumatol. Scandinav.* 1:127–134, 1955
280. Jeffrey, M. R., Anaemia of rheumatoid arthritis, *Ann. Rheumat. Dis.* 11:162–167, June 1952
281. Jeghers, H., and Robinson, L. J., Arthropathia psoriatica: report of a case and discussion of pathogenesis, diagnosis, and treatment, *J.A.M.A.* 108:949–952, March 1937

Bibliography

282. Jennison, J., Observations made on a group of employees with duodenal ulcer, *Am. J. M. Sc.* 196:654–662, Nov. 1938
283. Johnson, A., Shapiro, L. B., and Alexander, F., Preliminary report on a psychosomatic study of rheumatoid arthritis, *Psychosom. Med.* 9:295–300, Sept.–Oct. 1947
284. Jones, C. M., Benson, J. A., Jr., and Roque, A. L., Whipple's disease: report of a case with special reference to histochemical studies of biopsy material and therapeutic results of corticosteroid therapy, *New England J. Med.* 248:665–670, April 1953
285. Jones, R. L., Vasomotor and ocular phenomena in relation to rheumatoid arthritis, *Bristol Med.-Chir. J.* 20:328–332, Dec. 1902
286. Jones, R. Llewellyn, *Arthritis Deformans: Comprising Rheumatoid Arthritis, Osteo-arthritis, and Spondylitis Deformans.* 365 pp. William Wood, New York, 1909
287. Jonsson, E., and Berglund, K., Trauma and rheumatoid arthritis, *Acta med. Scandinav.* 135:255–262, 1949
288. Judd, E. S., and Hench, P. S., Coexistent chronic infectious (atrophic) arthritis and cholecystitis: results of cholecystectomy, *Minnesota Med.* 16:522–532, Aug. 1933
289. Keefer, C. S., Etiology of chronic arthritis, *New England J. Med.* 213:644–653, Oct. 1935
290. Keefer, C. S., and Myers, W. K., Differential diagnosis of acute arthritis, *M. Clin. North America* 16:929–942, Jan. 1933
291. Keefer, C. S., and Myers, W. K., Gonococcal arthritis: a clinical study of 69 cases, *Ann. Int. Med.* 8:581–594, Nov. 1934
292. Keefer, C. S., Myers, W. K., and Oppel, T. W., Streptococcal agglutinins in patients with rheumatoid (atrophic) arthritis and acute rheumatic fever, *J. Clin. Invest.* 12:267–277, March 1933
293. Keefer, C. S., and Spink, W. W., Gonococcic arthritis: pathogenesis, mechanism of recovery and treatment, *J.A.M.A.* 109:1448–1453, Oct. 1937
294. Kellgren, J. H., and Moore, R., Generalized osteoarthritis and Heberden's nodes, *Brit. M. J.* 1:181–187, Jan. 1952
295. Kelly, M., Chronic polyarthritis and monarticular trauma, *M. J. Australia* 2:197–198, Aug. 1951
296. Kersley, G. D., and Gibson, H. J., "The histopathology of rheumatoid arthritis, especially in the extra-articular manifestations," in C. H. Slocumb (ed.), *Rheumatic Diseases*, pp. 280–287. Saunders, Philadelphia, 1952
297. Key, J. A., Experimental arthritis: reactions of joints to mild irritants, *J. Bone & Joint Surg.* 11:705–738, Oct. 1929

298. Klauder, J. V., and Robertson, H. F., Symmetrical serous synovitis (Clutton's joints): congenital syphilis and interstitial keratitis, *J.A.M.A.* 103: 236–240, July 1934

299. Klemperer, P., Pollack, A., and Baehr, G., Diffuse collagen disease: acute disseminated lupus erythematosus and diffuse scleroderma, *J.A.M.A.* 119: 331–332, May 1942

300. Kling, D. H., Syphilitic arthritis with effusion, *Am. J. M. Sc.* 183:538–549, April 1932

301. Klinge, F., Die Eiweissüberempfindlichkeit (Gewebsanaphylaxie) der Gelenke; Pathogenese des Gelenkrheumatismus, *Beitr. path. Anat.* 83:185–216, Nov. 1929

302. Klinge, F., and Grzimek, N., Das Gewebsbild des fieberhaften Rheumatismus—VI. Der chronische Gelenkrheumatismus (Infectarthritis, Polyarthritis lenta) und über "rheumatische Stigmata," *Arch. path. Anat.* 284: 646–712, May 1932

303. Kinsella, R. A., Differential diagnosis of acute rheumatic fever, *J. Lab. & Clin. Med.* 22:26–29, Oct. 1936

304. Krida, A., Intermittent hydrarthrosis of the knee joint: a report of two cases apparently cured by synovectomy, together with pathological findings, *J. Bone & Joint Surg.* 31:449–462, April 1933

305. Kulka, J. P., Bocking, D., Ropes, M. W., and Bauer, W., Early joint lesions of rheumatoid arthritis, *A. M. A. Arch. Path.* 59:129–150, Feb. 1955

306. Lambert, J., "The arterial blood pressures in arthritic diseases," in T. S. P. Strangeways (ed.), *Bull. Comm. Study of Special Diseases*, vol. 2, pp. 11–82. Cambridge University Press, Cambridge, England, 1908

307. Lambert, J., "A report on some points in the etiology and onset of 195 cases of rheumatoid arthritis," in T. S. P. Strangeways (ed.), *Bull. Comm. Study of Special Diseases*, vol. 2, pp. 83–94. Cambridge University Press, Cambridge, England, 1908

308. Lane, C. G., and Crawford, G. M., Psoriasis: statistical study of 231 cases, *Arch. Dermat. & Syph.* 35:1051–1061, June 1937

309. Lane, J. E., Symmetrical synovitis of the knee in congenital syphilis (Clutton's joints), *Am. J. Syph.* 6:611–615, Oct. 1922

310. Lane, W. A., Chronic intestinal stasis, *Surg., Gynec. & Obst.* 11:495–500, Nov. 1910

311. Lang, S. J., Medical aspect of chronic arthritis, *Illinois M. J.* 67:470–473, May 1935

312. Latham, P. W., Acute rheumatism localized to a paralysed limb, *Lancet* 1:699–700, March 1914

313. Ledoux-Lebard, R., Radiodiagnostic, radiothérapie et radiumthérapie des ankyloses, *J. de radiol. et de électrol.* 1:217-222, April 1914
314. Lees, D., Gonococcal arthritis, with observations based on a series of 388 cases, *Brit. J. Ven. Dis.* 8:79-113; 192-204, April and July 1932
315. Lerman, J., and Means, J. H., The use of record forms and mechanical methods of analysis in the study of clinical data, *New England J. Med.* 208:1135-1143, June 1933
316. Lerman, J., Pierce, F. D., and Brogan, A. J., Gastric acidity in normal individuals, *J. Clin. Invest.* 11:155-165, Jan. 1932
317. Le Sage, A., Tuberculous rheumatism, *Canad. M. A. J.* 30:30-37, Jan. 1934
318. Lewis, B. G., Sinton, D. W., and Knott, J. R., Central nervous system involvement in disorders of collagen, *A. M. A. Arch. Int. Med.* 93:315-327, March 1954
319. Lewis-Faning, E., "The incidence and prevalence of adult rheumatism," Chapter 5 in E. Fletcher, *Medical Disorders of the Locomotor System Including the Rheumatic Diseases*, pp. 98-119. Williams & Wilkins, Baltimore, 1947
320. Lewis-Faning, E., Report on an enquiry into the aetiological factors associated with rheumatoid arthritis, *Ann. Rheumat. Dis.* 9:suppl. 94 pp. 1950
321. Lewis-Faning, E., and Fletcher, E., A statistical study of 1,000 cases of chronic rheumatism, *Post-Grad. M. J.* 21:137-146; 176-185, April and May 1945
322. Leys, D. G., and Swift, P. N., Pulmonary lesions in rheumatoid arthritis, *Brit. M. J.* 1:434-435, March 1949
323. Lindsay, J., "The relation of infective foci to rheumatoid arthritis. An analysis of 172 cases," in T. S. P. Strangeways (ed.), *Bull. Comm. Study of Special Diseases*, vol. 2, pp. 106-116. Cambridge University Press, Cambridge, England, 1908
324. Llewellyn, R. L. J., Discussion on climacteric arthritis, *Proc. Roy. Soc. Med.* (Sect. Balneol. and Climatol.) 20:511-513, Jan. 1927
325. Lockie, L. M., and Norcross, B. M., Juvenile rheumatoid arthritis, *Pediatrics* 2:694-698, Nov. 1948
326. Louis, P. C. A., *Researches on the Effects of Blood Letting in some Inflammatory Diseases, and on the Influence of Tartarized Antimony and Vesication in Pneumonitis.* Translated by C. G. Putnam with preface and appendix by James Jackson. 171 pp. Hilliard, Boston, 1836
327. Lövgren, O., Rheumatoid arthritis and the liver, *Ann. med. int. Fenniae* 42:42-51, 1953

328. Ludwig, A. O., Psychogenic factors in rheumatoid arthritis, *Bull. Rheumat. Dis.* 2:15–16, April 1952
329. Ludwig, A. O., Bennett, G. A., and Bauer, W., A rare manifestation of gout; widespread ankylosis simulating rheumatoid arthritis, *Ann. Int. Med.* 11:1248–1276, Jan. 1938
330. Ludwig, A. O., Short, C. L., and Bauer, W., Rheumatoid arthritis as the cause of increased cerebrospinal-fluid protein: study of 101 patients, *New England J. Med.* 228:306–310, March 1943
331. McCahey, J. F., Important factors in onset and course of arthritis complicating gonorrhea in the adult male, *Urol. & Cutan. Rev.* 37:217–222, April 1933
332. McClure, J. C., Toxic arthritis, *Quart. J. Med.* 3:61–72, Oct. 1909
333. McCrae, T., "Arthritis deformans," Chapter 25 in W. Osler and T. McCrae (ed.), *Modern Medicine, Its Theory and Practice*, vol. 5, pp. 895–946. Second edition. Lea & Febiger, Philadelphia, 1915
334. McEwen, C., Chasis, H., and Alexander, R. C., Agglutination and precipitation between hemolytic streptococci of various groups and sera of rheumatoid arthritis patients, *Proc. Soc. Exper. Biol. & Med.* 33:133–135, Oct. 1935
335. McEwen, C., and Thomas, E. W., Syphilitic joint disease, *M. Clin. North America* 22:1275–1286, Sept. 1938
336. McKittrick, L. S., and Miller, R. H., Idiopathic ulcerative colitis: review of 149 cases, with particular reference to the value of, and indications for surgical treatment, *Ann. Surg.* 102:656–673, Oct. 1935
337. Macalister, C. J., Some diseases simulating acute rheumatism and their probable relation to chronic rheumatoid arthritis, *Med. Surg. & Path. Reports, Royal South Hosp.*, Liverpool 1:153–161, 1901
338. Macalister, R., Rheumatoid arthritis and its relations to some other diseases, *Liverpool Med.-Chir. J.* 24:66, June 1904. Abstract
339. Mainland, D., Risk of fallacious conclusions from autopsy data on the incidence of diseases with applications to heart disease, *Am. Heart J.* 45:644–654, May 1953
339a. Mainland, D., Use of Case Records in the Study of Therapy and Other Features in Chronic Disease—I. Planning the Survey, *Ann. Rheumat. Dis.* 14:337–352, Dec. 1955
340. Maranon, G., *The Climacteric*. Translated by K. S. Stevens; edited by C. Culbertson. First American edition from second Spanish edition. 425 pp. Mosby, St. Louis, 1929
341. Marie, P., Sur la spondylose rhizomélique, *Rev. de méd.*, Paris 18:285–310, 1898

Bibliography

342. Marie, P., and Léri, A., Une variété de rhumatisme chronique: la main en lorgnette (Présentation de pièces et de coupes), *Bull. et mém. Soc. méd. d. hôp. de Paris*, series 3, 36:104–107, July 1913

343. Martin, G. M., Roth, G. M., Elkins, E. C., and Krusen, F. H., Cutaneous temperature of extremities of normal subjects and of patients with rheumatoid arthritis, *Arch. Phys. Med.* 27:665–682, Nov. 1946

344. Martin, L., Studies on metabolism and results of treatment in various forms of arthritis, *South. M. J.* 26:699–713, Aug. 1933

345. Massachusetts General Hospital: Medical Grand Rounds, Case no. 83, *Am. Pract. & Digest Treat.* 3:378–380, Feb. 1949

346. Master, A. M., Dublin, L. I., and Marks, H. H., The normal blood pressure range and its clinical implications, *J.A.M.A.* 143:1464–1470, Aug. 1950

347. Means, J. H., *The Thyroid and Its Diseases; Being an Account Based in Large Measure on the Experience Gained in the Thyroid Clinic of the Massachusetts General Hospital.* 602 pp. J. B. Lippincott, Philadelphia, 1937

348. Menkin, V., Biochemistry of inflammation, *Lancet* 1:660–662, May 1947

349. Menkin, V., Determination of the level of leukocytes in the blood stream with inflammation; thermostable component concerned in the mechanism of leukocytosis, *Blood* 4:1323–1337, Dec. 1949

350. Mettier, S. R., and Minot, G. R., The effect of iron on blood formation as influenced by changing the acidity of the gastroduodenal contents in certain cases of anemia, *Am. J. M. Sc.* 181:25–36, Jan. 1931

351. Meyer, A., in E. A. Strecker and F. G. Ebaugh, *Practical Clinical Psychiatry for Students and Practitioners*, p. 10. Blakiston, Philadelphia, 1930

352. Miall, W. E., Rheumatoid arthritis in males: an epidemiological study of a Welsh mining community, *Ann. Rheumat. Dis.* 14:150–158, June 1955

353. Miall, W. E., Caplan, A., Cochrane, A. L., Kilpatrick, G. S., and Oldham, P. D., An epidemiological study of rheumatoid arthritis associated with characteristic chest x-ray appearances in coal-workers, *Brit. M. J.* 2:1231–1236, Dec. 1953

354. Micheli, F., Sur la maladie de Still-Chauffard, *Acta rheumatol.* 3:11, Feb. 1931

355. Miller, J. L., Undulant fever, *Ann. Int. Med.* 8:570–580, Nov. 1934

356. Miller, J. L., Critical review of the literature on chronic rheumatism, *Arch. Int. Med.* 57:213–234, Jan. 1936

357. Miller, J. L., and Lewin, P., Evidence of the anaphylactic character of intermittent hydrarthrosis, *J.A.M.A.* 82:1177–1179, April 1924

358. Miller, S., "Hepatic efficiency in chronic rheumatic diseases: preliminary

communication," in C. W. Buckley (ed.), *Reports on Chronic Rheumatic Diseases*, vol. 1, pp. 53–54. H. K. Lewis, London, 1935

359. Moltke, O., Still's disease in adults: a contribution to the symptomatology of subchronic polyarthritis, *Acta med. Scandinav.* **80**:427–453, 1933
360. Moltke, O., and Ohlsen, A. S., Gastric achlorhydria in chronic and subchronic proliferative arthritis, *Lancet* **2**:1034–1038, Oct. 1936
361. Monroe, R. T., Chronic arthritis in hyperthyroidism and myxedema, *New England J. Med.* **212**:1074–1077, June 1935
362. Monroe, R. T., "Chronic arthritis," Chapter 15 in H. A. Christian (ed.), *Oxford Medicine*, vol. 4, pp. 367–404. Oxford University Press, New York, 1939
363. Moore, C. H., Clinical lectures in surgery: periodical inflammation of the knee-joint, *Lancet* **1**:485–486, April 1864
364. Moore, C. H., Two cases of periodical inflammation of the right knee-joint; with remarks, *Med.-Chir. Tr.* **50**:21–38. Published by the Royal Medical and Chirurgical Society, London, 1867
365. Moore, J. E., and Mohr, C. F., Incidence and etiologic background of chronic biologic false-positive reactions in serologic tests for syphilis: preliminary report, *Ann. Int. Med.* **37**:1156–1161, Dec. 1952
366. Morris, E. H., "Observations on the temperature and pulse rate in ninety-five cases of rheumatoid arthritis," in T. S. P. Strangeways (ed.), *Bull. Comm. Study of Special Diseases*, vol. 3, pp. 75–81. Cambridge University Press, Cambridge, England, 1910
367. Morrison, L. R., Cattogio, P. M., and Bauer, W., "Observations on the histopathology of the neuromuscular system in rheumatoid arthritis," in C. H. Slocumb (ed.), *Rheumatic Diseases*, pp. 304–307. Saunders, Philadelphia, 1952
368. Morrison, L. R., Short, C. L., Ludwig, A. O., and Schwab, R. S., The neuromuscular system in rheumatoid arthritis: electromyographic and histologic observations, *Am. J. M. Sc.* **214**:33–49, July 1947
369. Morse, J. L., *Clinical Pediatrics*. 848 pp. Saunders, Philadelphia, 1926
370. Motulsky, A. G., Weinberg, S., Saphir, O., and Rosenberg, E. F., Lymph nodes in rheumatoid arthritis, *A. M. A. Arch. Int. Med.* **90**:660–676, Nov. 1952
371. Mouriquand, G., Le ménopause dans ses rapports avec le rhumatisme chronique, *Lyon méd.* **154**:257–260, Sept. 1934
372. Movitt, E. R., and Davis, A. E., Liver biopsy in rheumatoid arthritis, *Am. J. M. Sc.* **226**:516–520, Nov. 1953
373. Mueller, E. E., and Mead, S., Electromyogram in rheumatoid arthritis, *Am. J. Phys. Med.* **31**:67–73, April 1952

Bibliography

374. Munro, J. M. H., Rheumatoid arthritis, its causation and treatment, *Brit. M. J.* 2:598–599, Oct. 1925
375. Myers, W. K., Etiology of rheumatoid (atrophic) arthritis, *M. Ann. District of Columbia* 5:203–206, July 1936
376. Myers, W. K., and Gwyen, H. B., Clinical features of gonococcal arthritis; observations in 85 cases, *M. Ann. District of Columbia* 4:194–197, July 1935
377. Naide, M., Sayen, A., and Comroe, B. I., Characteristic vascular pattern in patients with rheumatoid arthritis, *Arch. Int. Med.* 76:139–142, Sept. 1945
378. Nathan, P. W., Gonorrheal joint disease and its treatment, *New York Med. J.* 85:501–507, 1907
379. Neil, M. S., and Hartung, E. F., Precipitins for Streptococcus hemolyticus in rheumatoid arthritis serums, *J. Lab. & Clin. Med.* 22:881–889, June 1937
380. Nichols, E. H., and Richardson, F. L. Arthritis deformans, *J. Med. Research* 21:149–221, Sept. 1909
381. Nilsson, F., Anaemia problems in rheumatoid arthritis, *Acta med. Scandinav.* 130:1–193 (suppl. 210), 1948
382. Nissen, H. A., Atonic stasis: clinical and laboratory study of intestinal variations in chronic disease, *M. Clin. North America* 13:269–280, July 1929
383. Nissen, H. A., Chronic arthritis and its treatment, *New England J. Med.* 210:1109–1115, May 1934
384. Nissen, H. A., Tonsils as foci of systemic infection, *Tr. Am. Acad. Ophth.* 39:313–326, 1934; abstract, Arthritis and tonsillar infection, *New England J. Med.* 212:1027–1033, May 1935
385. Nissen, H. A., The significance of the life course (or level of activity) of the chronic arthritic, *Maine M. J.* 26:181–189, Dec. 1935
386. Nissen, H. A., and Spencer, K. A., Sugar tolerance in the arthritic, *New England J. Med.* 210:13–19, Jan. 1934
387. Nissen, H. A., and Spencer, K. A., Arteriosclerosis in the arthritic, *New England J. Med.* 210:92–97, Jan. 1934
388. Nissen, H. A., and Spencer, K. A., Arthritis and systemic involvement as exemplified in a group of dead arthritics, *New England J. Med.* 210:147–149, Jan. 1934
389. Nissen, H. A., and Spencer, K. A., Psychogenic problem (endocrinal and metabolic) in chronic arthritis, *New England J. Med.* 214:576–581, March 1936
390. Nobl, G., "Psoriasis," in *Handbuch der Haut- und Geschlechtskrankheiten*, vol. 7, part 1, pp. 180–288. Springer, Berlin, 1928
391. Nordin, G., Fatal case of psoriasis arthropathica, *Acta Dermat.-venereol.* 15:221–242, June 1934

392. Olch, I. Y., Menopausal age in women with cancer of the breast, *Am. J. Cancer* **30**:563-566, July 1937

393. Ord, W. M., Rheumatoid arthritis, regarded from a clinical point of view, *Tr. Clinical Soc.* **12**:90-97, Feb. 1879

394. Ord, W. M., Address on some of the conditions included under the general term "rheumatoid arthritis," *Brit. M. J.* **1**:155-158, 1880

395. Ormsby, O. S., *A Practical Treatise on Diseases of the Skin for the Use of Students and Practitioners.* Third edition. 1262 pp. Lea & Febiger, Philadelphia, 1927

396. Paget, J., On the relation between the symmetry and the diseases of the body, *Med.-Chir. Tr.* 2d series, **7**:30-41. Published by the Royal Medical and Chirurgical Society, London, 1842

397. Painter, C. F., Importance of early diagnosis and careful differentiation of types in chronic arthritis, *New England J. Med.* **208**:447-450, Feb. 1933

398. Palmer, R. S., Personal communication

399. Parker, F., and Keefer, C. S., Gross and histologic changes in the knee joint in rheumatoid arthritis, *Arch. Path.* **20**:507-522, Oct. 1935

400. Patterson, R. M., Craig, J. B., Waggoner, R. W., and Freyberg, R., Studies of the relationship between emotional factors and rheumatoid arthritis, *Am. J. Psychiat.* **99**:775-780, May 1943

401. Paul, J. R., Salinger, R., and Zuger, B., Relation of rheumatic fever to postscarlatinal arthritis and postscarlatinal heart disease: familial study, *J. Clin. Invest.* **13**:503-516, May 1934

402. Pemberton, R., *Arthritis and Rheumatoid Conditions: Their Nature and Treatment.* Second edition. 455 pp. Lea & Febiger, Philadelphia, 1935

403. Pemberton, R., and Peirce, E. G., Clinical and statistical study of chronic arthritis based on 1100 cases, *Am. J. M. Sc.* **173**:31-46, Jan. 1927

404. Pemberton, R., Studies on arthritis in the army based on four hundred cases—V. Roentgen-ray evidences, clinical considerations, treatment, summary, conclusions, and clinical abstracts of cases studied, *Arch. Int. Med.* **25**:351-404, April 1920

405. Pepper, O. H. P., The diagnosis of gonococcal arthritis with report of three cases in patients with chronic rheumatoid arthritis, *Ann. Int. Med.* **3**:328-334, Oct. 1929

406. Perla, D., and Gross, H., Atypical amyloid disease, *Am. J. Path.* **11**:93-112, Jan. 1935

407. Perrin, E. R., Cas curieux de contracture partielle intermittente à type octane, avec irritation violente et épanchement de sériosité dans plusiers articulations, *Union méd.*, series 3, **25**:821-823, 1878

Bibliography

408. Perry, H. M., Jr., and Schroeder, H. A., Syndrome simulating collagen disease caused by hydralazine (apresoline), *J.A.M.A.* 154:670–673, Feb. 1954
409. Pickard, N. S., Rheumatoid arthritis in children: clinical study, *Arch. Int. Med.* 80:771–790, Dec. 1947
410. Plenk, H. P., Psoriatic arthritis: report of a case, *Am. J. Roentgenol.* 64:635–639, Oct. 1950
411. Polland, W. S., Blood in cases of unexplained gastric anacidity, *J. Clin. Invest.* 12:599–611, May 1933
412. Polland, W. S., Histamine test meals: analysis of 988 consecutive tests, *Arch. Int. Med.* 51:903–919, June 1933
413. Polley, H. F., and Slocumb, C. H., Rheumatoid spondylitis: a study of 1035 cases, *Ann. Int. Med.* 26:240–249, Feb. 1947
414. Poncet, A., Rhumatisme tuberculeux ankylosant, *Bull. et mém. Soc. méd. d. hôp. de Paris*, series 3, 20:841–849, 1903
415. Porter, J. L., and Lonergan, R. C., Intermittent hydrarthrosis, *J. Bone & Joint Surg.* 14:631–639, July 1932
416. Portis, R. B., Pathology of chronic arthritis of children (Still's disease), *Am. J. Dis. Child.* 55:1000–1017, May 1938
417. Potter, T. A., Barkin, T., and Stillman, J. S., Occurrence of spondylitis in juvenile rheumatoid arthritis, *Ann. Rheumat. Dis.* 13:364, Dec. 1954. Proc.
418. Price, A. E., and Schoenfeld, J. B., Felty's syndrome: report of a case with complete postmortem findings, *Ann. Int. Med.* 7:1230–1239, April 1934
419. Pringle, G. L. K., Discussion of V. Coates, Clinical types of so-called multiple infective arthritis, *Proc. Roy. Soc. Med.* (Sect. Balneol. and Climatol.) 18:18, Jan. 1925
420. Pringle, G. L. K., Endocrine imbalance and its relation to chronic arthritis, *Brit. M. J.* 1:751–752, May 1928
421. Pringle, G. L. K., "The endocrine factor in atrophic arthritis," in *Proceedings of a Conference on Rheumatic Diseases Held at Bath, 10th and 11th of May, 1928*, pp. 234–235. Published by the Hot Mineral Baths Committee of the Bath City Council, 1928
422. Rackemann, F. M., *Clinical Allergy, Particularly Asthma and Hay Fever: Mechanism and Treatment.* 617 pp. Macmillan, New York, 1931
423. Ragan, C., The general management of rheumatoid arthritis, *J.A.M.A.* 141:124–127, Sept. 1949
424. Ragan, C., "Intermittent Hydrarthrosis," Chapter 34, in *Comroe's Arthritis and Allied Conditions*, pp. 629–634. Fifth edition, edited by J. L. Hollander et al. Lea & Febiger, Philadelphia, 1953

425. Rawls, W. B., Ressa, A. A., Gruskin, B., and Gordon, A. S., Thyroid activity in chronic arthritis, *Ann. Int. Med.* 11:1401–1406, Feb. 1938
426. Rawls, W. B., Weiss, S., and Collins, V. L., Liver function in rheumatoid (chronic infectious) arthritis: preliminary report, *Ann. Int. Med.* 10:1021–1027, Jan. 1937
427. Ray, M. B., *Rheumatism in General Practice: a Clinical Study.* 414 pp. H. K. Lewis, London, 1934
428. Raymond, Recherches expérimentales sur la pathogénie des atrophies musculaires consécutives aux arthrites traumatiques, *Rev. de méd., Paris* 10:374–392, 1890
429. Reimann, H. A., Focal infection and systemic disease: critical appraisal; the case against indiscriminate removal of teeth and tonsils, *J.A.M.A.* 114:1–6, Jan. 1940
430. Rentschler, E. B., Vanzant, F. R., and Rowntree, L. G., Arthritic pain in relation to changes in weather, *J.A.M.A.* 92:1995–2000, June 1929
431. Reynolds, W. E., Short, C. L., and Bauer, W., The course of rheumatoid arthritis, *Bull. Rheumat. Dis.* 5:77–78, Nov. 1954
432. Richardson, W., Note on the racial incidence in portal cirrhosis, *New England J. Med.* 218:257–258, Feb. 1938
433. Robichaux, E. C., Uncomplicated exudative synovitis (with report of two cases), *Ann. Int. Med.* 1:513–516, Jan. 1928
434. Robinson, D., Rheumatoid arthritis, *Canad. M. A. J.* 50:223–230, March 1944
435. Rogoff, B., and Freyberg, R. H., Family incidence of rheumatoid spondylitis, *Ann. Rheumat. Dis.* 7:40–41, March 1948. Proc.
436. Rolleston, H., "The history of chronic rheumatism," in R. G. Gordon (ed.), *A Survey of Chronic Rheumatic Diseases*, pp. 3–14. Oxford University Press, London, 1938
437. Romanus, R., Pelvo-spondylitis ossificans in the male (ankylosing spondylitis, morbus Bechterew-Marie-Strümpell) and genito-urinary infection; the aetiological significance of the latter and the nature of the disease based on a study of 117 male patients, *Acta med. Scandinav.* 145:1–368 (suppl. 280), 1953
438. Ropes, M. W., Unpublished data
439. Ropes, M. W., and Bauer, W., Medical progress; rheumatoid arthritis; its varied clinical manifestations, *New England J. Med.* 233:592–596; 618–623, Nov. 1945
440. Ropes, M. W., and Bauer, W., *Synovial Fluid Changes in Joint Disease.* 150 pp. Harvard University Press, Cambridge 1953

Bibliography

441. Ropes, M. W., and Bauer, W., Unpublished data
442. Ropes, M. W., Perlmann, G. E., Kaufman, D., and Bauer, W., The electrophoretic distribution of proteins in plasma in rheumatoid arthritis, *J. Clin. Invest.* **33**:311–318, March 1954
443. Rosenberg, E. F., "The visceral lesions of rheumatoid arthritis," Chapter 12 in *Comroe's Arthritis and Allied Conditions*, pp. 171–185. Fifth edition, edited by J. L. Hollander *et al.* Lea & Febiger, Philadelphia, 1953
444. Ross, D. N., Oral and intravenous iron therapy in the anaemia of rheumatoid arthritis, *Ann. Rheumat. Dis.* **9**:358–362, Dec. 1950
445. Rowntree, L. G., and Adson, A. W., Bilateral lumbar sympathetic ganglionectomy and ramisectomy for polyarthritis of the lower extremities, *J.A.M.A.* **88**:694–696, March 1927
446. Roy, L. M. H., Alexander, W. R. M., and Duthie, J. J. R., Nature of anaemia in rheumatoid arthritis—I. Metabolism of iron, *Ann. Rheumat. Dis.* **14**: 63–72, March 1955
447. Rydén, E., Chronic polyarthritis and trauma, *Acta med. Scandinav.* **114**: 442–469, 1943
448. Sanes, K. I., "The age of menopause: a statistical study," in *Tr. Am. M. A.* (Sect. Obst., Gynec., and Abdom. Surg.), pp. 258–284. American Medical Assn. Press, Chicago, 1918
449. Sargent, F., II, and Sargent, V. W., Season, nutrition, and pellagra, *New England J. Med.* **242**:447–453; 507–514, March 1950
450. Sashin, D., Spanbock, J., and Kling, D. H., Gold therapy in rheumatoid arthritis, *J. Bone & Joint Surg.* **21**:723–734, July 1939
451. Schlesinger, H., Intermittent effusions in joints, *Wien. klin. Wchnschr.* **39**: 68, Jan. 1926; abstracted in *J.A.M.A.* **86**:728, March 1926
452. Schnell, A., Clinical features of rheumatic infection in the old, *Acta med. Scandinav.* **106**:345–351, 1941
453. Schwartz, H. J., The complement-fixation test in the differential diagnosis of acute and chronic gonococcic arthritis, *Am. J. M. Sc.* **144**:369–386, Sept. 1912
454. Sclater, J. G., An analysis of 388 cases of rheumatoid arthritis, *Ann. Rheumat. Dis.* **3**:195–206, Dec. 1943
455. Scott, S. G., *A Monograph on Adolescent Spondylitis or Ankylosing Spondylitis: the Early Diagnosis and Its Treatment by Wide-Field X-Ray Irradiation* (Published under the Auspices of the Nuffield Wide-Field X-Ray Therapy Research; Research no. 1). 132 pp. Oxford University Press, New York, 1942
456. Selye, H., *Textbook of Endocrinology*, pp. 135 and 260. *Acta Endocrinologica*. Montreal, 1947

457. Service, W. C., Hydroarthrosis of allergic origin, *Am. J. Surg.* 37:121–122, July 1937
458. Shapiro, M. J., Modern conception of chronic arthritis, *Minnesota Med.* 16:719–728, Dec. 1933
459. Sharpe, J. C., Intermittent hydrarthrosis associated with undulant fever, *Ann. Int. Med.* 9:1431–1436, April 1936
460. Sherman, M. S., Non-specificity of synovial reactions, *Bull. Hosp. Joint Dis.* 12:110–125, 1951
461. Sherman, M. S., Psoriatic arthritis: observations on clinical roentgenographic and pathological changes, *J. Bone & Joint Surg.* 34:831–852, Oct. 1952
462. Shlionsky, H., and Blake, F. G., Arthritis psoriatica; report of a case, *Ann. Int. Med.* 10:537–546, Oct. 1936
463. Short, C. L., Arthritis in the Mediterranean Theater—I. Incidence of joint disease: clinical description of rheumatoid arthritis, *New England J. Med.* 236:383–391, March 1947
464. Short, C. L., and Bauer, W., Cincophen hypersensitiveness: a report of four cases and a review, *Ann. Int. Med.* 6:1449–1464, May 1933
465. Short, C. L., and Bauer, W., Treatment of rheumatoid arthritis with fever induced by diathermy: follow-up study, *J.A.M.A.* 104:2165–2168, June 1935
466. Short, C. L., and Bauer, W., The course of rheumatoid arthritis in patients receiving simple medical and orthopedic measures, *New England J. Med.* 238:142–148, Jan. 1948
467. Short, C. L., and Bauer, W., Unpublished data
468. Short, C. L., Beckman, W. W., and Bauer, W., Medical progress: gold therapy in rheumatoid arthritis, *New England J. Med.* 235:362–368, Sept. 1946
469. Short, C. L., Dienes, L., and Bauer, W., Rheumatoid arthritis: comparative evaluation of commonly employed diagnostic tests, *J.A.M.A.* 108:2087–2091, June 1937
470. Simpson, N. R. W., and Stevenson, C. J., An analysis of 200 cases of ankylosing spondylitis, *Brit. M. J.* 1:214–216, Feb. 1949
471. Singer, H. A., and Levy, H. A., Relationship of Felty's and allied syndromes to sepsis lenta, *Arch. Int. Med.* 57:576–600, March 1936
472. Slocumb, C. H., Report on diagnosis and treatment of rheumatic diseases in Europe, *Minnesota Med.* 19:436–440. July 1936
473. Slocumb, C. H., "Intramuscular fibrositis, secondary and primary," in R. L. Cecil and H. G. Wolff (ed.), *A Textbook of Medicine*, pp. 1421–1426. Seventh edition. Saunders, Philadelphia, 1947

Bibliography

474. Smith, A. D., Monarticular arthritis simulating tuberculosis: clinical and pathologic study of 24 cases, *Arch. Surg.* **25**:54–64, July 1932
475. Smith, G. V. S., "The ovaries," in R. H. Williams (ed.), *Textbook of Endocrinology,* pp. 349–449. Saunders, Philadelphia, 1950
476. Smith, M., Nature of atrophic arthritis and its treatment, *Am. Med.* **36**:622–630, Oct. 1930
477. Smith, M., A study of 102 cases of atrophic arthritis—I. Introduction; statistical data, *New England J. Med.* **206**:103–110, Jan. 1932
478. Smith, M., A study of 102 cases of atrophic arthritis—II. Constitutional defects, *New England J. Med.* **206**:160–173, Jan. 1932
479. Smith, M., A study of 102 cases of atrophic arthritis—III. Etiologic factors, *New England J. Med.* **206**:211–216, Feb. 1932
480. Smith, W., Incidence of certain rheumatic diseases in occupations, *Acta rheumatolog.* **4**:33–34, Dec. 1932
481. Smyth, C. J., "Bone absorption in rheumatoid arthritis: the opera-glass hand (la main en lorgnette)," in C. H. Slocumb (ed.), *Rheumatic Diseases,* pp. 196–208. Saunders, Philadelphia, 1952
482. Smyth, C. J., Freyberg, R. H., and Peck, W. S., Roentgen therapy for rheumatic disease, *J.A.M.A.* **116**:1995–2001, May 1941
483. Snorrason, E., Rheumatoid arthritis and occupation, *Acta med. Scandinav.* **140**:355–358, 1951
484. Sokoloff, L., The heart in rheumatoid arthritis, *Am. Heart J.* **45**:635–643, May 1953
485. Sokoloff, L., Wilens, S. L., Bunim, J. J., and McEwen, C., Diagnostic value of histologic lesions of striated muscle in rheumatoid arthritis, *Am. J. M. Sc.* **219**:174–182, Feb. 1950
486. Sokolow, M., and Snell, A. M., Atypical features of rheumatic fever in young adults, *J.A.M.A.* **133**:981–989, April 1947
487. Sorsby, A., and Gormaz, A., Iritis in the rheumatic affections, *Brit. M. J.* **1**: 597–600, April 1946
488. Soto-Hall, R., and Haldeman, K. O., The diagnosis of neuropathic joint disease (Charcot joint): an analysis of forty cases, *J.A.M.A.* **114**:2076–2078, May 1940
489. Spackman, E. W., Bach, T. F., Scull, C. W., and Pemberton, R., Complete roentgen ray studies of the gastro-intestinal tract in 400 arthritics, *Am. J. M. Sc.* **202**:68–77, July 1941
490. Spender, J. K., On some of the rarer complications of rheumatoid arthritis, *Brit. M. J.* **1**:905–907, 1892

491. Spender, J. K., and Garrod, A. E., "Rheumatoid arthritis," in T. C. Allbutt (ed.), *A System of Medicine by Many Writers*, vol. III, pp. 73–96. Macmillan, New York, 1898

492. Spink, W. W., and Keefer, C. S., Diagnosis, treatment, and end results in gonococcal arthritis: study of 70 cases, *New England J. Med.* 218:453–456, March 1938

493. Spitzy, Sur chronischen Arthritis des Kindes, *Ztschr. f. orth. Chir.* 2:1903. As cited by R. L. Jones in *Arthritis Deformans*, etc., p. 340. William Wood, New York, 1909

494. Stecher, R. M., and Hauser, H., Heberden's nodes; roentgenological and clinical appearance of degenerative joint disease of the fingers, *Am. J. Roentgenol.* 59:326–337, March 1948

495. Stecher, R. M., Hersh, A. H., and Solomon, W. M., Heredity of gout and its relationship to familial hyperuricemia, *Ann. Int. Med.* 31:595–614, Oct. 1949

496. Stecher, R. M., Hersh, A. H., Solomon, W. M., and Wolpaw, R., The genetics of rheumatoid arthritis: analysis of 224 families, *Am. J. Human Genet.* 5:118–138, June 1953

497. Stecher, R. M., Solomon, W. M., and Wolpaw, R., "Heredity in rheumatoid arthritis and ankylosing spondylitis," in C. H. Slocumb (ed.), *Rheumatic Diseases*, pp. 66–67. Saunders, Philadelphia, 1952

498. Steinbrocker, O., *Arthritis in Modern Practice: the Diagnosis and Management of Rheumatic and Allied Conditions.* 606 pp. Saunders, Philadelphia, 1941

499. Stenstam, T., On the occurrence of keratoconjunctivitis sicca in cases of rheumatoid arthritis, *Acta med. Scandinav.* 127:130–148, 1947

500. Stephens, C. A. L., Borden, A. L., Holbrook, W. P., and Hill, D. F., The use of folic acid in the treatment of anemia of rheumatoid arthritis: a preliminary report, *Ann. Int. Med.* 27:420–432, Sept. 1947

501. Sterne, E. H., and Schneider, B., Psoriatic arthritis, *Ann. Int. Med.* 38:512–522, March 1953

502. Stewart, J., Introduction to a discussion on the relation of rheumatoid arthritis to diseases of the nervous system, tuberculosis, and rheumatism, *Brit. M. J.* 2:1225–1229, Oct. 1897

503. Stiles, M. H., Basal metabolic rate in low grade chronic illness: statistical analysis of 166 cases, *Am. J. Clin. Path.* 11:871–877, Dec. 1941

504. Still, G. F., On a form of chronic joint disease in children, *Med.-Chir. Tr.* 80:47–59. Published by the Royal Medical and Chirurgical Society of London, 1897

Bibliography

505. Still, G. F., "Rheumatoid arthritis in children," in T. C. Allbutt (ed.), *A System of Medicine*, vol. 4, pp. 102–107. Macmillan, New York, 1897
506. Stockman, R., The causes and treatment of chronic rheumatism, *Brit. M. J.* 1:477–479, Feb. 1904
507. Stockman, R., *Rheumatism and Arthritis.* 132 pp. W. Green and Son, Edinburgh, 1920
508. Stoner, W. C., Importance of intensive program in management of arthritic patient, *J. Lab. & Clin. Med.* 15:1291–1294, Sept. 1930
509. Strangeways, T. S. P., "A case of so-called rheumatoid arthritis due to pneumococcal infection," in T. S. P. Strangeways (ed.), *Bull. Comm. Study of Special Diseases*, vol. 4, pp. 87–89. Edinburgh, 1914
510. Strangeways, T. S. P., and Burt, J. B., "A report on some points in the etiology and onset of 200 cases of so-called rheumatoid arthritis," in T. S. P. Strangeways (ed.), *Bull. Comm. Study of Special Diseases*, vol. 1, pp. 55–78. Cambridge University Press, Cambridge, England, 1907
511. Strümpell, A., Bemerkung über die chronische ankylosirende Entzündung der Wirbelsäule und der Hüftgelenke, *Deutsche Ztschr. Nervenh.* 11:338–342, Nov. 1897
512. Sundt, H., Still's disease and tuberculosis, *Mitt. a. d. Kustenhospital in Stavern, Norwegen*. 321 pp. Reviewed in *Acta rheumatol.* 10:16, Aug. 1938
513. Sury, B., *Rheumatoid Arthritis in Children: a Clinical Study.* 94 pp. Ejnar Munksgaards, Copenhagen, 1951
514. Swaim, L. T., Chronic arthritis, *J. Bone & Joint Surg.* 20:426–445, July 1922
515. Swaim, L. T., Chronic arthritis: further metabolism studies, *J.A.M.A.* 93:259–263, July 1929
516. Swaim, L. T., and Spear, L. M., Studies of basal metabolism in chronic arthritis, *Boston Med. & Surg. J.* 197:350–357, Sept. 1927
517. Sydenham, T., as cited by R. L. Jones in *Arthritis Deformans*, etc., p. 21. William Wood, New York, 1909
518. Symes, J. O., *The Rheumatic Diseases.* 241 pp. John Lane, London, 1905
519. Talbott, J. H., *Gout and Gouty Arthritis.* 92 pp. Grune & Stratton, New York, 1953
520. Talkov, R. H., Discussion of family incidence of rheumatoid spondylitis, by B. Rogoff and R. H. Freyberg, *Ann. Rheumat. Dis.* 7:40–41, March 1948
521. Talkov, R. H., Bauer, W., and Short, C. L., Rheumatoid arthritis associated with splenomegaly, *New England J. Med.* 227:395–399, Sept. 1942

522. Talkov, R. H., and Bennett, G. A., Attempts to induce subcutaneous nodules in rheumatoid arthritis patients, *J. Clin. Invest.* 25:935, Nov. 1946. Proc.
523. Taussig, A. E., Still's disease with hyperglobulinemia, *J. Lab. & Clin. Med.* 23:833–838, May 1938
524. Taylor, G. D., Ferguson, A. B., Kasabach, H., and Dawson, M. H., Roentgenologic observations on various types of chronic arthritis, *Arch. Int. Med.* 57:979–998, May 1936
525. Teissier, J., and Roque, G. "Rhumatismes chroniques," in P. Brouardel, A. Gilbert, and J. Girode, *Traité de médicine et de thérapeutique*, vol. 3, pp. 468–515. J. B. Baillière et Fils, Paris 1897
526. Thomas, B. A., Gonorrheal arthritis, *J.A.M.A.* 89:2174–2177, Dec. 1927
527. Thomas, G. W., Psychic factors in rheumatoid arthritis, *Am. J. Psychiat.* 93:693–710, Nov. 1936
528. Thomson, F. G., "Endocrine factors in some forms of arthritis," in *Proceedings of a Conference on Rheumatic Diseases held at Bath, 10th and 11th of May, 1928*, pp. 232–233. Published by the Hot Mineral Baths Committee of the Bath City Council, 1928
529. Thomson, F. G., Rheumatoid and climacteric arthritis, *Brit. M. J.* 1:1171–1172, June 1936
530. Thomson, F. G., and Gordon, R. G., *Chronic Rheumatic Diseases: Their Diagnosis and Treatment*. 202 pp. Oxford University Press, London, 1926
531. Thompson, H. E., Wyatt, B. L., and Hicks, R. A., Chronic atrophic arthritis, *Ann. Int. Med.* 11:1792–1805, April 1938
532. Thompson, M., Personal communication
533. Toone, E. C., Jr., and Irky, W. R., Evaluation of phenylbutazone (butazolidin) in the treatment of rheumatoid spondylitis: report of 50 cases, *Ann. Int. Med.* 41:70–78, July 1954
534. Traeger, C. H., Fibrositis, *M. Clin. North America* 21:1797–1806, Nov. 1937
535. Traut, E. F., and Vrtiak, E. G., A statistical study of allergy in arthritis, *Ann. Int. Med.* 13:761–767, Nov. 1939
536. Trousseau, A., *Lectures on Clinical Medicine Delivered at the Hôtel-Dieu, Paris*, vols. 1–5. Translated from the edition of 1868. The New Sydenham Society, London, 1868–1872
537. Tuft, L., *Clinical Allergy*. 711 pp. Saunders, Philadelphia, 1937
538. Turner, L. W., and Lansbury, J., Low diastolic pressure as a clinical feature of rheumatoid arthritis and its possible etiologic significance, *Am. J. M. Sc.* 227:503–508, May 1954
539. Turner, T. B., Race and sex distribution of lesions of syphilis in 10,000 cases, *Bull. Johns Hopkins Hosp.* 46:159–184, Feb. 1930

Bibliography

540. Tyson, T. L., Spondylitis ankylopoietica, *M. Clin. North America* 21:1755–1761, Nov. 1937

541. Unger, L., *Bronchial Asthma.* 724 pp. C. C. Thomas, Springfield, Illinois, 1945

542. van der Hoeve, J., Scleromalacia perforans, *Arch. Ophth.* 11:111–118, Jan. 1934

543. Vanzant, F. R., Normal range of gastric acidity from youth to old age: analysis of 3,746 records, *Proc. Staff Meet., Mayo Clin.* 6:297–300, May 1931

544. Verhoeff, F. H., and King, M. J., Scleromalacia perforans: report of case in which eye was examined microscopically, *Arch. Ophth.* 20:1013–1035, Dec. 1938

545. von Bechterew, W., Von der Verwachsung oder Steifigkeit der Wirbelsäule, *Deutsche Ztschr. Nervenh.* 11:327–337, Nov. 1897

546. Vrtiak, E. G., and Jordan, E. P., Clinical study of chronic arthritis, *J.A.M.A.* 94:863–867, March 1930

547. Wagner, L. C., Chronic bone abscesses (Brodie) simulating symptoms of arthritis, *M. Clin. North America* 21:1763–1769, Nov. 1937

548. Wainwright, C. W., and Janeway, C. A., Diagnosis of acute arthritis, *Internat. Clin.* 3:55–63, Sept. 1937

549. Waldo, H., The paralysis of osteo-arthritis, *Bristol Med.-Chir. J.* 12:90–94, 1895

550. Warren, C. F., Hinton, W. A., and Bauer, W., Significance of gonococcus complement fixation test as diagnostic aid in study of arthritis, *J.A.M.A.* 108:1241–1247, April 1937

551. Warren, S. L., Differential diagnosis of gonococcal arthritis, *J. Lab. & Clin. Med.* 22:44–47, Oct. 1936

552. Wassmann, K., Rheumatoid arthritis and psoriasis: statistical statements, *Ann. Rheumat. Dis.* 8:70–71, March 1949

553. Waterhouse, R., The superficial lymph glands in rheumatoid arthritis, *St. Bartholomew's Hosp. Reports* 43:107–113, 1907

554. Waterhouse, R., Still's disease and rheumatoid arthritis, *Proc. Roy. Soc. Med.* (Sect. Dis. Child.) 24:95–98, Oct. 1931

555. Wehrbein, M. L., Gonococcus arthritis; study of 610 cases, *Surg., Gynec. & Obst.* 49:105–113, July 1929

556. Weil, M.-P., La maladie dite de "Chauffard-Still" correspond-elle à une entité clinique véritable? *Presse méd.* 45:1627–1628, Nov. 1937

557. Weinberger, H. J., and Bauer, W., Diagnosis and treatment of Reiter's syndrome, *M. Clin. North America* 39:587–599, March 1955

558. Weismann-Netter, R., Hydrarthrose périodique: guérison par le tartrate d'ergotamine, *Bull. et mém. Soc. med. de hôp. de Paris.* 53:909–914, July 1929

559. Weiss, E., Psychogenic rheumatism, *M. Clin. North America* 39:601–612, March 1955

560. Weiss, S., Gallbladder disease and arthritis, *Rev. Gastroenterol.* 11:116–120, March–April 1944

561. Weissenbach, R. J., and Françon, F., Le syndrome de Chauffard-Still rhumatisme chronique fibreux déformant progressif avec adénopathies et splenomégalie, sa place en nosalgie, *Presse méd.* 39:1197–1200, Aug. 1931

562. Wetherby, M., Chronic arthritis: a clinical analysis of three hundred and fifty cases, *Arch. Int. Med.* 50:926–944, Dec. 1932

563. Whitman, R., A report of final results in two cases of polyarthritis in children of the type first described by Still, together with remarks on rheumatoid arthritis, *Med. Rec.* 63:601–605, April 1903

564. Wichmann, R., *Der chronische Gelenk-Rheumatismus und seine Beziehungen zum Nerven system, nach eigenen Beobachtungen.* Louis Heuser, Berlin, 1890

565. Wile, U. J., and Butler, M. G., A critical survey of Charcot's arthropathy. Analysis of eighty-eight cases, *J.A.M.A.* 94:1053–1055, April 1930

566. Willard, J. H., and Strawbridge, R. R., Gallbladder infections as a factor in arthritis, *M. Clin. North America* 24:1709–1716, Nov. 1940

567. Wilson, M. G., *Rheumatic Fever: Studies of the Epidemiology, Manifestations, Diagnosis, and Treatment of the Disease During the First Three Decades.* 595 pp. Commonwealth Fund, New York, 1940

568. Wolfson, W. Q., Beierwaltes, W. H., Robinson, W. D., Duff, I. F., Jones, J. R., Knorpp, C. T., Siemienski, J. S., and Eya, M., "Corticogenic hypothyroidism: its incidence, clinical significance and management during prolonged treatment with ACTH or cortisone," in J. R. Mote (ed.), *Proceedings of the Second Clinical ACTH Conference*, vol. 2, pp. 95–121. Blakiston, New York, 1951

569. Wong, R. T., Band-shaped opacity of the cornea associated with juvenile atrophic arthritis: report of a case, *Arch. Ophth.* 26:21–24, July 1941

569a. Woodmansey, A., and Beattie, J. W., Effect of cortisone and certain other steroids on the peripheral vasculature in arthritis, *Ann. Rheumat. Dis.* 14:293–297, Sept. 1955

570. Woodmansey, A., Collins, D. H., and Ernst, M. M., Vascular reactions to the contrast bath in health and in rheumatoid arthritis, *Lancet* 2:1350–1353, Dec. 1938

Bibliography

571. Wyatt, B. L., *Chronic Arthritis and Rheumatoid Affections with Recovery Record*. 166 pp. William Wood, New York, 1930

572. Young, A. G., The occurrence of allergic reactions in arthritic patients, *New England J. Med.* 214:779–782, April 1936

573. Young, D., and Schwedel, J. B., The heart in rheumatoid arthritis: a study of thirty-eight autopsy cases, *Am. Heart J.* 28:1–23, July 1944

574. Yule, G. U., and Kendall, M. G., *An Introduction to the Theory of Statistics*. Fourteenth edition. Hafner, New York, 1950

575. Zeller, J. W., discussion in Medical Grand Rounds, Massachusetts General Hospital: postrheumatic arthritis, *Am. Pract. & Digest Treat.* 1:189, Feb. 1950

576. Ziff, M., Brown, P., Badin, J., and McEwen, C., A hemagglutination test for rheumatoid arthritis with enhanced sensitivity using the euglobulin fraction, *Bull. Rheumat. Dis.* 5:75–76, Oct. 1954

Index

Index

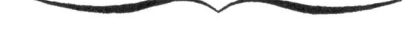

f = figure.   fn = footnote.   t = table.

Abdominal pain
  frequency in patients and controls, 25.1 t, 25.2
Activity of disease
  classification of patients by, 43.1 t, 43.3
  definition, 4.27
  relation to: age at admission, 18.2, 43.2; anemia, 38.3; bronchial asthma, 20.20; constitutional symptoms, 21.8; duration of arthritis before admission, 18.5, 43.2; extent of joint involvement, 34.5; fever, 26.9; high basal metabolism, 41.5; lymphadenopathy, 30.4; subcutaneous nodules, 33.1 t, 33.3; various disease attributes, 43.2; vasomotor symptoms and signs, 22.11
Age of patients
—At onset
  compared with age distribution of population, 1.21, 6.1, 6.1 f, 6.1 t, 6.2, 6.2 f, 6.2 t, 6.7
  in other diseases, 6.7
  in persons over 60 years, 6.6
  in population studies, 6.7, 6.9
  in previous studies, 6.1, 6.4–6.6
  relation to: age at admission, 18.2;

Age of patients, at onset (cont.)
  menopause, 6.7, 6.9; sex, 5.1, 5.1 t, 6.3
—On hospital admission
  compared with age distribution of Massachusetts population, 18.1, 18.1 f, 18.1 t, 18.2 f, 18.2 t
  median in males and females, 18.1
  relation to: activity of disease, 18.2, 43.2; age at onset, 18.2; constitutional symptoms, 21.4; duration of arthritis before admission, 18.5; fever, 26.3; influence of cold, moisture, and heat on course, 20.10; influence of strain on course, 20.4; prognosis, 18.2, 44.5 t, 44.6; severity of disease, 18.2, 43.5; sex, 18.2; subsequent course, 18.2, 44.5 t, 44.6; various disease attributes, 18.2, 18.3 t
  sex ratio, 18.1
Age distribution, 2.118
Albuminuria. *See under* Urinary findings, abnormal
Allergic diseases
  family history, 9.1 t, 9.2
  frequency: in patients and controls,

Allergic diseases (cont.)
9.2, 9.2 t; in patients compared with population, 9.3; in previous studies, 9.3, 9.4
influence on course, 20.9
Amyloidosis, 2.119, 39.1
Anacidity, gastric. See Gastric anacidity
Anemia, 2.119
characteristics, 38.4
definition, 4.23
frequency: in patients, 38.1 t, 38.2; in previous studies, 38.3
pathogenesis, 38.4, 38.10
relation to: activity and course of arthritis, 38.3, 38.4, 38.10; duration of arthritis before admission, 38.3, 38.3 t; fever, 38.3; gastric anacidity, 38.3, 40.3 t, 40.5; iron absorption and metabolism, 38.4; plasma volume, 38.4; prognosis, 38.3; severity of disease, 38.2 t, 38.3; sex, 38.1 t, 38.2; subsequent course, 38.3; type of onset, 15.4, 38.3; various disease attributes, 38.3
Anorexia, 2.118
—As constitutional symptom
frequency in patients and controls, 21.1 t, 21.2
relation to: low basal metabolism, 41.3; nervousness and/or emotional upsets, 21.4; prodromal anorexia, 21.3; type of onset, 15.4; various disease attributes, 21.3 t, 21.4
Anthropometric studies
relation to severity of disease, 43.8
Appetite loss. See Anorexia
Asthma, bronchial
influence on activity of disease, 20.9, 20.20
See also Allergic diseases

Basal metabolism
—High
frequency: in control series, 41.1 t, 41.2; in patients, 41.1 t, 41.2, 41.5; in previous studies, 41.1, 41.2 t, 41.5

Basal metabolism, high (cont.)
relation to: activity of disease, 41.5; various disease attributes, 41.5
—Low
due to hypothroidism, 41.7, 41.9
extra-thyroid causes, 41.7
frequency: in control series, 41.1 t, 41.2; in patients, 41.1 t, 41.2; in previous studies, 41.1, 41.2, 41.2 t
metabolic rate below minus 20, 41.4
relation to: age, 41.3; duration of arthritis before admission, 41.3; malnutrition, 41.4; severity of disease, 41.4; sex, 41.3; various disease attributes, 41.4; vasomotor symptoms and signs, 41.4; weakness and anorexia, 41.3
—Methods of determination in patients, 41.2
Blood
—Leukocytosis, 2.119
frequency in patients, 38.4 t, 38.5
pathogenesis, 38.6
relation to: splenomegaly, 38.7; various disease attributes, 38.5
significance, 38.6
—Leukopenia, 2.119
frequency in patients, 38.4 t, 38.7
in Felty's syndrome, 2.29, 2.30
relation to: duration of arthritis before admission, 38.7; splenomegaly, 2.29, 30.6, 38.7, 38.10
—Red-cell count. See under Anemia
—White-cell count, differential
increase in: eosinophils, 38.4 t, 38.8, 38.10; lymphocytes, 38.4 t, 38.8; monocytes, 38.4 t, 38.8; polymorphonuclears, 38.4 t, 38.8
—See also under Anemia
Blood pressure
—Findings: in patients and controls, 28.1, 28.1 t, 28.2, 28.2 t, 28.3 t; in previous studies, 28.1, 28.4 t
—High, 28.3 fn
in controls, 28.2
in patients, 28.5

Index

Blood pressure (cont.)
—Low
as clinical feature of rheumatoid arthritis, 28.8
in patients, 28.4
in previous studies, 28.1, 28.3, 28.4
possible causes, 28.6
—Relation to: age and sex, 28.1, 28.2, 28.2 t, 28.3 t
Bowel disorders, 25.1
Bronchiectasis
frequency in patients, 24.4
Brucellosis
arthritis of, 2.85
with intermittent hydrarthrosis, 2.86
with joint disease resembling rheumatoid arthritis, 2.85, 2.115
Bursitis, 2.118

Cardio-respiratory symptoms
frequency in patients, 24.1, 24.1 t
Childbirth, as precipitating factor
frequency: in patients, 14.25, 14.27; in previous studies, 14.26, 14.27
Climacteric arthritis. *See* Menopausal arthritis
Clonus, 23.10
Clubbing
diagnostic value, 32.3
frequency in patients, 32.3
Clutton's joints. *See under* Syphilitic arthritis, congenital
Cold extremities. *See under* Vasomotor symptoms
Cold influencing course. *See under* Course before hospital admission, factors influencing
Colitis, ulcerative
accompanying rheumatoid arthritis, 2.106
arthritis of: as an independent entity, 2.105, 2.116; differentiated from rheumatoid arthritis, 2.105; pathologic findings, 2.105
patients with, included in study, 2.106

Colon, abnormalities of
frequency of diverticula, 36.3
relation to: age, 36.3; duration of arthritis before admission, 36.3; severity of disease, 36.3; sex, 36.3
results of roentgenograms: in patients, 36.1 t, 36.2; in previous studies, 36.1, 36.2
significance of changes, 36.4
Connective tissue diseases
concept, 2.111
differentiation of individual examples, 2.111, 2.115
patients with, excluded from study, 2.112
relationships among, 2.111
simulating rheumatoid arthritis, 2.112, 2.113
subcutaneous nodules in, 2.122
Constipation
frequency in patients and controls, 25.1 t, 25.2
Constitutional symptoms
absence as criterion for nonspecific "infectious" arthritis, 16.13, 16.14
associations among, 21.4
definition, 4.14
frequency in patients and controls, 21.1 t, 21.2
psychogenic factors in their production, 21.8
relation to: activity of disease, 21.8; age on admission, 21.4; course before admission, 21.4; monarticular onset, 21.4; muscular atrophy, 21.4; neurologic symptoms, 23.3; prodromal symptoms, 21.1; prognosis, 21.4; severity of disease, 21.4; sex, 21.4; spondylitis, 21.4; subsequent course, 21.4; unilateral onset, 21.4; various disease attributes, 21.3 t, 21.4; vasomotor signs, 21.4; vasomotor symptoms, 21.4, 22.4
See also Anorexia, Headache, Weakness, Weight loss (as constitutional symptoms), *and under* Weight of patients

Controls
  age and sex distribution, 3.4
  collection of data on, 3.7
  selection, 1.4, 3.4
  source, 3.5
  use in previous studies, 1.6, 1.11, 1.23
Course before hospital admission
—Factors influencing
  allergic diseases, 20.9
  asthma, bronchial, 20.9
  childbirth, 19.12
  cold, moisture, and heat
    frequency: in patients, 20.9 t, 20.10; in previous studies, 20.14
    relation to: age on admission, 20.10; sex, 20.10, 20.11 t, 20.12; various disease attributes, 20.12; vasomotor symptoms, 20.10 t, 20.11, 20.12, 20.17
  enumerated, 20.1
  exposure, 19.12
  frequency in previous studies, 20.14
  infection, 19.12, 20.15
    frequency, 20.5
    relation to: infection as a precipitant, 20.7, 20.7 t, 20.20; influence of strain on course, 20.3 t, 20.4, 20.5 t, 20.7; prognosis, 20.4 t, 20.6; severity of disease, 20.4 t, 20.6; type of onset, 20.6 t, 20.7; various disease attributes, 20.6
  menstruation, 20.8, 20.8 t, 20.16
  operation, 19.12
  pregnancy, 2.123, 20.8, 20.16
  season, 20.12 t, 20.13
  strain, 19.12, 20.4, 20.15
    frequency, 20.3
    relation to: age on admission, 20.4; duration of arthritis, 20.4; influence of infection on course, 20.3 t, 20.4, 20.5 t, 20.7; prognosis, 20.2 t, 20.4; severity of disease, 20.2 t, 20.4; sex, 20.1 t, 20.4; spondylitis, 20.4; strain as a precipitant, 20.4; type of onset, 20.4

Course before hospital admission (cont.)
—Intermittent
  as criterion for nonspecific "infectious" arthritis, 16.13, 16.14
  average duration of arthritis of patients with, 19.7 t
  classification, 19.8–19.10
  definition, 4.13, 19.1
  duration, 19.10
  exacerbations: average number, 19.7 t; average time in, 19.5 t; degree, 19.4 t; duration, 19.10, 19.11; factors associated with, 19.12; monthly distribution, 19.6 f, 19.8 t; number, 19.10; patients subdivided according to length of, 19.6 t; proportion of course spent in, 19.5 t, 19.7; seasonal distribution, 19.10 t, 19.13; severity, 19.11
  frequency, 19.2
  graphic presentation, 19.1 f–19.5 f, 19.5, 19.6
  individual patterns, 19.4
  months of onset in patients, 19.8 f, 19.11 t
  relation to: duration of arthritis before admission, 18.3; fever, 19.2, 26.5; monarticular onset, 19.2
  remissions: average time in, 19.5 t; duration, 19.10, 19.11; monthly distribution, 19.7 f, 19.9 t; patients subdivided according to length of, 19.6 t; proportion of course spent in, 19.5 t, 19.7; seasonal distribution, 19.10 t, 19.13
—Progressive
  definition, 4.13, 19.1
  frequency, 19.2
  relation to: primary involvement of small joints, 19.2; shorter duration of arthritis, 19.2
—Relation to: age at onset, 19.2, 19.2 t, 19.3, 44.8; constitutional symptoms, 21.4; duration of arthritis before admission, 18.5, 19.3 t; influence of strain on course, 20.4; onset near

Index

Course before hospital admission, relation to (cont.)
  menopause, 12.4; primary joint involvement, 16.11, 16.11 t, 44.8; prodromal symptoms, 13.10, 13.10 t; prognosis, 19.3; severity of disease, 19.3, 43.4; sex, 19.1 t, 19.2; spondylitis, 42.4; subsequent course, 19.3; type of onset, 15.5, 15.5 t, 15.7, 19.3, 44.8; various disease attributes, 44.8; vasomotor symptoms, 22.5
—See also under Prognosis
Course following hospital admission
—Definition of improvement, 4.28
—Method of study: duration of observation, 44.1 t, 44.3; improvement, 44.10, 44.16; limitations, 44.10; selection of patients, 44.2; used in evaluation, 44.3, 44.4
—Relation to: age at onset, 44.6; age on admission, 18.2, 44.5 t, 44.6; anemia, 38.3; constitutional symptoms, 21.4; course before admission, 19.3; duration of arthritis before admission, 18.5, 18.8, 44.6 t, 44.7, 44.7 t; fever, 26.4; joint effusion, 34.2; joint redness, 34.2; onset near menopause, 12.4; postmenopausal state, 12.4; presence of focal infection, 37.3 t, 37.4; prodromal symptoms, 13.10; sex, 44.3 t, 44.5; sex, with spondylitis excluded, 44.4 t, 44.5; spondylitis, 42.3, 42.3 t, 44.5; subcutaneous nodules, 33.4 t, 33.5; treatment of focal infection, 37.3 t, 37.4; type of onset, 15.5; various disease attributes, 44.8 t, 44.9; vasomotor symptoms, 22.5
—Results: in previous studies, 44.12; in 1937 tabulation, 44.9 t, 44.11; in 1947 tabulation, 44.2 t, 44.4, 44.9 t, 44.11; in 1954 tabulation, 44.9 t, 44.11
—See also under Prognosis
Cyanosis. See under Vasomotor symptoms
Cylindruria. See under Urinary findings, abnormal

Dampness. See under Course before hospital admission, factors influencing
Data
—Analysis
  comparisons: among attributes of patients, 3.1 t–3.9 t, 3.12–3.15, 3.22; between patients and controls, 3.10, 46 t
  interpretation of numerical comparisons, 3.9
  statistical "impressions," 3.11
  variables: association, 3.16–3.19; hidden, 3.17, 3.19, 3.20; spurious associations, 3.20; spurious independence, 3.22
—Collection
  categories used: for controls, 3.7; for patients, 3.6
  checklist of findings: on controls, 3.7; on patients, 3.1 f, 3.6
  follow-up studies, 1.4, 3.8
  observers responsible for, 3.6
Degenerative joint disease
  clinical features of rheumatoid arthritis associated with, 1.18
  co-existence with rheumatoid arthritis, 2.5, 2.115
  distinguished from rheumatoid arthritis: clinically, 1.7, 1.9, 1.21, 2.4; pathologically, 1.9, 2.4
  not distinguished from rheumatoid arthritis, 1.10, 1.13, 1.15, 1.19, 2.5
  pathologic lesions assigned to rheumatoid arthritis, 2.4
  spinal symptoms due to, 42.2
  synovial fluid, 2.119
  synovial and periarticular inflammation, 2.5
Diabetes
  frequency in rheumatoid arthritis, 10.7
Diarrhea
  frequency in patients and controls, 25.1 t, 25.2
Differential white-cell count. See Blood, white-cell count, differential

Duration of arthritis before hospital admission
  classification, 18.4
  definition, 4.12
  relation to: activity of disease, 18.5, 43.2; age at onset, 18.5; age on admission, 18.5; anemia, 38.3, 38.3 t; course before admission, 18.5, 19.2, 19.3 t; gastric anacidity, 40.5; infection as a precipitant, 14.10, 18.5; influence of strain on course, 20.4; intermittent course before admission, 18.3; leukopenia, 38.7; low basal metabolism, 41.3; primary joint involvement, 16.2 t, 16.3; prodromal symptoms, 13.6, 18.3, 18.5; prognosis, 18.5, 44.6 t, 44.7, 44.7 t; roentgenographic changes in colon, 36.3; severity of disease, 18.5, 43.4; sex, 18.3, 18.3 f, 18.4 f, 18.4 t, 18.5; spondylitis, 42.3; subcutaneous nodules, 33.3; subsequent course, 18.5, 18.8, 44.6 t, 44.7, 44.7 t; type of onset, 15.3, 15.3 t, 18.5; various disease attributes, 18.3 t, 18.4; vasomotor symptoms, 22.5

Edema of extremities
  frequency in patients and controls, 32.1, 32.1 t
  from extraneous causes, 32.1
  in previous studies, 32.1
  pathogenesis, 32.2, 32.5
  relation to: involved joints, 32.1; various disease attributes, 32.1
Endocarditis
  frequency in patients and controls, 24.4 t, 24.5
  in rheumatoid arthritis, 1.7, 2.6, 2.8–2.10, 2.115, 24.7
Eosinophilia. *See under* Blood, white-cell count, differential
Exacerbations
  distribution: by months, 19.6 f, 19.8 t;

Exacerbations, distribution (cont.)
  occurrence in same quarter of year, 19.15, 19.19; seasonal, 19.10 t, 19.13, 19.14, 19.19
See also under Course before hospital admission, intermittent
Exposure, as precipitating factor
  frequency: in patients, 14.1 t, 14.16; in previous studies, 14.14 t, 14.19
  relation to: age at onset, 14.17; other precipitants, 14.18; prognosis, 14.13 t, 14.17; sex, 14.12 t, 14.17; spondylitis, 14.17; type of onset, 14.17
  significance, 14.19 fn
  types, 14.11 t, 14.16
Eyes
—Abnormalities in patients and controls, 29.1, 29.1 t
—Inflammatory lesions, 2.118, 29.2, 29.2 t
  iritis
    frequency: in patients, 29.2, 29.2 t; in previous studies, 29.2, 29.2 t
    in juvenile rheumatoid arthritis, 2.27
    lateral distribution, 29.3
    relation to: onset of arthritis, 29.3; spondylitis, 2.15, 29.2 t, 29.3 t, 29.4, 29.6
    varying severity, 29.3
  keratoconjunctivitis sicca, 29.2, 29.2 t, 29.6
  gastric acidity in, 40.8
  keratopathy, 29.2
    in juvenile rheumatoid arthritis, 2.27
  scleritis, 29.2 t
  scleromalacia perforans, 29.2, 29.2 t

Family history
  genetic mechanisms, 8.10
  multiple cases of rheumatoid arthritis in single families, 8.5
  of diseases other than rheumatoid arthritis, 8.1 t, 8.3; rheumatic disease in general, 8.2 t, 8.3 t, 8.9; rheumatic fever, 8.2 t, 8.3 t, 8.8, 8.12

Index

Family history (cont.)
  of rheumatoid arthritis
    as aid in diagnosis, 8.6
    in patients and controls, 8.2 t, 8.4
    relation to: age at onset, 8.4 t, 8.6; type of onset, 8.5 t, 8.6
  of rheumatoid spondylitis, 8.7
  relative influence of environment, contagion, and heredity, 8.10, 8.12
  results in previous studies, 8.3 t, 8.4
  validity of data, 8.1, 8.2
Fasciitis, 2.118
Fatigue. See Weakness, as a constitutional symptom
Felty's syndrome
  as independent entity, 2.30
  as variant of rheumatoid arthritis, 2.29, 2.116
  inclusion of patients with, in study, 2.30
Fever, 2.118
  classification, 26.1 t, 26.2
  definition, 4.18
  effect of antipyretic agents, 26.9
  frequency: in patients, 26.1 t, 26.2; in previous studies, 26.6
  pathogenesis, 26.7
  relation to: activity of disease, 26.9; age at onset, 26.3; age on admission, 26.3; anemia, 38.3; course before admission, 19.2, 26.5; joint effusion, 34.2; primary joint involvement, 16.12, 26.3; prognosis, 26.4; severity of disease, 26.2 t, 26.4; sex, 26.3; spondylitis, 26.3; subsequent course, 26.4; tachycardia, 27.1 t, 27.4; type of onset, 15.4, 26.5; various disease attributes, 26.3, 26.4; vasomotor symptoms, 22.5; weight loss, 21.4, 26.3
Fibrositis
—Primary, 2.107, 2.109
  as psychosomatic disorder, 2.109
  differentiated from rheumatoid arthritis, 2.110, 2.115
—Secondary, 2.107, 2.108, 2.115

Flatulence
  frequency in patients and controls, 25.1 t, 25.2
Focal infection
  absence in patients, 37.4
  frequency: in patients, 37.1 t, 37.3; in patients and controls, 37.6
  location in patients, 37.2 t, 37.3
  methods of investigation, 37.2
  previous treatment in patients, 37.3
  relation to prognosis, 37.3 t, 37.4
  results of treatment in relation to: infection as a precipitant, 37.5; type of onset, 37.5
  significance, 37.6
  subsequent course in relation to treatment, 37.3 t, 37.4, 44.2
  See also under Gallbladder disease; Colon, abnormalities of

Gallbladder
—Disease
  frequency: in patients, 35.1; in previous studies, 35.1
  results of treatment in rheumatoid arthritis, 35.2
—Roentgenograms
  findings in patients, 35.1 t
Gastric anacidity
  definition, 4.24
  frequency: in control series reported in literature, 40.1 t, 40.3; in patients, 40.1 t, 40.3; in previous studies, 40.1, 40.4
  in keratoconjunctivitis sicca, 40.8
  methods employed for determination, 40.2
  relation to: age, 40.1 t, 40.2 t, 40.3, 40.5; anemia, 38.3, 40.3 t, 40.5; duration of arthritis before admission, 40.5; severity of disease, 40.5; sex, 40.1 t, 40.3, 40.5; various disease attributes, 40.6
Gastric crises, 25.3

Gastro-intestinal symptoms
  frequency: in patients and controls, 25.1 t, 25.2; in previous studies, 25.3
  pathogenesis, 25.5, 25.7
Glomerulitis
  as autopsy finding in rheumatoid arthritis, 39.1, 39.6
Goiter, non-toxic
  frequency: in patients and controls, 41.3 t, 41.6; in previous studies, 41.6
Gonococcal arthritis
  as self-limiting disease, 2.88, 2.93
  chronic progressive forms, 2.89, 2.90, 2.93, 2.115
  co-existence with rheumatoid arthritis, 2.91, 2.95
  diagnosis, 2.88
  follow-up studies, 2.93
  frequency, 2.87
  pathologic findings, 2.92
  patients with, excluded from study, 2.87, 2.94
  phalangeal arthritis, 2.90
  polyarticular, 2.88
  proliferative synovitis, 2.92
  resembling rheumatoid arthritis, 2.88
Gonorrhea, genito-urinary
  evidence for, in patients, 2.1 t, 2.96, 2.97
  history of, in patients and controls, 10.3 t, 10.5
  precipitating rheumatoid arthritis, 2.88, 2.90, 2.93, 2.95
Gouty arthritis
  chronic resembling rheumatoid arthritis, 2.3, 2.115
  clinical resemblance to atypical rheumatoid arthritis, 2.3
  co-existence with rheumatoid arthritis, 2.3, 39.6
  distinguished: from acute and chronic rheumatism, 2.2; from rheumatoid arthritis, 2.2, 2.3, 2.115
  hyperuricemia, 2.2, 2.119
  roentgenographic changes resembling those in rheumatoid arthritis, 2.3
Granuloma annulare, 2.122

Hay fever. *See under* Allergic diseases
Headache, as constitutional symptom, 21.2
Heart disease
  frequency in patients and controls, 24.4 t, 24.5
Heat, associated with remissions, 19.12
  See also under Course before hospital admission, factors influencing
Hepatitis
  as systemic manifestation of rheumatoid arthritis, 10.4
  frequency in patients and controls, 10.4
  in past, as cause of altered liver function, 10.4
Herpes zoster, 31.6
Hypertension
  relation to rheumatoid arthritis, 28.5, 28.8
  See also Blood pressure, high
Hypertrophic arthritis. *See under* Degenerative joint disease
Hypotension. *See* Blood pressure, low

Illnesses other than rheumatoid arthritis
  frequency: in patients and controls, 10.1–10.3, 10.1 t, 10.2 t; in previous studies, 10.4 t, 10.7
  relation to: prognosis, 10.9; severity of disease, 10.9; spondylitis, 10.9
Infection
  —As precipitating factor, 1.7
  as criterion for nonspecific "infectious" arthritis, 16.13, 16.14
  combined with other precipitants, 14.14
  frequency: in controlled study, 14.15; in patients, 14.1 t, 14.10; in previous studies, 14.10 t, 14.15
  relation to: age at onset, 14.11; duration of arthritis before admission, 14.10, 18.5; influence of infection on course, 20.7, 20.7 t, 20.20; prognosis, 14.11; sex, 14.11; spondylitis, 14.11; strain, 14.6 t, 14.7, 14.11; type of onset, 14.8 t, 14.10, 15.3, 18.5; weakness, 21.4

Index

Infection, as precipitating factor (cont.)
  time before onset, 14.13
  types, 14.9 t, 14.12
  —*See also* Focal infection *and under*
    Course before hospital admission,
    factors influencing
"Infectious" arthritis, nonspecific
  as stage of rheumatoid arthritis, 2.102,
    2.103, 2.116, 16.15, 16.19
  criteria for identification, 2.101, 16.13,
    16.14
  differentiated from arthritis due to
    specific infectious agents, 2.65
  inter-relationships among criteria for,
    16.13–16.15, 16.13 t
  patients with, included in study, 2.104
  relation to: prognosis, 2.103, 16.15; rheumatoid arthritis, 2.65
  roentgenograms, 2.102
  synonyms, 2.101, 2.102
Infectious arthritis, specific
  caused by pyogenic bacteria, 2.65
  co-existence with rheumatoid arthritis,
    2.63, 2.66
  differentiated from rheumatoid arthritis,
    2.63, 2.115
  occurrence of chronic progressive form,
    2.63
  patients with, excluded from study, 2.64
  synovial fluid, 2.119
Injuries
  frequency in patients and controls, 10.1,
    10.2, 10.5 t, 10.8
  relation to: prognosis, 10.9; severity of
    disease, 10.9; spondylitis, 10.9
  See also Precipitating factors
Intermittent hydrarthrosis
  as manifestation of rheumatoid arthritis, 2.52, 2.116
  causation, 2.51
  description, 2.50
  familial occurrence, 2.52
  frequency, 2.49
  idiopathic type, 2.48, 2.53
  in association with brucellosis, 2.86
  joint pathology, 2.52

Intermittent hydrarthrosis (cont.)
  patients with, included in study, 2.53
  symptomatic type, 2.48, 2.53
Iron utilization. *See under* Anemia;
    Tongue, atrophy

Jaundice
  in course of rheumatoid arthritis, 2.123,
    19.12
Joint involvement
—Extent
  classification of patients by, 34.5, 43.1 t,
    43.3
  definition, 4.22
  relation to: activity of disease, 34.5;
    prognosis, 34.5; severity of disease,
    43.1; various disease attributes,
    34.5, 34.5 t
—Primary, 2.118
  classification, 16.2
  differences in, 16.19
  distribution, 16.1 t, 16.2; in previous
    studies, 16.5
  frequency: in individual joints, 16.4 t,
    16.5; in knees, feet, and hands, 16.5,
    16.5 t
  in arms compared with legs, 16.6, 16.6 t
  in large joints
    as criterion for nonspecific "infectious"
      arthritis, 16.14
    compared with small joints, 16.3 t, 16.4
    definition, 4.10, 16.2
    frequency in patients, 16.1 t
  in small joints
    definition, 4.9, 16.2
    frequency in patients, 16.1 t
    relation to prognosis, 44.8
  in spine
    definition, 16.2
    frequency in patients, 16.1 t, 16.8
  in spondylitis, 16.4, 16.8, 16.8 t
  monarticular
    as criterion for nonspecific "infectious"
      arthritis, 16.14
    definition, 4.11, 16.2
    frequency: in individual joints, 16.7,

Joint involvement, primary,
  monarticular (cont.)
    16.7 t; in patients, 16.1 t, 16.7; in previous studies, 16.7
  persistence, 16.7
  relation to: constitutional symptoms, 21.4; course before admission, 16.7, 44.8; prognosis, 16.7, 44.8
  with remission, 16.7
  relation to: age at onset, 16.10, 16.10 t; course before admission, 16.11, 16.11 t, 19.2; duration of arthritis before admission, 16.2 t, 16.3; fever, 16.12, 26.3; lymphadenopathy, 16.12, 30.4; onset near menopause, 16.12; precipitating factors, 16.12; prodromal symptoms, 16.12; prognosis, 16.11, 16.11 t; sex, 16.5, 16.9, 16.9 t; subcutaneous nodules, 16.12, 33.3; type of onset, 15.4, 16.12; vasomotor symptoms, 22.5
—Primary, bilateral
  frequency: in patients, 17.2; in previous studies, 17.4
—Primary, lateral distribution, 16.1
  in patients, 17.1 t
  relation to: age at onset, 17.3, 17.4 t; age on admission, 17.3; prodromal symptoms, 17.3, 17.5 t; prognosis, 17.3, 17.6 t; severity of disease, 17.3, 17.6 t; sex, 17.3, 17.3 t
—Primary, unilateral
  as criterion for nonspecific "infectious" arthritis, 16.14
  duration, 17.2, 17.2 t
  frequency in patients, 17.2
  relation to: constitutional symptoms, 21.4; type of onset, 15.4, 17.3
—Symmetrical, 2.118, 17.1
  causation theories: neural, 17.5; Paget's, 17.8; reflex, 17.6
  in arthritides other than rheumatoid arthritis, 17.7
  mechanism, 17.11
—Unilateral
  relation to subcutaneous nodules, 33.3

Joints
—Deformity, 2.118
—Examination, 2.118
  frequency of various articular signs in patients, 34.1, 34.1 t
  relation of effusion and redness to various disease attributes, 34.2, 34.2 t
—Individual, involvement of, 34.4, 34.4 t
—Roentgenograms, 2.121
  absence of changes: in patients, 34.3; in previous studies, 34.3
  relation to: prognosis, 34.3; various disease attributes, 34.3, 34.3 t
Juvenile rheumatoid arthritis
  arrested growth, 2.20
  as clinical entity, 2.19, 2.20
  as pathologic entity, 2.20
  as variant of rheumatoid arthritis, 2.116
  differences from adult rheumatoid arthritis, 2.22, 2.27
  frequency, 2.18
  inclusion of patients with, in study, 2.27
  lymphadenopathy, 2.20, 2.22, 2.25
  pathologic findings, 2.20, 2.24
  pericarditis, 2.20, 2.25
  pleurisy, 2.20, 2.25
  splenomegaly, 2.20, 2.22, 2.25, 30.4 t, 30.5
  use of term "Still's disease," 2.26

Keratoconjunctivitis sicca. See under Eyes, inflammatory lesions
Keratopathy. See under Eyes, inflammatory lesions

Life course
  utilized in the study of rheumatoid arthritis, 1.19
Liver
  altered function, 10.4, 30.7, 30.10
  enlargement in patients and controls, 30.1 t, 30.7
  histopathology, 30.7, 30.10
Liver palms, 31.5
Lungs
  findings on examination in patients and controls, 24.1, 24.2 t

Index

Lungs (cont.)
  roentgenograms, 24.1, 24.3 t
Lymphadenopathy, 2.25, 2.28, 2.118
  criteria, 30.2
  definition, 4.20
  frequency: in patients and controls, 30.1 t, 30.2; in previous studies, 30.2
  histopathology, 2.28, 30.8
  in juvenile rheumatoid arthritis, 2.20, 2.22, 2.25
  relation to: activity of disease, 30.4; age in females, 30.3; involved joints, 30.8, 30.10; joint effusion, 34.2; primary joint involvement, 16.12, 30.4; prognosis, 30.4; sex, 30.2 t, 30.3; splenomegaly, 30.5 t, 30.6; type of onset, 15.4, 30.4; various disease attributes, 30.4; weight on admission, 30.3, 30.3 t; weight loss, 30.3
  significance, 30.8
Lymphocytosis. See under Blood, white-cell count, differential

Menopausal arthritis
  as form of degenerative joint disease, 2.59–2.61, 2.115
  definition, 2.57, 2.116
  differentiated from rheumatoid arthritis involving knees, 2.61
  in classification of arthritides, 2.56
  pathologic changes, 2.60
  synonyms, 2.56 fn
Menopause
—Age in patients and controls, 12.1, 12.1 t, 12.2 t
—Artificial
  in patients and controls, 12.1, 12.1 t
  relation to onset of arthritis, 12.2, 12.2 f, 12.6
—Definition, 4.5
—Patients near, given hormonal tests, 12.6
—Post-menopausal state
  relation to: prognosis, 12.4; severity of disease, 12.4; subsequent course, 12.4

Menopause (cont.)
—Relation to: course before admission, 12.4; onset of arthritis, 2.57, 6.7, 6.9, 12.1–12.3, 12.1 f, 12.3 t, 12.4 t, 15.4; primary joint involvement, 16.12; prognosis, 12.4, 12.5 t; severity of disease, 12.4, 12.5 t; subsequent course, 12.4
"Menopause arthralgia," 2.58
Menstruation
  influence on course, 20.8, 20.8 t, 20.16
Metabolism, basal. See Basal metabolism
Miners
  frequency of rheumatoid arthritis, 11.1
Moisture. See under Course before hospital admission, factors influencing
Muscular atrophy, 2.118
  pathogenesis, 23.11, 23.13
  relation to: age, 23.7; constitutional symptoms, 21.4; exaggerated tendon reflexes, 23.8; prognosis, 23.9; sex, 23.7; various disease attributes, 23.6 t, 23.9
  symmetrical distribution, 17.11
  See also under Neurologic signs
Myxedema
  occurrence in rheumatoid arthritis, 10.7, 41.6

Nails
—Atrophy of
  associated with atrophy of skin, 31.3
  frequency: in patients, 31.1; in previous studies, 31.1
  pathogenesis, 31.9
  relation to: prognosis, 31.3; various disease attributes, 31.1 t, 31.3
—Psoriasis of, 2.31, 2.34, 2.37, 2.39, 2.42, 2.43, 2.46, 2.47, 2.116
National origin
  compared: with hospital population, 7.1; with Massachusetts population, 7.1, 7.1 t, 7.2, 7.2 t
  Scandinavian, 7.2
Nausea. See under Gastro-intestinal symptoms

Negroes
  frequency of rheumatoid arthritis, 7.2
Nervousness and/or emotional upsets
  frequency: in patients and controls, 23.4, 23.4 t; in previous studies, 23.5
  relation to: constitutional symptoms, 21.4, 23.4; neurologic signs, 23.8; neurologic symptoms, 23.3, 23.3 t; prodromal symptoms, 13.9, 13.9 t, 23.4; prognosis, 23.4; sex, 23.4, 23.4 t; spondylitis, 23.4; strain as precipitant, 14.5 t, 14.6, 23.4; various disease attributes, 23.4; vasomotor symptoms, 22.4, 23.4
Neural theory of origin of rheumatoid arthritis, 23.10
Neurologic signs, 2.118
  frequency: in patients and controls, 23.5 t, 23.7; in previous studies, 23.10
  relation to: age, 23.7; nervousness and/or emotional upsets, 23.8; neurologic symptoms, 23.8; prognosis, 23.8; sex, 23.7; various disease attributes, 23.8
Neurologic symptoms, 2.118
  associations among, 23.3
  definition, 4.17
  frequency: in patients and controls, 23.1 t, 23.2; in previous studies, 23.10
  relation to: age, 23.2 t, 23.3; constitutional symptoms, 23.3; nervousness and/or emotional upsets, 23.3, 23.3 t; prognosis, 23.3; sex, 23.3; spondylitis, 23.3; various disease attributes, 23.3; vasomotor symptoms and signs, 23.3
  tinnitus as characteristic symptom, 23.2
Neuropathic arthritis, 2.76, 17.5
Nodules
—Subcutaneous, 2.118
  determining factors in location, 33.2, 33.8
  frequency: in patients and controls, 33.1; in previous studies, 33.1
  in connective tissue diseases, 2.122

Nodules, subcutaneous (cont.)
  in rheumatic fever, 2.122
  "nodule formers," 33.6
  pathologic findings, 2.122
  relation to: activity of disease, 33.1 t, 33.3; age, 33.2; duration of arthritis before admission, 33.3; primary joint involvement, 16.12, 33.3; prognosis, 33.4 t, 33.5; severity of disease, 33.3 t, 33.5; sex, 33.2; spondylitis, 2.15, 33.4, 42.3; subsequent course, 33.4 t, 33.5; type of onset, 15.4, 33.2 t, 33.3; unilateral joint involvement, 33.3; various disease attributes, 33.3
  symmetrical distribution, 17.1, 17.11
—Visceral, 33.6
Non-protein nitrogen, blood
  frequency of elevation in patients, 39.1 t, 39.4

Occupation
  distribution: at onset of arthritis, 11.1 t, 11.2, 11.3; in previous study, 11.1 t
  frequency of rheumatoid arthritis in miners, 11.1
  indoor contrasted with outdoor, 11.1, 11.2
  involving exposure to damp, 11.1
  of patients compared with population, 11.2 t, 11.3, 11.3 t
  relation to: prognosis, 11.4, 11.5 t; severity of disease, 11.4, 11.5 t; spondylitis, 11.4, 11.4 t
  responsible for mental or physical stress, 11.1
Onset of arthritis
—Acute
  as criterion for nonspecific "infectious" arthritis, 16.13, 16.14
  definition, 4.8, 15.1
  frequency: in patients, 15.2; in previous studies, 15.2
  results of treatment of focal infection in patients, 37.5
—Definition, 4.4, 13.3

Index

Onset of arthritis (cont.)
—Distribution: by months, 19.8 f, 19.11 t, 19.13, 19.19; frequency in March, 19.12 t, 19.13; seasonal, 19.10 t, 19.13, 19.14, 19.19
—Gradual
definition, 15.1
—Type, 2.118
relation to: age at onset, 15.2 t, 15.3; anemia, 15.4, 38.3; anorexia, 15.4, 21.4; course before admission, 15.5, 15.5 t, 15.7, 19.2, 19.3, 44.8; duration of arthritis before admission, 15.3, 15.3 t, 18.5; exposure as precipitant, 14.17; fever, 15.4, 26.5; infection as precipitant, 14.8 t, 14.10, 15.3, 18.5; infection influencing course, 20.6 t, 20.7; lateral distribution of primary joint involvement, 15.4, 17.3; lymphadenopathy, 15.4, 30.4; onset near menopause, 15.4; primary joint involvement, 15.4, 16.12; prodromal symptoms, 15.4; prognosis, 15.5, 15.6 t, 44.8; severity of disease, 15.5, 15.6 t, 43.4; sex, 15.1 t, 15.3; splenomegaly, 15.4, 30.6; spondylitis, 15.4, 42.4; strain as precipitant, 14.6, 15.3; strain as influence on course, 20.4; subcutaneous nodules, 15.4, 33.2 t, 33.3; subsequent course, 15.5; vasomotor symptoms, 22.5; weakness, 15.4, 21.4

Operation
—As precipitating factor
combined with other precipitants, 14.20
frequency: in patients, 14.1 t, 14.20; in previous studies, 14.21
relation to various disease attributes, 14.20
types, 14.15 t, 14.20
—Frequency in patients and controls, 10.1, 10.2, 10.5 t, 10.8
—Gynecologic, 10.6 t, 10.8, 10.12
—Relation to: prognosis, 10.9; remission, 19.12; severity of disease, 10.9; spondylitis, 10.9

Osteo-arthritis. *See under* Degenerative joint disease
Osteo-arthropathy, pulmonary, 32.3
as cause of joint pain, 2.76
Osteomyelitis
as cause of joint pain, 2.76

Palindromic rheumatism, 2.54
Paresthesias. *See under* Vasomotor symptoms
Parotitis, pneumococcal
concurrent with rheumatoid arthritis, 2.67
Pathologic findings
in subcutaneous nodules, 2.122
in synovial tissue, 2.122
Patients
collection of data on, 1.4, 3.6
relation to population sample, 3.3
removal of 7 from study, 3.1
residences, 3.2
selection, 1.3, 1.4, 2.11, 3.1, 3.3, 18.3
Peptic ulcer. *See* Ulcer, peptic
Periarteritis nodosa
simulating rheumatoid arthritis, 2.112
Pericarditis, 1.7, 2.118, 24.2
in juvenile rheumatoid arthritis, 2.20, 2.25
Peritonitis, 24.2
Plasma volume. *See under* Anemia
Pleurisy, 2.118
frequency in patients and controls, 10.4, 24.2
in juvenile rheumatoid arthritis, 2.20, 2.25
Pneumococcal arthritis, 2.66
Pneumonia
frequency in patients and controls, 10.3 t, 10.5, 10.6
Pneumonitis
as systemic manifestation of rheumatoid arthritis, 10.6, 24.1, 24.7
Post-rheumatic fibrous rheumatism, 2.9
Precipitating factors, 2.118
definition, 4.7

Precipitating factors (cont.)
  frequency in patients, 14.1 t, 14.2
  relation to: alterations in course of disease, 14.32; duration of arthritis before admission, 14.2 t, 14.3; primary joint involvement, 16.12, 16.12 t; prodromal symptoms, 13.11, 13.12 t, 13.14; vasomotor symptoms, 22.5
  See also under Childbirth, Exposure, Infection, Operation, Strain, *and* Trauma (as precipitating factors)
Pregnancy
  influence on course, 2.123, 19.12, 20.8, 20.16
  onset of arthritis during, 14.25, 14.26
Prodromal symptoms, 2.118
  definition, 4.6, 13.3
  early descriptions, 13.1
  in patients and controls, 13.1 t, 13.4, 13.5
  in patients without arthritis, 13.14
  in relatives of patients, 13.14
  list of those mentioned in literature, 13.2 fn
  marking disease onset, 1.9, 13.2, 13.11, 13.14
  patients with, forming a sub-type of rheumatoid arthritis, 1.17
  relation to: age at onset, 13.6 t, 13.7; constitutional symptoms, 21.1, 21.3, 21.4; course before admission, 13.10, 13.10 t; duration of arthritis before admission, 13.2 t–13.4 t, 13.6, 18.3, 18.5; exacerbations, 13.14; lateral distribution of arthritis at onset, 17.3, 17.5 t; nervousness and/or emotional upsets, 13.9, 13.9 t; precipitating factors, 13.11, 13.12 t, 13.14; primary joint involvement, 16.12; prognosis, 13.10, 13.10 t, 13.11 t; remissions, 13.14; severity of disease, 13.10, 13.11 t; sex, 13.5 t, 13.7; spondylitis, 13.7 t, 13.8; strain as precipitant, 13.8 t, 13.9; subsequent course, 13.10; type of onset, 15.4; vasomotor symptoms, 22.4

Prodromal symptoms (cont.)
  selected list studied, 13.3
  synonyms, 13.1
Prognosis
  determined by: course before admission, 44.8, 44.8 t; severity of disease on admission, 44.8, 44.8 t; subsequent course, 44.8, 44.8 t
  method of study: improvement, 44.10; limitations, 44.10
  relation to: absence of roentgenographic changes, 34.3; age at onset, 44.6, 44.8; age on admission, 18.2, 44.5 t, 44.6, 44.8; anemia, 38.3; atrophy of nails, 31.3; atrophy of skin, 31.2; constitutional symptoms, 21.4; course before admission, 19.3; duration of arthritis before admission, 18.5, 44.6 t, 44.7, 44.7 t, 44.8; duration of failure to improve, 44.11; exposure as precipitant, 14.13 t, 14.17; extent of joint involvement, 34.5; fever, 26.4; focal infection, 37.3 t, 37.4; illnesses other than rheumatoid arthritis, 10.9; infection as precipitant, 14.11; infection influencing course, 20.4 t, 20.6; injuries, 10.9; joint effusion, 34.2; joint redness, 34.2; lateral distribution of arthritis at onset, 17.3, 17.6 t, 44.8; lymphadenopathy, 30.4; monarticular onset, 16.7, 44.8; muscular atrophy, 23.9; nervousness and/or emotional upsets, 23.4; neurologic signs, 23.8; neurologic symptoms, 23.3; nonspecific "infectious" arthritis, 2.103, 16.14, 16.15; occupation, 11.4, 11.5 t; onset in small joints, 44.8; onset near menopause, 12.4, 12.5 t; operations, 10.9; postmenopausal state, 12.4; primary joint involvement, 16.11, 16.11 t; prodromal symptoms, 13.10, 13.10 t, 13.11 t; sex, 44.3 t, 44.4 t, 44.5; splenomegaly, 30.6; spondylitis, 42.3, 42.3 t, 44.5; strain as precipi-

Index

Prognosis, relation to (cont.)
  tant, 14.6; strain as influence on course, 20.2 t, 20.4; subcutaneous nodules, 33.4 t, 33.5; tachycardia, 27.3; type of onset, 15.5, 15.5 t, 15.6 t, 44.8; various disease attributes, 44.8; vasomotor symptoms, 22.5
  results in previous studies, 44.12
  See also under Course before hospital admission; Course following hospital admission; Severity of disease
Proteins, plasma, 2.119
Psoriasis
  arthropathy secondary to, 2.32, 2.42
  as manifestation of rheumatoid arthritis, 2.32, 2.44
  clinical features resembling those of rheumatoid arthritis, 2.40
  co-existence with rheumatoid arthritis due to constitutional or hereditary tendency, 2.32, 2.45
  frequency: in patients and controls, 31.2 t, 31.6; of arthritis in, 2.43
  of nails, 2.31, 2.34, 2.37, 2.39, 2.42, 2.43, 2.46, 2.47, 2.116
  patients with, included in study, 2.47
  relation to rheumatoid arthritis, 2.31–2.33, 2.46
  sharing common etiology with rheumatoid arthritis, 2.32, 2.40, 2.41
"Psoriatic arthritis"
  as independent entity, 2.32, 2.34, 2.39, 2.116
  bony destruction, 2.36
  criteria for diagnosis, 2.31
  joint lesions, 2.35, 2.36
  pathology: of arthritis, 2.38; of skin lesions, 2.34
  relation between course of arthritis and of psoriasis, 2.42
  skin lesions, 2.34
  terminal interphalangeal joint involvement, 2.37, 2.42, 2.43, 2.116
  See also under Nails, psoriasis of
Psychogenic rheumatism. *See* Fibrositis

Pulse rate. *See* Tachycardia
Purpura, 31.5

Raynaud's syndrome. *See under* Vasomotor symptoms
Reflexes
  absent, 23.10
  exaggerated, 23.6–23.8, 23.10
    relation to muscular atrophy, 23.8
  See also under Neurologic signs
  plantar, 23.10
  spread of, 23.10
Reiter's syndrome, 2.98
  as variant of rheumatoid arthritis, 2.99
  resembling rheumatoid arthritis, 2.99
Remissions
  associated with: freedom from strain, 19.12; heat, 19.12; increased rest, 19.12; jaundice, 19.12; operation, 19.12; pregnancy, 19.12
  distribution: by months, 19.7 f, 19.9 t, 19.13; occurrence in same quarter of year, 19.15; seasonal, 19.10 t, 19.13
  See also under Course before admission, intermittent
Renal function tests, 39.3, 39.6
Rest, increased, associated with remission, 19.12
Rheumatic fever
  distinguished from chronic rheumatism, 2.6
  frequency in patients and controls, 10.4
  pathologic changes resembling those in rheumatoid arthritis, 2.6
  preceding chronic progressive arthritis, 1.14, 2.6
  preceding onset of rheumatoid arthritis, 1.6, 1.7, 2.6
  relation to arthritis of scarlet fever, 2.80
  relation to rheumatoid arthritis, 2.6, 2.10, 2.12; clinical differentiation, 2.10; clinical and pathologic differentiation, 2.9, 2.115; co-existence with, 2.7; criteria for differentiation, 2.10

Rheumatic fever (cont.)
  sex distribution compared with rheumatoid arthritis, 5.2
  simulated by acute "atypical" rheumatoid arthritis, 2.7, 2.10
  subcutaneous nodules, 2.122
  with articular features of rheumatoid arthritis, 2.7, 2.9, 2.10
Rheumatoid arthritis
  as a disease entity, 2.124
  as a systemic disease, 1.17
  diagnosis, 2.116, 2.117
  diagnostic laboratory test, 2.117, 2.120
  geographic prevalence, 7.4
  nervous system involvement, 23.10, 23.13
  prevalence in various occupations, 11.6
  racial prevalence, 7.4
  variants, 2.1, 2.115, 2.116

Scarlet fever
—Arthritis of
  chronic, 2.83
  differentiated from rheumatoid arthritis, 2.83
  forms, 2.79
  frequency, 2.79
  post-scarlatinal form, 2.82
  resembling rheumatic fever, 2.80
  suppurative form, 2.81
—Preceding onset of rheumatoid arthritis, 2.83, 2.84
Scleritis, 29.2 t
Scleroderma
  sex distribution, 5.4
  simulating rheumatoid arthritis, 2.113
Scleromalacia perforans, 29.2, 29.2 t
Season
  influence on course, 20.12 t, 20.13
Sedimentation rate, 2.119
Serologic tests
  hemagglutination reaction, 2.120
  streptococcal agglutination, 2.120
Severity of disease
  classification of patients by, 43.1 t, 43.3
  definition, 4.26, 43.1
  relation to: age on admission, 18.2; ane-

Severity of disease, relation to (cont.)
  mia, 38.2 t, 38.3; anthropometric studies of patients, 43.8; constitutional symptoms, 21.4; course before admission, 19.3, 43.4; disease attributes unrelated to definition of severity, 43.2 t, 43.5; duration of arthritis before admission, 18.5, 43.4; exposure as precipitant, 14.13 t, 14.17; extent of joint involvement, 34.5, 43.1; fever, 26.2 t, 26.4; gastric anacidity, 40.5; illnesses, operations, and injuries, 10.9; infection influencing course, 20.4 t, 20.6; lateral distribution of arthritis at onset, 17.3, 17.6 t; low basal metabolism, 41.4; occupation, 11.4, 11.5 t; onset near menopause, 12.4, 12.5 t; post-menopausal state, 12.4; prodromal symptoms, 13.10, 13.11 t; roentgenographic changes in colon, 36.3; strain influencing course, 20.2 t, 20.4; subcutaneous nodules, 33.3 t, 33.5; type of onset, 15.5, 15.6 t, 43.4; various disease attributes, 43.2 t, 43.4, 43.5, 44.8, 44.8 t; vasomotor symptoms, 22.5
See also under Prognosis
Sex distribution
—In rheumatoid arthritis, 2.118
  compared to that in persons with other diseases, 5.4; with disseminated lupus erythematosus, 5.4; with rheumatic fever, 5.2; with scleroderma, 5.4; with syphilis, 5.2
  endocrine influence, 5.3
  explanations, 5.3, 5.6; constitutional susceptibility as explanation, 5.4
  findings in previous studies, 5.1 t; of rheumatoid arthritis in population, 5.6
  genetic basis, 5.3
  influence of hospitalization, 5.1
  relation to: age at onset, 5.1, 5.1 t, 6.3; vasomotor instability, 5.3
—In rheumatoid spondylitis, 5.2

Index

Sjögren's syndrome. *See under* Eyes, inflammatory lesions, keratoconjunctivitis sicca

Skin
—Atrophy, 2.118
  as systemic manifestation of rheumatoid arthritis, 31.4
  description, 31.1
  frequency in patients and controls, 31.1
  histopathology in, 31.4, 31.9
  mentioned in previous studies, 31.1
  relation to: prognosis, 31.2; various disease attributes, 31.1 t, 31.2
  symmetrical distribution, 17.11
  theories of causation, 31.4
  with atrophy of nails, 31.3
—Diseases
  frequency in patients and controls, 31.2 t, 31.6
  herpes zoster, 31.6
  psoriasis, 31.6
  vitiligo, 31.6
—Manifestations of rheumatoid arthritis
  erythematous rashes, 31.5
  liver palms, 31.5
  purpura, 31.5
—Pigmentation, 2.118
  frequency in patients, 31.5
  mentioned in previous studies, 31.5
  symmetrical distribution, 17.11
Spinal arthritis. *See* Spondylitis, rheumatoid
Splenomegaly, 2.25, 2.28, 2.118
  definition, 4.21
  frequency: in adults compared with children, 30.4 t, 30.5; in patients and controls, 30.1 t, 30.5; in previous studies, 30.4 t, 30.5
  from extraneous causes, 2.29, 30.5
  in Felty's syndrome, 2.29, 2.30
  in juvenile rheumatoid arthritis, 2.20, 2.22, 2.25, 30.4 t, 30.5
  pathology in rheumatoid arthritis, 2.29, 30.8
  relation to: leukocytosis, 38.7; leukopenia, 2.29, 30.6, 38.7, 38.10;

Splenomegaly, relation to (cont.)
  lymphadenopathy, 30.5 t, 30.6; prognosis, 30.6; type of onset, 15.4; various disease attributes, 30.6
  significance, 30.8
Spondylitis, ankylosing. *See* Spondylitis, rheumatoid
Spondylitis, rheumatoid
  age distribution, 2.15, 42.3
  as disease entity, 2.13, 2.16, 42.5, 42.8
  as variant of rheumatoid arthritis, 2.13, 2.16, 42.5
  Bechterew's disease as form of, 2.13
  classification of patients with, by joints involved, 42.1 t, 42.2
  compared with peripheral rheumatoid arthritis, 42.2 t, 42.5
  definition, 4.25
  diagnostic criteria, 42.2
  earliest post-mortem study, 2.13
  effects of treatment, 2.15, 42.5
  in juvenile rheumatoid arthritis, 42.6
  iritis, 2.15, 29.2 t, 29.3 t, 29.4, 29.6
  joint involvement: peripheral, 2.14; primary, 16.8, 16.8 t
  laboratory tests, 2.15, 42.5
  pathologic findings: in muscles, 2.15, 42.5, 42.8; in peripheral and spinal joints, 2.14
  patients with, included in study, 2.16, 2.116, 42.5
  relation to: constitutional symptoms, 21.4; course before admission, 42.4; duration of arthritis before admission, 42.3; exposure as precipitant, 14.17; fever, 26.3; history of illnesses, operations, and injuries, 10.9; indoor or outdoor occupation, 11.4, 11.4 t; infection as precipitant, 14.11; joint effusion, 34.2; joint redness, 34.2; nervousness and/or emotional upsets, 23.4; neurologic symptoms, 23.3; prodromal symptoms, 13.7 t, 13.8; prognosis, 42.3, 42.3 t, 44.5; strain as precipitant, 14.6; strain influencing course, 20.4;

Spondylitis, rheumatoid,
relation to (cont.)
subsequent course, 42.3, 42.3 t, 44.5;
type of onset, 15.4, 15.4 t, 42.4;
various disease attributes, 42.2 t,
42.3, 42.4; vasomotor symptoms,
22.4
sex distribution, 2.15, 5.2, 42.3
spinal involvement of minor degree,
42.1 t, 42.2, 42.6, 42.8
subcutaneous nodules, 2.15, 33.4, 42.3
valvular heart disease, 42.4
Still-Chauffard syndrome
as variant of rheumatoid arthritis, 2.28,
2.116
patients with, included in study, 2.30
Still's disease. *See* Juvenile rheumatoid
arthritis
Strain
—As precipitating factor
combined with other precipitants, 14.7
frequency: in controlled studies, 14.9;
in patients, 14.1 t, 14.4; in previous
studies, 14.5, 14.7 t, 14.8
relation to: age at onset, 14.4 t, 14.6;
history of nervousness and/or emotional upsets, 14.5 t, 14.6; infection,
14.6 t, 14.7, 14.11; influence of
strain on course, 20.4; prodromal
symptoms, 13.8 t, 13.9; prognosis,
14.6; sex, 14.6; spondylitis, 14.6;
type of onset, 14.6; weakness, 21.4
types, 14.3 t
—Freedom from, associated with remissions, 19.12
—*See also under* Course before hospital
admission, factors influencing
Subsequent course. *See* Course following
hospital admission
Symptoms, constitutional. *See* Constitutional symptoms
Synovial fluid, 2.119
Syphilis
patients with, included in study, 2.78
sex distribution compared with rheumatoid arthritis, 5.2

Syphilitic arthritis
categories, 2.74; congenital, 2.75; polyarticular, 2.77; neuropathic, 2.76;
simulating rheumatoid arthritis,
2.74, 2.77; tertiary, 2.76
treponemata in synovial fluid, 2.77
Syphilitic periostitis
as cause of bone and joint pain, 2.76

Tachycardia, 2.118
definition, 4.19
frequency: in patients, 27.2; in previous
studies, 27.2
mechanism, 27.5, 27.7
persistent and marked, 27.4
relation to: fever, 27.1 t, 27.4; prognosis,
27.3; various disease attributes, 27.3;
vasomotor symptoms, 22.5; vasomotor symptoms and signs, 27.3
variability of pulse rate, 27.4
Tendonitis, 2.118
Tenosynovitis
symmetrical distribution, 17.1, 17.11
Thyroid disorders
frequency in patients and controls,
41.3 t, 41.6
histopathology of thyroid in rheumatoid
arthritis, 41.7, 41.9
relation to rheumatoid arthritis, 41.6,
41.9
See also under Basal metabolism;
Myxedema; Thyrotoxicosis
Thyrotoxicosis
frequency: in patients and controls,
10.4, 41.3 t, 41.6; in previous
studies, 41.6
Tinnitus. *See under* Neurologic symptoms
Tongue, atrophy, 31.7
relation to: iron utilization, 31.7; vitamin deficiency, 31.7
Trauma, as precipitating factor
combined with other precipitants, 14.23
frequency: in patients, 14.1 t, 14.22; in
previous studies, 14.16 t, 14.24
relation to various disease attributes,
14.23

Index

Trauma, as precipitating factor (cont.)
  significance, 14.22, 14.24
  types, 14.22
Treatment
  by hospitalization, 44.2
  conservative, 44.2
  diagnostic value of response, 2.123
  of focal infection, 37.4, 44.2
  with blood transfusions, 44.2
  with fever, 44.2
  with simple medical and orthopedic measures, 44.2
Tremor
  origin, 23.10
  See also under Neurologic signs and Neurologic symptoms
Tuberculosis, pulmonary
  frequency in patients, 24.3
  in rheumatoid arthritis, 2.71, 2.73, 24.3
  patients with, included in study, 2.73
Tuberculous arthritis
  co-existence with rheumatoid arthritis, 2.70, 2.73
  confused with rheumatoid arthritis, 2.68
  diagnosis, 2.68
  differentiated from monarticular rheumatoid arthritis, 2.69, 2.70
  polyarticular, 2.70, 2.73
"Tuberculous rheumatism"
  diagnosis, 2.72
  evidence against recognition, 2.73, 2.115
Twitching. See under Neurologic symptoms

Ulcer, peptic
  frequency: in patients and controls, 10.7, 25.4; in rheumatoid arthritics and general population, 25.4, 25.7
Unitarian theory, 1.10, 1.16, 2.5
Uric acid, blood
  elevation, 2.3; in patients, 39.1 t, 39.4; in previous studies, 39.4
Urinary findings, abnormal
  frequency of albuminuria and cylindruria: in patients, 39.1 t, 39.2; in previous studies, 39.1, 39.3

Urinary findings, abnormal (cont.)
  quantitative measurements, 39.3, 39.6
  relation to various disease attributes, 39.2
Urticaria
  relation to rheumatoid arthritis, 9.6
Uveitis. See under Eyes, inflammatory lesions, iritis

Variants of rheumatoid arthritis. See Rheumatoid arthritis, variants
Varicosities
  frequency in patients and controls, 32.1, 32.1 t
Vascular spasm. See Vasomotor symptoms
Vasomotor signs, 2.118
  definition, 4.16, 22.6
  frequency: in patients and controls, 22.3 t, 22.6; in previous studies, 22.8
  measurements: in extremities, 22.9; in extremities in relation to climatic changes, 20.20
  mechanism, 22.11
  relation to: activity of disease, 22.11; age, 22.4 t, 22.5 t, 22.6; constitutional symptoms, 21.4; female sex distribution of rheumatoid arthritis, 5.3, 22.9; joint redness, 34.2; low basal metabolism, 41.4; neurologic symptoms, 23.3; pathogenesis of rheumatoid arthritis, 22.9; sex, 22.4 t, 22.5 t, 22.6; tachycardia, 27.3; various disease attributes, 22.7; vasomotor symptoms, 22.7
Vasomotor symptoms, 2.118
  definition, 4.15
  frequency: in patients and controls, 22.1 t, 22.3; in previous studies, 22.8
  listed, 22.2
  mechanism, 22.11
  mechanism of paresthesias, 22.2, 22.11
  relation to: activity of disease, 22.11; age, 22.2 t, 22.3, 22.4; constitutional symptoms, 21.4, 22.4; course before admission, 22.5; duration of arthritis before admission, 22.5; female sex distribution of rheuma-

Vasomotor symptoms,
  relation to (cont.)
    toid arthritis, 5.3, 22.9; fever, 22.5; influence of cold, moisture, and heat on course, 20.10 t, 20.11, 20.12, 20.17; joint redness, 34.2; low basal metabolism, 41.4; nervousness and/or emotional upsets, 22.4; neurologic symptoms, 23.3; pathogenesis of rheumatoid arthritis, 22.9; precipitating factors, 22.5; primary joint involvement, 22.5; prodromal symptoms, 22.4; prognosis, 22.5; severity of disease, 22.5; sex, 22.2 t, 22.3; spondylitis, 22.4; subsequent course, 22.5; tachycardia, 22.5, 27.3; type of onset, 22.5; vasomotor signs, 22.7

Vertigo. *See under* Neurologic symptoms

Villous arthritis, chronic. *See* Menopausal arthritis

Vitiligo, 31.6

Vomiting
  frequency in patients and controls, 25.1 t, 25.2
  See Gastro-intestinal symptoms

Weakness, 2.118
—As constitutional symptom
  frequency in patients and controls, 21.1 t, 21.2

Weakness, as constitutional symptom (cont.)
  relation to: infection as precipitant, 21.4; low basal metabolism, 41.3; nervousness and/or emotional upsets, 21.4; prodromal weakness, 21.3, 21.4; strain as precipitant, 21.4; type of onset, 15.4; various disease attributes, 21.3 t, 21.4

Weight loss, 2.118
—As constitutional symptom
  frequency in patients and controls, 21.1 t, 21.2
  possible causes, 21.6, 21.8
  relation to: fever, 21.4, 26.3; lymphadenopathy, 30.3; prodromal weight loss, 21.3; various disease attributes, 21.3 t, 21.4
  time in relation to onset, 21.2 t, 21.3
  See also under Weight of patients

Weight of patients
  compared with average weight, 21.4 t, 21.5
  relation to: history of weight loss, 21.5; lymphadenopathy, 30.3, 30.3 t
  results in previous studies, 21.5
  See also under Weight loss, as constitutional symptom

Whipple's disease, 25.7

White-cell count. *See* Blood, white-cell count

Table 47

Master table showing the nature of the associations found among 39 factors studied with reference to rheumatoid arthritis

	1	2	3	4	5	6	7	8	9	10	11	12	13	14	15	16	17	18	19	20	21	22	23	24	25	26	27	28	29	30	31	32	33	34	35	36	37	38	39
1 Sex (male)	0	0	−	−	−	0	0	−	0	0	0	+	0	0	−	−	0	−	−	0	0	0	0	−	0	−	0	0	0	0	+	0	0	0	−	−	0	0	0
2 Age at onset under 40	0	−	0	−	−	0	+	0	0	0	+	+	0	+	0	0	0	−	−	+	+	+	0	0	0	0	0	−	0	0	+	0	0	0	0	0	+	0	0
3 Family history of rheumatoid arthritis	0	−	0	0	0	0	0	0	0	0	0	0	0	0	0	0	0	0	0	0	0	0	0	0	0	0	0	0	0	0	−	0	0	0	0	0	0	0	0
4 Prodromal symptoms	−	−	0	0	+	0	0	0	0	0	0	0	−	0	+	0	0	+	0	0	+	0	0	0	0	0	0	0	0	−	0	−	0	0	0	0	0	0	0
5 Strain before onset	−	0	+	+	0	0	0	0	0	0	0	−	−	0	+	+	0	+	0	0	0	0	0	0	0	+	0	0	0	+	0	0	0	+	0	0	0	0	0
6 Infection before onset	0	0	0	0	0	0	+	0	0	0	0	0	−	0	0	+	0	0	0	0	0	0	0	0	0	+	+	−	0	−	0	0	0	0	+	0	0	0	0
7 Onset acute	0	+	0	0	0	+	0	0	0	0	0	+	−	−	+	0	0	0	0	0	0	0	0	0	0	0	0	0	+	+	0	0	+	0	0	0	0	0	0
8 Onset in small joints	−	0	0	0	0	0	0	0			0	0	0	−	0	0	0	0	0	0	0	0	0	0	0	0	0	0	0	0	0	0	0	0	0	0	0	0	0
9 Onset in large joints	0	0	0	0	0	0	0		0		0	0	0	+	0	0	0	0	0	0	0	0	0	0	0	0	0	0	0	0	0	0	0	0	0	0	0	0	0
10 Onset monarticular	0	0	0	0	0	0	0			0	0	0	0	0	0	−	0	0	0	0	0	0	0	0	0	0	0	0	0	0	0	0	0	0	−	0	0	−	0
11 Onset unilateral	+	+	0	−	0	0	0	0	0	0	0	0	0	0	0	0	0	0	0	0	+	0	0	0	0	0	0	0	0	0	0	0	0	0	0	0	0	0	+
12 Age on admission under 40	+	0	0	−	−	0	+	0	0	0	0	0	−	+	0	0	0	0	0	0	0	0	0	−	−	0	0	−	0	0	0	0	0	0	0	−	+	−	+
13 Duration before admission (longer)	0	0	0	0	0	−	−		0		0	0	0	+	0	0	0	+	+	0	0	0	0	0	0	0	+	+	0	0	0	0	0	0	0	+	+	+	−
14 Intermittent course before admission	0	0	0	0	0	0	+	−	+	0	+	+	0	0	0	+	0	+	+	+	+	+	+	0	0	0	0	+	+	0	0	0	0	0	0	0	0	0	0
15 Weakness	−	0	+	+	+	0	0	0	0	+	0	0	+	0	0	0	+	+	+	0	0	0	+	+	+	+	0	+	0	0	0	0	0	0	0	0	0	0	0
16 Anorexia	−	0	0	0	0	0	+	0	0	−	0	0	0	0	+	+	0	+	+	0	0	0	+	+	+	+	+	+	0	0	0	0	0	0	0	+	+	+	0
17 Weight loss	0	0	0	0	0	0	0	0	0	0	−	0	0	0	0	0	0	0	0	0	+	+	+	+	+	0	+	+	0	0	+	+	0	0	0	0	0	+	0
18 Cold extremities	−	0	0	+	+	0	0	0	0	0	0	0	0	+	+	+	0	+	+	+	+	+	+	+	+	+	+	+	0	0	0	0	0	0	0	+	0	0	0
19 Paresthesias	−	0	0	0	0	0	0	0	0	−	0	0	0	+	0	+	0	+	+	+	0	0	+	+	0	+	+	+	0	0	0	0	0	0	0	0	0	0	0
20 Cyanosis	0	+	0	0	0	0	0	0	0	0	0	0	0	0	0	0	0	0	+	+	0	0	0	0	0	0	0	0	0	0	0	0	0	0	0	0	0	0	0
21 Vascular spasm	0	+	0	+	0	0	0	0	0	+	0	0	0	+	+	0	+	+	+	+	+	+	0	+	0	+	+	+	0	0	0	0	0	0	0	0	0	0	0
22 Vasomotor signs	0	+	0	0	0	0	0	0	0	0	0	0	0	0	0	0	0	+	0	0	+	0	0	+	+	0	0	0	0	0	0	0	0	0	−	0	0	0	0

		1	2	3	4	5	6	7	8	9	10	11	12	13	14	15	16	17	18	19	20	21	22	23	24	25	26	27	28	29	30	31	32	33	34	35	36	37	38	39	
23	Muscular twitching	0	0	0	0	0	0	0	0	0	0	0	0	0	0	0	0	0	0	0	0	0	0	0	+	+	+	0	0	0	0	0	0	0	0	0	0	0	0	0	23
24	Vertigo	0	−	0	0	0	0	0	0	0	0	0	0	0	0	0	0	0	0	0	0	0	+	+	0	+	+	+	0	0	0	0	0	0	0	0	0	0	0	0	24
25	Tremor (subjective)	0	0	0	0	0	0	0	0	0	0	0	0	0	0	0	0	0	0	0	0	0	+	+	+	+	+	+	+	0	0	0	0	0	0	0	0	0	+	−	25
26	Nervousness and/or emotional upsets	−	0	0	0	0	+	0	0	0	0	0	−	0	0	−	0	0	+	+	0	0	+	+	+	+	+	+	0	0	0	0	0	0	0	0	0	0	0	0	26
27	Exaggerated reflexes	0	0	0	0	0	0	0	0	0	0	0	0	0	0	0	+	+	+	+	0	0	0	0	0	0	+	+	0	0	0	0	0	0	0	0	0	+	0	0	27
28	Muscular atrophy	0	−	0	0	0	0	−	0	0	0	0	0	0	0	0	+	+	+	0	0	0	+	0	0	+	+	0	0	0	0	+	0	+	0	0	0	0	+	−	28
29	Fever	0	0	0	0	0	0	+	0	0	0	0	0	0	+	0	0	0	0	0	0	0	0	0	0	0	0	0	0	0	+	0	0	0	0	0	0	0	+	0	29
30	Tachycardia	0	0	0	0	0	−	0	+	0	0	0	0	0	0	0	0	0	0	0	0	0	0	0	0	0	0	0	0	0	0	0	0	+	0	0	0	0	0	0	30
31	Lymphadenopathy	+	+	−	0	0	0	0	0	0	0	0	0	0	0	0	0	0	0	0	0	0	0	0	−	0	0	0	+	0	0	0	0	+	0	0	0	0	0	0	31
32	Splenomegaly	0	0	0	0	0	0	0	0	0	0	0	0	0	0	0	+	+	0	0	0	0	0	0	0	0	0	0	+	+	0	+	0	0	0	0	0	0	0	0	32
33	Nodules	0	0	0	0	0	0	+	0	0	0	0	0	0	0	0	0	0	0	0	0	0	0	0	0	0	0	0	0	+	0	0	0	0	0	0	0	0	0	0	33
34	Anemia	0	0	0	0	0	+	0	0	0	0	0	0	0	0	0	0	0	0	0	0	0	0	0	0	0	0	0	0	0	0	0	0	0	0	0	0	−	+	0	34
35	Gastric anacidity	−	0	0	0	0	0	0	0	0	0	0	0	0	0	0	0	0	0	0	0	0	−	0	0	0	0	0	0	0	0	0	0	0	+	0	0	0	0	0	35
36	Low basal metabolism	−	0	0	0	0	0	0	0	0	0	0	−	0	0	0	+	+	0	0	0	0	0	0	0	0	0	0	0	0	0	0	0	0	0	0	0	0	0	0	36
37	Spondylitis (males)	0	+	0	0	0	0	0	0	0	0	0	+	+	0	0	+	+	0	0	−	0	0	0	0	0	+	0	0	0	0	0	0	0	0	0	0	0	0	−	37
38	Total severity (increased)	0	0	0	0	0	0	0	0	0	0	0	−	+	0	0	+	+	+	0	0	0	0	+	+	+	+	0	+	+	0	+	0	+	0	0	0	0	+	−	38
39	Improvement (after discharge)	0	0	0	0	0	0	0	0	0	0	0	+	−	0	0	0	0	0	0	0	0	0	0	0	−	0	−	−	0	0	0	0	0	0	0	0	−	−	0	39
		1	2	3	4	5	6	7	8	9	10	11	12	13	14	15	16	17	18	19	20	21	22	23	24	25	26	27	28	29	30	31	32	33	34	35	36	37	38	39	

A positive association is designated by +, a negative association by −, and an absence of association by 0.

Where the association is listed as positive or negative, the result is statistically significant at the 5 per cent level (see pars. 3.9 and 3.15).

The degree of association has been omitted when (1) a positive association is obvious: age at onset under 40 and age on admission under 40, onset unilateral and onset monarticular; (2) a negative association is obvious: spondylitis with onset in small or large joints, monarticular or unilateral; and (3) the factors are mutually exclusive: onset in small or large joints or monarticular.

Bei Fragen zur Produktsicherheit wenden Sie sich bitte an:
If you have any questions regarding product safety,
please contact:

Walter de Gruyter GmbH
Genthiner Straße 13
10785 Berlin
productsafety@degruyterbrill.com